Dec. 28, 2005

Milk

A ticking bomb inside your body

Russell Eaton, HND

Foreword by Dr. Amy Lanou

Published by
DeliveredOnline.com

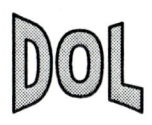

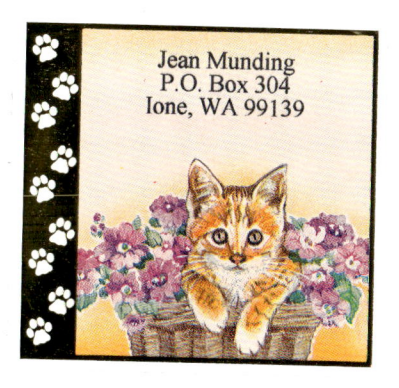

DOL

Jean Munding
P.O. Box 304
Ione, WA 99139

509 442 0715

Title	The Milk Imperative
Subtitle	*A ticking bomb inside your body*
Author	Russell Eaton
Published by	Deliveredonline.com
	Wokingham, United Kingdom
Email	mailto@deliveredonline.com
Email relating to this book:	milkimperative@milkimperative.com
Website relating to this book:	www.milkimperative.com
Copyright	© 2005 Russell Eaton
Edition	August 2005

ISBN 1-903339-16-2

Printed in the United Kingdom and in the United State of America. All rights reserved. No part of this publication may be reproduced, stored in a retrieval system, or transmitted in any form by any means, electronic, mechanical, photocopying, recording, or otherwise (except brief extracts for the purpose of review) without permission of the publisher and copyright owner. Disclaimer: This book examines the latest available data relating to dairy milk and its role or otherwise in the human diet. The text is written in plain language. It is not intended as medical guidance and should not be substituted for a physician's advice. Neither the publisher nor the author can be held legally responsible for the consequences of any errors, omissions, or advice given in this book.

The first half of this book tells the shocking truth about dairy milk. New discoveries are revealing a startling picture:

> ➢ **How dairy milk causes calcification, the biggest cause of illness in the world today.**

> ➢ **Why just about anybody who consumes dairy milk suffers from lactose intolerance and milk allergy – it's just a matter of degree.**

> ➢ **Why nearly all pasteurized milk contains a cocktail of harmful hormones, allergens, antibiotics, bad fats, cholesterol, toxins, cow blood, bacteria, viruses, PCB's, dioxins, heavy metals, and more!**

> ➢ **Why dairy milk is the biggest cause of anemia in infants and children, caused by a small, but relentless loss of blood.**

> ➢ **Why dairy milk is so bad for infants and children in all stages of development.**

> ➢ **Why low-fat dairy milk is more harmful and more fattening than whole milk.**

> ➢ **Plus a unique way to lose surplus body fat using *The NDM Plan* – this never fails!**

A special message for women: Osteoporosis is a terrible and painful disease that usually catches people by surprise. About one out of every two women will suffer from osteoporosis if they do nothing about it! This book gives vital new information on how to avoid osteoporosis, whether or not you consume dairy milk. Act now before it's too late.

A special message for men: Prostate cancer is the most common type of cancer for men. It's a terrible disease that affects sleep, makes you impotent and progressively becomes more painful, affecting your back and lower body. This book proves beyond any doubt that dairy milk is the biggest single cause of prostate cancer. Act now before it's too late.

Recipes next page ▶

The second half of this book provides a big selection of recipes for non-dairy milk. This means there is no need to give up milk – just switch from dairy to non-dairy and watch your health improve dramatically

Every recipe is quick and easy to make:

- All recipes completely non-dairy and non-animal.
- Suit virtually any dietary regimen.
- Delicious and non-fattening.
- Enjoy a big variety of flavours and textures.
- Save time and money – every recipe in the book can be made in under ten minutes if everything is to hand – never buy milk again.
- Super-nutritious, as packed with vitamins, minerals, lots of energy, soluble fibre, health-promoting oils, life-giving enzymes, easily digested protein, and much more.
- Ideal as part of any weight-loss regimen as nutritious, filling, and non-fattening – the fats in non-dairy milk get used by the body as energy or nutrition instead of being stored as surplus body fat.
- Many mouthwatering smoothie recipes – all completely non-dairy.

Non-dairy milk recipes for making at home

- No special milk-making machine required
- Make any recipe in less than 10 minutes

Almond Milk *Pea Milk*
Brazil Nut Milk *Peanut Milk*
Cashew Nut Milk *Pecan Nut Milk*
Chestnut Milk *Pine Nut Milk*
Coconut Milk *Pumpkin Seed Milk*
Corn Milk *Sesame Seed Milk*
Green Pea Milk *Soybean Milk*
Hazelnut Milk *Sunflower Seed Milk*
Hemp Seed Milk *Tiger Nut Milk*
Macadamia Milk *Walnut Milk*
Oat Milk *Blended Milks*

And Many Sprouted Seed Milks

Plus

A host of recipes for making mouth-watering smoothies or ice-cream, using non-dairy milk and the left-over okara, for maximum nutritional benefit

Plus

The Low G.I. Workout [tm]
– the ***only*** way to exercise for optimum good health and bones. *Discover the revolutionary new way to exercise that is changing people's lives*

Contents

Foreword by Dr. Amy Lanou	8
Introduction	10
PART ONE: ALL ABOUT DAIRY MILK	17
Dairy Milk Effect on Health	17
Dairy Milk Effect on Osteoporosis	45
Dairy Milk Effect on Calcification	83
Dairy Milk Effect on Protein	96
Dairy Milk Effect on Young People	103
Dairy Milk Effect on Weight Loss	122
Dairy Milk and Related Products	135
Dairy Milk Effect on Physical Fitness	143
Dairy Milk and So Called Myths	155
PART TWO: ALL ABOUT NON-DAIRY MILK	167
Why Choose Non-Dairy Milk?	167
Almond Milk	178
Brazil Nut Milk	179
Cashew Nut Milk	182
Chestnut Milk	184
Coconut Milk	186
Corn Milk	188
Grain Milks	190
Green Pea Milk	191
Hazelnut Milk	192
Hemp Seed Milk	194
Macadamia milk	197
Oat Milk	199
Peanut Milk	200
Pecan Nut Milk	202
Pine nut milk	204
Pumpkin Seed Milk	206
Sesame Seed Milk	208
Soy milk	210
Sprouted Seed Milk	212
Sunflower Seed Milk	215
Tiger Nut Milk	216
Walnut Milk	219
PART THREE: NON-DAIRY MILK RECIPES	222
Recipe Tips & Tricks	222
The Master Recipe	226
Blended Milks	236

Non-Dairy Smoothies & Ice-Cream	240
Bibliography & Notes	243
Appendix One: Vitamins & Minerals	249
Appendix Two: The Root Cause of Osteoporosis	253
Appendix Three: Estrogen Myths	259
Appendix Four: The Calcium Yo-Yo Effect	263
Appendix Five: Dairy Milk and Prostate Cancer	269
Appendix Six: Milk Recipe List	272
Appendix Seven: The Missing Link	274
About the Author	277
Staying in touch with *The Milk Imperative*	278
Index	279
The Master Recipe (Summary)	282

Foreword by Dr. Amy Lanou

For years, the dairy industry's milk-mustache and other advertisements have pushed the notion that milk drinking helps children grow strong bones. Scientists have known for a long time that countries with the highest dairy product consumption, such as the United States and Finland, suffer from high osteoporosis and hip fracture rates. And findings from studies in women, children, and adolescents have also raised questions about the use of dairy products in the promotion of bone health.

The *World Health Organization* recommendations for preventing osteoporosis acknowledge this "calcium paradox." The agency advises that individuals 50 years of age or older, from countries with a high fracture incidence, only consume a minimum of 400–500 mg of calcium daily, far less than the current—and inflated—U.S. government recommendations, which range from 800 to 1,300 mg of calcium daily for all ages.

In ***The Milk Imperative*** the author, Russell Eaton, explodes the myth that osteoporosis is about insufficient calcium. Why is it that high dairy milk consumers (and hence, high calcium consumers) have a greater incidence of osteoporosis? This "calcium paradox" has intrigued doctors for many years, but new research is revealing a remarkable and intriguing answer to this paradox. In this book Russell Eaton takes you on a tour de force that lays bare the truth about dairy milk in a way that is likely to change your view of milk forever.

As a nutrition scientist I have spent many years overseeing nutrition education and programs for healthier diets. In early 2005 I published a study showing that currently available evidence does not support the notion that dairy milk consumption promotes bone health in young people. ***The Milk Imperative*** shows how dairy milk is harmful to health from just about any perspective. Eaton makes a compelling argument that today's pasteurized milk, in all its guises, has virtually no redeeming features at all, and serves only to cause disease and poor health.

I remember well the day that I began learning about the dangers of milk consumption. Dr. T. Colin Campbell, now professor emeritus at Cornell University, was giving a lecture on milk in his Vegetarian Nutrition class. He showed slide after slide of data showing that milk and its constituents – milk protein (mainly casein), and milk fat (mostly saturated), and milk sugar (lactose) – were strongly linked to increased risks of heart disease, cancer, inflammatory disorders, and digestive problems. I was startled and appalled that I had spent more than 10 years in higher education as a student of human nutrition at two of the best schools in the US and had been teaching nutrition to college students for about 4 years – and I hadn't heard this information before! It was a life-changing discovery. My own diet changed, as did the way I taught nutrition. My students and I are all healthier for it.

The Milk Imperative offers you this same opportunity. In it, Russell Eaton breaks new ground by bringing together the latest findings on dairy milk and revealing them in a very readable fashion that turns many pre-conceptions on their head – get ready for a roller-coaster ride! Anybody reading this extraordinary book will take away the profound message that by simply switching from dairy to non-dairy milk we will make a dramatic and long-lasting improvement to our health.

The Milk Imperative is a book I recommend to everybody because its message is a critically important one. If you do consume dairy milk, take this opportunity to try going dairy-free for at least a month. You'll be surprised at how easy it is. You may also find that this book will change your life in a remarkable way. If you already avoid dairy milk, or if you have a family, this book shows how best to keep osteoporosis at bay and how to stay slim and healthy. Many non-dairy milk recipes in the second half of the book provide a wide choice of nutritious and tasty alternatives to dairy milk.

Amy Lanou, Ph.D., is senior nutrition scientist for the *Physicians Committee for Responsible Medicine* (PCRM), a Washington D.C. based nonprofit organization dedicated to promoting preventive medicine, especially better nutrition, and higher standards in research. Dr. Lanou is also the author of *Healthy Eating for Life for Children* (John Wiley & Sons, Inc.; Feb. 2002). Amy Lanou has taught nutrition at Ithaca College and Cornell University. She received her B.S. in Nutrition Science from the University of California at Davis and her Ph.D. in Human Nutrition from Cornell University, USA.

Introduction

The root cause of osteoporosis

It used to be thought that osteoporosis was a *disease of calcium insufficiency* and that is why, for generations, we have been told to drink our milk and eat our cheese. Then it was thought that osteoporosis was a *disease of excessive calcium loss*, and we were told to avoid dairy milk because the protein in milk robbed the body of calcium.

The first theory is now known to be incorrect because there is no shortage of calcium in all kinds of foods and we only need less than half a gram a day for healthy bones. Also, you cannot get away from the fact that the highest milk-consuming countries also have the highest incidence of osteoporosis. Furthermore, even people with osteoporosis have a normal amount of calcium in the blood as the bloodstream is compelled to always carry a certain 'default' level.

The second theory that it is a *disease of excessive calcium loss* is also not correct: The protein in dairy milk does indeed rob the body of minerals, but it doesn't rob enough calcium from the bones or from dairy milk to prevent calcium being absorbed into the bone matrix. Many studies show that calcium in dairy milk does indeed increase bone density.

For many years doctors have faced a conundrum: How can it be that dairy milk causes osteoporosis when at the same time dairy milk increases bone density? The close correlation between osteoporosis and dairy milk consumption cannot be denied. Hip fracture rates and the incidence of osteoporosis are highest in countries with the highest consumption of dairy milk. Less developed countries such as Romania and Poland have the same high rates of osteoporosis as other high milk-consuming countries such as the USA and Sweden.

Doctors know that osteoporosis cannot be a *disease of calcium insufficiency* because they can see that their patients have been eating a calcium-rich diet all their lives. Doctors also know that osteoporosis cannot be a *disease of excessive calcium loss* because they see that dairy milk consumers have strong bone mineral density. So what is going on?

When confronted with such conundrums, some doctors resort to saying that 'other factors such as smoking, lack of exercise, the menopause, etc. are to blame.' But this is stating the obvious – it is well known that different factors can affect osteoporosis. The point here is that dairy milk is the biggest *dietary cause* of osteoporosis. Furthermore, *diet per se* is the major factor in the vast majority of cases of osteoporosis.

How then do we explain the apparent contradiction that dairy milk increases bone density while also causing osteoporosis? Until now there has been no answer to this riddle. Now, for the first time, this riddle can be answered: Osteoporosis is not a *disease of calcium insufficiency*. Nor is it a *disease of excessive calcium loss*, it is a *disease of bone-making cell insufficiency*.

In a nutshell, osteoporosis is not about a lack of calcium in the diet or in the bones, it's about a lack of bone-making cells.

To be more specific, it is a disease caused by the in and out movement of calcium in the bones, thus aging the bones before their time. By understanding and addressing this, better and more effective solutions can be found to prevent and treat osteoporosis, which is after all a terrible and painful disease. Dairy milk is a major, if not the principal, dietary cause of osteoporosis and this book shows why this is the case and how to avoid this shocking and unnecessary disease.

'The myth that osteoporosis is caused by calcium deficiency was created to sell dairy products and calcium supplements. There's no truth to it. American women are among the biggest consumers of calcium in the world, and they still have one of the highest levels of osteoporosis in the world. And eating even more dairy products and calcium supplements is not going to change that fact.' Source: Dr. John McDougall, The McDougall Program for Women (2000).

'Milk, it now seems clear, is not the solution to poor bone density. To the contrary, it's part of the problem.' Source: Dr. Charles Attwood, M.D., author of *Dr. Attwood's Low-Fat Prescription for Kids*.

The shocking truth about nanobacteria

New discoveries in medicine, and in particular groundbreaking research into nanobacteria, are dramatically changing the way we view the world of human health. Until recently, we were unaware that nanobacteria even existed. Today, scientists know that nanobacteria are all around us; in rain clouds, on pastures, and in our bodies.

Nanobacteria are important because they're at the root of all the major diseases in the world today. As explained in this book, there is a direct and strong link between nanobacteria and calcification of the human body. And calcification causes a greatly impaired quality of life, and an almost endless list of diseases including heart disease, cancer, and diabetes.

The roles played by dairy milk, nanobacteria and calcification are examined in detail in *Part One* as all three play a part in a shocking story that is still unfolding.

In **Parts Two and Three** you have a big choice of non-dairy milk recipes that you can make at home quickly and easily, plus detailed nutritional information on different milks. Appendix six gives a complete *Milk Recipe Index* of all the recipes in the book.

Why make milk at home?

Because it is better for your health and you save money. But an even more important reason for making home-made milk is the avoidance of dairy milk.

Whether or not you are vegan, vegetarian, or a meat-eater, you should avoid dairy milk for one simple reason: *Dairy milk is bad for you!* This topic is explored in Part One of this book as it is important to appreciate just how bad for health dairy milk really is.

Milk Allergy

Many people are either allergic to dairy milk (and other types of animal milk) or they suffer from lactose intolerance. (Allergies and lactose intolerance are different things). An allergic reaction is the body's response to a foreign body (antigen), typically proteins. In the case of animal milk allergy, the human body cannot tolerate the protein molecules designed for another animal species.

Allergy to animal milk is a well-studied form of food allergy (particularly dairy milk). There are both *immediate* and *delayed* patterns of animal milk allergy. Immediate type allergy tends to be obvious and shows up on skin tests. Delayed patterns of milk allergy are not obvious and tend to produce chronic disease that is seldom diagnosed.

Often, infant milk allergy is thought to be a specific and limited condition which children "outgrow." This idea can be misleading: many children continue to have chronic symptoms from animal milk, and although the original problem may disappear, the pattern of illness changes and confuses parents and physicians.

The symptoms of animal milk allergy can manifest in the skin, the digestive system, or the respiratory system.

Skin reactions may include an itchy red rash, hives, eczema, allergic "shiners" (black eyes), and swelling of lips, mouth, tongue, face or throat.

Digestive system reactions might include nausea, vomiting, diarrhea, gas, bloating, or abdominal cramps.

Respiratory system reactions can include a runny nose, sneezing, watery eyes, itchy eyes, nasal congestion, wheezing, shortness of breath, or coughing; or even anaphylactic shock.

Some people (particularly children) may have reddish ear lobes or a glazed look in their eyes. Other symptoms that may be attributed to animal milk allergy are bed wetting, lethargy, and inattentiveness.

'*At least 50% of all children in the USA are allergic to cow's milk, many undiagnosed. Dairy products are the leading cause of food allergy, often* revealed by diarrhea, constipation, and fatigue. Many cases of asthma and sinus infections are reported to be relieved and even eliminated by cutting out dairy.[1] Although the majority of people become allergic as infants, dairy milk allergy can be acquired later in life. Furthermore, you never outgrow dairy milk allergy, you just hide it better.

In fact, virtually everybody is either allergic or sensitive to animal milk. It's a matter of degree. If you are allergic the symptoms are strong, if you are sensitive the symptoms are weak (sometimes not obvious enough for the person to make a connection between the symptom and the cause).

For example, many people suffer regularly from mild headaches, fatigue, lethargy, respiratory ailments, shortness of breath and other symptoms, not realizing that they are caused by consuming animal milk in its various forms.

Lactose Intolerance

Lactose intolerance is different because it is caused by sugar molecules rather than protein molecules. Lactose is present in all animal milks. Thus, goat's milk cannot successfully be substituted for dairy milk in cases of lactose intolerance, *but non-dairy milks can.*

With lactose intolerance the body is unable to digest lactose properly, causing varying degrees of nausea, cramps, bloating, gas, and diarrhea, which begin about 30 minutes to 2 hours after eating or drinking foods containing lactose. The severity of symptoms varies depending on the amount of lactose each individual consumes or can tolerate. Lactose intolerance usually develops over time, getting worse as you get older. Technically, what happens is that lactose is broken down by bacteria in the lower intestines into glucose and galactose. As a result of eating this lactose, bacteria then produce their own body wastes which combine with glucose and galactose to ferment into gas and toxins causing bloating and cramps.

In the USA, for example, between 30 and 50 million people are regarded by the medical profession as being lactose intolerant. Certain ethnic and racial populations are more widely affected than others. As many as 75 percent of all African Americans and American Indians and 90 percent of Asian Americans are lactose intolerant. The condition is least common among persons of northern European descent.

Health professionals are aware that lactose intolerance is a major problem, but getting the word out to the public at large is an uphill struggle when confronted with a worldwide billion dollar industry intent on protecting dairy interests. For example, in mid 2005 the *Physicians Committee for Responsible Medicine,* USA, launched an advertising campaign on the public transit system in Washington DC to find people willing to join a

Class Action lawsuit against the milk industry. The objective of the Class Action is to force the milk industry to put warning labels on milk cartons alerting people to the symptoms of lactose intolerance.

There are dozens of studies showing how lactose in dairy milk causes human illness. Here are just three:

Lactose intolerance is widespread and... may co-exist in adults with irritable bowel syndrome and in children with recurrent abdominal pain. Management consists primarily of dietary change.[30]

Lactose malabsorption and lactase deficiency are chronic organic pathologic conditions... introduction of a lactose-free diet relieves symptoms in most patients who remain unaware of the relationship between food intake and symptoms.[31]

Females with lactose malabsorption not only showed signs of irritable bowel syndrome but also signs of premenstrual syndrome and mental derpression.[32]

Non-dairy milk

As with animal milk *allergy*, virtually everybody is either lactose *intolerant* or lactose sensitive – it's just a matter of degree. That's the bad news. The good news is that plant milks, as described in this book, do not produce milk protein allergies or lactose intolerance.

That is why the health benefits of plant, seed, and nut-based milks (referred to as '*plant milks*' or '*non-dairy milks*' in this book) go far beyond the provision of vitamins, minerals and other nutrients: plant milks help prevent a multitude of symptoms and illnesses commonly caused by animal milk.

Part Two of the book is about non-dairy milk, including nutritional tables on many different types of milk. **Part Three** is dedicated to non-dairy milk recipes, including smoothies and ice-cream. All the milk recipes are based on one master recipe template. This way, you will find it very easy to follow and remember any recipe.

Once you start making your own non-dairy milk you will never want to have dairy milk again. You will discover that non-dairy milk is absolutely delicious, nutritious, and ideal for shedding surplus body fat. Plant milks are generally low in harmful fats and carbohydrates, and by making the milk at home *you* control what goes into the milk. Most recipes involve no cooking at all, and some just a bare minimum, so the natural goodness of the ingredients is maintained.

Also, the wonderful *milk-by-product* that you get from making milk is yet another big advantage. This *milk-by-product* (referred to as 'okara') can be added to just about any dish you may be cooking such as soup, casseroles, vegetable bakes, lasagna, home-made bread, and even sweet desserts like cakes, cookies, pastries, and ice-cream. However, you can if you wish, just freeze the okara for future use, or not use it at all, and just enjoy the milk itself.

> *Okara is an added plus! The okara pulp that remains after extracting the milk is a wonderful, versatile, high fibre and nutritious-rich food. Okara has little taste and takes on the taste of the food it is mixed with, so it can be used in many ways in different recipes.*

Whether you live alone or with a family, making home-made milk is quick and easy and it can be kept fresh in the refrigerator just like any other milk. Alternatively, you may freeze the home-made milk and use it at a future date. If freezing, be sure to divide the milk into several bags or containers so that the frozen milk can be used up gradually over time.

The Recipes

The many recipes in the book (*Part three*) are simple to follow and no special apparatus is needed apart from a standard food blender (also known as a 'liquidizer'). A grinder or grain/coffee mill is also required (usually supplied as an attachment to a blender). By trying all the recipes you will quickly get to know your favourite ones for making on a regular basis. Unlike dairy milk, the beauty of home-made milk is that you can enjoy a variety of milks with different tastes. Once you start using home-made milk instead of dairy milk, you will notice a big improvement in health and well-being.

You can, of course, buy commercially made non-dairy milk which is becoming more widely available in supermarkets and health stores. This can be a good way to bridge the gap between giving up dairy milk and making your own non-dairy milk. The big advantage of making milk at home, apart from the cost-saving, is that you control the ingredients, you have greater variety, and less processing is involved.

A note on milk-making machines: The recipes in this book are designed for use with a blender combined with a simple straining method. But most of these same recipes can be adapted for use with a milk-making machine. The advantage of a milk-making machine is that once switched on you can just leave it and come back later to find the milk ready made. The disadvantages are:

- More hassle: the same preparatory work applies, whichever method is used, but with a milk-making machine you have the additional burden of having to take apart and clean all the component parts.

- Not as effective at extracting milk (nothing can beat the human hand and a nylon stocking when it comes to straining the milk!).

- Some milk recipes cannot be made using a milk-making machine, and very often a blender is more effective than the limited mixing capability of a milk-making machine.

- The okara (left-over residue) tends to end up too soggy when using a milk-making machine, making it more difficult to freeze or use in other recipes.

- When adding condiments (e.g. vanilla extract, maple syrup, salt, etc.) you cannot check the taste of the mixture while you are making it in the machine.

- Biggest drawback: It is difficult to control the heating/boiling process, and as a result, the nutritional value of the milk can be affected (vitamins and plant oils are easily destroyed with heat). None of the milk recipes in this book involve any boiling, and all the nutrients are kept intact.

When making milk, I personally find it much easier and quicker to *not use* a milk-making machine, even though I have one.

Under 10 minutes
Assuming you have everything you need, and you have prepared the basic ingredient, it will take no more than 10 minutes to make non-dairy milk from any recipe in this book

For the sake of simplicity, every recipe has been designed to give approximately 2 pints (just over 1 litre or 1 US quart) of milk volume. To change the volume simply adjust the proportions of each ingredient.

As you will see, home-made non-dairy milk is truly bursting with vitamins, minerals, antioxidants, phytochemicals, enzymes, and other super-healthy nutrients. If you want to lose weight or maintain your ideal body weight, home-made milk, as part of a healthy life style, provides an ideal form of nutrition.

Appendix One gives a nutritional summary of all the main vitamins and minerals. This provides a quick reference if you want to know what each nutrient does (and which foods provide good nutritional sources). And appendix six give an *at a glance* list of all the recipes in the book.

Whether or not you consume dairy milk, please do read *Part One* – it reveals a shocking and fascinating side to a food product that is consumed by millions of people everyday.

PART ONE: ALL ABOUT DAIRY MILK

***

Dairy Milk Effect on Health

Is dairy milk good for you?

In the distant past when food was scarce and everyday was a fight for survival, dairy milk (and derivative products such as butter and cheese) fulfilled an important role in everyday nutrition. When faced with starvation, just about any kind of food, including dairy milk, is better than nothing! But in today's world, when not faced with starvation, dairy milk is bad for human health in every respect (as explained later). If, after reading this chapter, you are not convinced, you are invited to enter 'dairy milk' in Google and check the results on Internet.

If dairy milk is not good for you why do so many people believe the opposite?

Because for generations people have been brought up to believe that dairy milk is basically a good food. We've been conditioned since childhood to think of milk as 'nature's most perfect food'. Of course in the past, when faced with a daily possibility of starvation, raw dairy milk was highly prized. Just about any kind of food, plant, animal, or insect, is good for you if the only alternative is literal starvation. The belief in the goodness of dairy milk is very strong in human society: *'If my own milk is good for my baby, dairy milk must also be good.'* This belief, albeit false, has cascaded down the generations, from mother to child. Because of this, many people continue to believe in the goodness of dairy milk even though countless scientific studies have proved that it is bad for human health, with absolutely no redeeming features at all.

If dairy milk is bad for health why is it so widely available?

Because it is a vast industry, employing millions of people worldwide. Dairy milk producers in all countries tend to be well represented in their communities. Very often a dairy milk producer will be part of a large farming or food business, or a consortium of dairy farmers, providing employment locally and nationally.

In the USA, for example, the dairy industry has a powerful hold on the nutrition industry and it pays huge numbers of dietitians, doctors, and researchers to push dairy, spending more than $300 million annually, just at the national level, to retain a market for its products.

The dairy industry is a truly huge big business, with sales of over $11 billion for milk and $16 billion for cheese annually in the USA alone. Virtually all countries have vested interest lobby groups that campaign continuously to promote dairy milk. Just the annual advertising budget for milk *in the USA alone* is $180 million! The dairy industry has infiltrated schools, bought off sports stars, celebrities, and politicians, pushing all the while an agenda based on profit, rather than public health.

Dr. Walter Willett, a veteran nutrition researcher at the *Harvard School of Public Health* studied 80,000 women over a twelve year period. He says that calcium consumption *'has become like a religious crusade, overshadowing true preventive measures such as physical exercise. To hear the dairy industry tell it, if you consume three glasses of milk daily, your bones will be stronger, and you can rest safely knowing that osteoporosis is not in your future.'*

Despite the dairy industry funding study after study to try to prove its claims, Dr. John McDougall (Physician and nutrition expert, USA), upon examining all the available nutritional studies and evidence, concludes:

'The primary cause of osteoporosis is the high-protein diet most Americans and Europeans consume today. As one leading researcher said, eating a high-protein diet is like pouring acid rain on your bones.'

Remarkably enough, as explained in this book, if dairy milk has any effect, both clinical and population evidence strongly show dairy milk as *causing*, rather than preventing osteoporosis. That the dairy industry would lull unsuspecting women and children into complacency by telling them, essentially, *'drink more milk and your bones will be fine'* may make good business sense, but it does the public a grave disservice.

Dairy farmers tend to be influential and can lobby hard to make sure that their milk is sold successfully. This, coupled with the widespread misconception that milk is a good thing to consume, helps to perpetuate the demand for and widespread consumption of dairy milk. But although dairy milk is widely consumed in many countries (particularly America and Europe), most human beings in the world cannot drink it because the lactose in dairy milk makes them ill.

Another factor often ignored is the fact that pharmaceutical companies spend millions of dollars developing and promoting unnecessary calcium and vitamin D supplements – this bolsters the image that calcium, and by association dairy milk, is good for bones. Pharmaceutical companies risk losing billions of dollars in profits: they sell drugs and calcium supplements to treat the symptoms of osteoporosis. If they cure the source of the disease, they would no longer make any money. They also have a vested interest in providing veterinary products and chemicals to a huge dairy industry. This is why pharmaceutical companies are happy to cooperate with dairy companies to promote the myth that milk is good for bones. There may not be any conspiracy for the two industries to work together, but they both lobby hard to promote the idea that taking more calcium is good for bones. As explained in the next chapter, taking more calcium actually promotes osteoporosis!

If dairy milk is bad for you, why do dieticians continue to recommend it?

Some dieticians may recommend the consumption of milk, particularly if allied to the vast dairy or pharmaceutical industries. But increasingly, many dieticians now recognize that dairy milk is bad for you. Nobody (not even dieticians) recommend dairy milk for infants under one year old. Any dieticians who still recommend dairy milk may be sincere and well-meaning, but nevertheless are either ill-informed, out-of-date, or allied to the farming and dairy industries. Consider the following:

• A dietician, like most people, is brought up from childhood believing in the goodness of dairy milk. This belief is based on false logic that goes like this: *Our bones are made of calcium. Milk is rich in calcium. Therefore milk is good for our bones. Therefore milk is good for our health. Therefore all of us should drink lots of milk.* This is false logic because it is based on one aspect of nutritional content rather than on the biological effect of dairy milk consumption.

• The belief in the goodness of dairy milk gets reinforced daily by the widespread availability and consumption of dairy milk (how can everybody be wrong?).

• At medical school the dietician gets taught by manuals and tutors that mostly come from a previous generation; from a generation that believed in the goodness of milk.

• Dieticians get bombarded with pseudo-scientific evidence that dairy milk/calcium is good for health. This 'evidence' comes from sponsored studies, seminars, exhibitions, advertising, etc. all funded by the dairy and pharmaceutical industries.

- The dietician is unlikely to examine the latest scientific evidence proving that milk is bad for you, particularly as the world around you continues to consume dairy milk with complete abandon. If you have spent all your life believing that dairy milk is good for human consumption, it is very difficult to then accept and promote the opposite view, particularly if your job is on the line.

Why is dairy milk bad for you?

The answer is manifold, as explained below.

▶ **Contamination.** Dairy milk causes a multitude of diseases. Dairy milk and its derivative dairy products contain no fibre or complex carbohydrates and are mostly laden with saturated fat and rancid cholesterol. Dairy products are contaminated with cow's blood and pus cells, which often do not get neutralized through pasteurization. Virtually all dairy cows are given drugs, hormones and antibiotics to make them produce plenty of milk for as long as possible. Also, the grass (if any) and food they eat is frequently contaminated with filth and farm waste, giving rise to E.coli, salmonella, and listeria, leading to food poisoning and illness in humans who consume dairy milk.

In a major study in the USA over 76% of pasteurized milk transported by bulk tankers was found to be contaminated with coli bacteria.[29] At best a coli bacteria infection will make you feel very ill for about a week and may require hospitalization. At worst, coli bacteria infections such as E.coli have been known to kill people.

In addition to farm waste, dairy cows are increasingly being fed disease-ridden commercial and domestic waste as a way of cutting down on land-fill costs. *'Feeding waste products* [to cows] *has some positive economic impacts for the milk producer. If they can buy waste products for less than they can buy traditional feed ingredients, it will reduce their cost of milk production. The alternative of feeding much of the material to livestock would be to landfill it, and that has some significant costs to society'*[89]

Furthermore, feedgrains destined for livestock (including dairy cows) are usually sprayed heavily with herbicides and pesticides. These are hydrocarbons whose chronic ingestion may raise the risk of birth defects or cancer.

These pesticides, herbicides, hormones, drugs and antibiotics get passed into the milk and *do not get eliminated with pasteurization.* Furthermore, all lactating mammals eliminate some of their toxic waste through their milk!

▶ **Disease.** Dairy milk and dairy products are linked to a long list of illnesses. In particular, antigenic proteins in cow's milk can 'leak' into the bloodstream of a milk consumer through the intestinal lining and incite allergic reactions in lungs and joints – exacerbating asthma and rheumatoid arthritis.

Here is a letter received by Robert Cohen, author of '*Milk – The Deadly Poison*' and '*Milk A-Z*'. Regarded as an arch enemy of the dairy industry and despised by most dairy farmers, the letter was sent to Robert Cohen in January 2002 by a long-time dairy farmer:

You and I have stood on different sides of the fence for a number of years, but I've got a story to tell you, and an apology to offer. Catherine (my wife of 21 years) and I both grew up on dairy farms. We've been raising Holsteins as long as we can remember. Cath is just 42 years old, but she is crippled with **rheumatoid arthritis**. *There is no record of this disease in her family, but she has been in pain for the past two years, much of it bedridden.*

We've tried traditional and alternative therapies and medicines, but she only got a little short term relief. We even tried acupuncture. Try finding an acupuncturist in the rural Midwest! It was expensive, and didn't really work. Catherine's pain has been unbearable at times.

Despite there being no information on the internet linking dairy consumption to **rheumatoid arthritis**, *and nothing in medical journals (I've searched online Medline), we made a resolution together to discontinue drinking our own milk, and not eat cheese or any other dairy product for six months, just to see if there would be some improvement.*

I have to tell you this. Catherine feels like she's been to Lourdes. She's cured. There is some pain, but most is gone. I've had changes too which I'll discuss another time. I thank you, and curse you at the same time. Milking cows is my livelihood. I've always believed that what I was doing was the right thing. I'm not going to sell my cows and sell my farm. I love the business. I just don't feel that good about it anymore. You were right about the arthritis. I don't know about the cancer and heart attacks, but you have given us a miracle that doctors were not able to provide. It did not take us three to six months to learn the truth. It took just three weeks. I've ridiculed your work in the past. Please accept my apology. Your friend, Tom.

Here are a few comments from physicians and scientists regarding diseases caused by dairy milk:

Certain foods trigger the symptoms of **rheumatoid arthritis**, *and eliminating these foods sometimes causes even long-standing symptoms to improve or even remit entirely. It's important to avoid the problem foods completely, as even a small amount can cause symptoms. All dairy products should be avoided: skim or whole milk, goat's milk, cheese, yogurt, cream, etc.* [48]

Milk's biological purpose is to promote rapid growth in infant cows. It makes biological sense that its nutrients and hormonal effects might also promote the growth of cancer cells. [39]

There is a colossal amount of information linking the consumption of milk to arthritis...and a multitude of other problems as documented by Hannah Allen, Alec Burton, Viktoras Kulvinsdas, F.M. Pottenger, Herbert M, Shelton, and N.L. Walker, among others. [40]

From 1988 to 1993 there were over 2,700 articles dealing with [dairy] milk recorded in the "Medicine" archives... There is no lack of scientific information on the subject. I reviewed over 500 articles. They were only slightly less than horrifying...none of the authors spoke of cow's milk as an excellent food. The main focus seemed to be on intestinal colic, intestinal irritation, bleeding, anemia, allergic reactions, viral infection with bovine leukemia, childhood diabetes, contamination of milk by blood and pus cells, as well as a variety of chemicals and insecticides were also discussed. [60]

The list of ailments cited by medical literature in relation to dairy milk is almost too long to publish. Here are just a few in no particular order: constipation, obesity, heart disease, several types of cancer (including ovarian, lung, and breast cancer), colitis, tonsillitis arthritis, sinusitis, asthma, infant anemia, leukemia, diabetes, gastrointestinal bleeding, atherosclerosis, salmonella, diarrhea, abdominal cramps, migraine, colds, and many other diseases.

Prostate cancer, for example, is strongly associated with dairy milk as evidenced by many studies (please see appendix five).

And let's not forget BSE (known as 'mad cow disease'). The fact that humans can catch BSE from eating cooked cow's meat has been proven. When it comes to BSE and dairy milk, the jury is still out!

Several cases of mad cow disease have been reported in North America in 2004-05. The USA Consumer's Union states:

Mad cow disease is a fatal, brain-wasting affliction, which can be passed on to humans by eating tainted beef. Consumers Union has serious concerns about the effectiveness of the U.S. mad cow surveillance program including its failure to use the most sensitive and up-to-date testing methods that are used in Europe and Japan. Just as troublesome is the fact that the government does not have mandatory recall authority and refuses to publicize the names of the retailers that are selling the tainted meat. Source: www.consumersunion.org.

> **Dairy milk contains many protein-allergens that cause allergic reactions. The two main allergens are whey and casein, and an individual may be allergic to either or both. The casein is the curd that forms when milk is left to sour, and the whey is the watery residue which is left after the curd is removed.**

Irritable Bowel Syndrome (IBS) deserves a special mention. It is estimated that about a quarter of all adults suffer periodically from IBS, causing a multitude of digestive disorders. Stress used to be thought of as a major cause of IBS, but it is now thought that dairy milk is the biggest cause.

The lactose intolerance, indigestible protein, and antibiotics in the milk, all combine to provide a ready-made cocktail for IBS. *Some kinds of bacteria in dairy milk are able to survive pasteurization, causing Johne's Disease, Crohns Disease, and IBS.* [3] By simply giving up dairy milk, most people find that IBS disappears.

Ear infections are another major cause of disease from dairy milk: *Milk allergies …are the leading cause of chronic ear infections that plague up to 40% of all children under the age of six.*[9] *Cows milk allergy is associated with recurrent otitis media (ear infection) during childhood.*[10] *Concerning ear infections, you just don't see this painful condition among infants and children who aren't getting cow's milk into their systems.*[11]

Cow's milk is the primary cause of recurrent ear infections in children. It has also been linked to insulin dependent diabetes, rheumatoid arthritis, infertility, and leukemia. Source: Dr. Joseph Mercola (licensed Osteopathic physician and board-certified in family medicine, www.mercola.com).

In May 2005 it was reported that dairy milk increases the risk of getting Parkinson's Disease (a degenerative disease of the brain). The study in Hawaii followed 7,594 men. During the course of the 30-year study 128 developed Parkinson's. The researchers found that men who consumed 16 oz of milk a day were 2.3 times more likely to develop Parkinson's than those who drank no milk at all. *'Findings suggest that milk intake is associated with an increased risk of Parkinson's disease.'* [98]

In the book *Killers Within* the authors reveal that *Staphlococcus Aureus* is the most common infection of dairy cows. Typical symptoms in humans include nausea, vomiting, diarrhea, abdominal cramps, and fever. Bacterial toxins are easily passed from cows to humans in milk, and are not destroyed by pasteurization. On page 30, the authors write: *'Staphlococcus Aureus bacteria are so virulent that very few are needed to do the job…it's the most successful of all bacterial pathogens and the number one cause of hospital infections in the world.'* [138]

Last, but not least, TB (tuberculosis) is widespread in dairy cows in all parts of the world. The incidence of infection in cows is chronic and it varies tremendously from farm to farm, and from country to country, but it would be rare for a dairy farm to have no cows infected with TB. In fact, pasteurization was originally introduced because of the widespread incidence of bovine TB.

The milk industry is quick to say that bovine TB is killed with pasteurization. But consider this:

(i) *A cow with TB may swallow her own saliva and this, with the infected material coughed up from the lungs, then passes through the whole digestive tract, and remains as an active form of infection. Particles of infected dust or manure may contaminate the milk, or it may be infected directly from the tubercular udder.*[44]

(ii) Sometimes farm workers and veterinarians are known to catch TB from cows. This is not unusual because coughs and sneezes from cows can easily infect people nearby with TB. These people can then unwittingly infect other people.

(iii) *Some strains of mycobacteria, similar to those that are associated with TB have been found to survive pasteurization.*[43]

(iv) TB incidence in humans is increasing worldwide and it is easily transmissible between persons. Ask yourself this: Do you really want to ingest body fluids (i.e. milk) from diseased animals?

▶ **Galactose.** A type of sugar, galactose is found in small amounts in many foods, including fruit and vegetables. Dairy milk, however, is super-rich in galactose. Weight for weight, dairy milk typically has 20 to 30 times more galactose than, say, cheddar cheese or lentils, and 500 times more than an orange. For a list of foods showing their galactose content go to www.galactosemia.org.

The human body can use galactose in small amounts by converting it into energy. But the *very large* amounts provided by dairy milk cannot be broken down and used as energy and become toxic. Hence, the large surplus amounts of galactose provided by dairy milk end up causing illness in several ways. Note that here we are not talking about people allergic to galactose – people allergic to galactose can actually die from consuming dairy milk or any galactose rich food. ***Galactose-rich dairy milk is bad for anybody, whether or not allergic to galactose!***

For example, several studies show that galactose from dairy milk increases the risk of cataracts in the eyes:

• *This patient presented with cataracts and galactosuria that developed upon drinking milk...The mechanism that produces galactose-related **cataracts** is understood fairly well...Diet is the foundation of therapy.*

Elimination of lactose and galactose sources suffices for definitive therapy.[149]

- *Galactose is toxic in high doses or if insufficiently removed, and causes tissue damage above certain levels in humans. Galactose reaches high levels in human plasma following milk ingestion. Galactose increases atheromatous plaque formation in Baboons and other experimental animals, causes **cataracts** in rats (and possibly in humans), and is related to the onset of diabetes in humans (Gordon, 1999).*

Another study shows a strong link between galactose and infertility in women.[148] Many other studies show a close association between galactose and a variety of diseases, arising from dairy milk consumption. Doctors even have a name for galactose when it causes disease: *galactosemia.*

The dairy industry tries to get round the problem of galactose by marketing lactose-reduced milk. Unfortunately, such milk only encourages a greater consumption of an extremely unhealthy product in many other ways. Note that compared to whole milk, evaporated milk contains twice as much, and goat's milk has about 10% more galactose.

A book on this subject titled *Milk and mortality*[147] lists dozens of studies showing strong associations between galactose from dairy milk and disease.

▶ **Bovine sex hormones.**

Progesterone is the single most important hormone made by the female human body. It is critically important for the health of virtually every cell and organ in the body. Because progesterone is a master hormone, it is used as a precursor for the production of other important hormones, such as estrogen and cortisone.

*Progesterone production, however, can be suppressed by environmental antagonists, such as the hormones found in most commercially grown meats & **dairy products**, pesticides, petro-chemicals, prescription hormones and stress.* Source: www.progesterone.com.

The natural progesterone produced by a woman's body is known to protect against breast cancer. But dairy milk increases the risk of breast cancer in women by suppressing her progesterone. This happens because bovine sex hormones interfere with a woman's body chemistry. (Women produce varying levels of progesterone throughout their lives, whether or not pregnant, as it is so vital).

Also, dairy milk interferes with the production of oxytocin in the woman's body. The hormone oxytocin is known to protect against breast cancer, yet another reason for avoiding dairy milk. [150]

Men do not require progesterone as it is a female sex hormone. Nevertheless, bovine sex hormones can also interfere with a man's body chemistry leading to cancer.

About 80% of milk is obtained from pregnant cows *before* birth. The other 20% is obtained in the period between giving birth and the next forced pregnancy. Virtually all dairy cows (including 'organic' dairy cows) are kept in a state of almost continuous pregnancy so as to maximize milk production. This continuous state of pregnancy produces milk rich in bovine sex hormones which survive pasteurization.

Milk and dairy products contain the female sex hormones estrogen and progesterone. [142] *It is reasonable to hypothesize that estrogens or progesterone in milk and dairy products may be associated with the development of testicular cancer.* [143]

Dairy farming involves milking the cows even when pregnant, and this practice is associated with higher levels of estrogen and progesterone in milk, which in turn may increase risk of premature sexual development [in humans] *and also breast cancer.* [144]

▶ **Pus.** How does a cow make milk? A dairy cow filters 10,000 quarts (about 11,000 litres) of blood through her udder each day and uses dead white blood cells to manufacture her milk. Put another way: dairy milk is mainly pus with hormones, and just about every cupful of pasteurized dairy milk contains pus. Humans make breast milk differently: the hormone prolactin makes the breasts produce milk.

The milk industry tries to argue that pus in milk (euphemistically referred to as *somatic cells*) is not harmful, but the evidence contradicts this.

It is estimated that about one-third of cows being milked at any one time are stressed and infected. Milk from these cows contains large amounts of bacteria, viruses, and pus. As a consequence, farmers must treat their herds with increased amounts of antibiotics. In an extensive study, Pam Ruegg, a University of Wisconsin mastitis researcher, examined more than a million records, and concluded that the higher the herd's pus cell count, the greater the risk of antibiotic residues in milk. So pus goes hand in hand with antibiotics which do not get neutralized by the pasteurization process.

The Milk Development Council [in the UK] *charges farmers £0.04 per litre to pay for its research on milk marketing, but it does not investigate safety or levels of diseases such as mastitis, which causes dead cells from pus residue to pass into milk.*[59]

Any lactating mammal excretes toxins through her milk. This includes antibiotics, pesticides, chemicals and hormones. Also, all cow's milk contains blood! The [US] *inspectors are simply asked to keep it under* certain limits. You may be horrified to learn that the USDA allows milk to contain from one to one and a half million pus cells per milliliter (1/30 of an ounce). [60]

The dairy industry knows that there is a problem with pus in milk. Accordingly, it has developed a system known as the "somatic cell count" to measure the amount of pus in milk. The somatic cell count is the standard used to gauge milk quality. The higher the somatic cell count, the more pus in the milk.

Any milk with a somatic cell count higher than 200 million per litre should not enter the human food supply, according to the American dairy industry. Therefore, anyone living in a region where the somatic cell count is higher than 200 million shouldn't be drinking milk. There is only one problem—virtually every state in the USA is producing milk with pus levels so high that it shouldn't enter the human food supply! Even the US national average, at 322 million, is well above the industry's limit.

▶ **Antibiotics.** Dairy cows are given antibiotics to fend off disease and make them produce more milk. Here is an extract from *Dr. Neil Barnard, The Physicians Committee on Responsible Medicine, USA*:

'Milk is extracted from cows that are kept producing milk with the help of hormones, long after they need it for their calves. The cows are fed commercially created feeds that may include hay, grain, cardboard, and wood shavings They are regularly plied with large amounts of antibiotics to treat or fend off infections, which then find their way into the milk.'

Antibiotics from dairy milk (including penicillin) are bad for humans because they weaken the immune system and make you more prone to disease. This happens because the continual exposure to small levels of antibiotics in milk causes a modification of "good" bacteria in the intestine leading to vitamin and mineral deficiencies and a greater tendency to contract infections. This also leads to drug-resistant strains of bacteria inside your body, making you less capable of responding to medication.

Also, trace amounts of penicillin found in most pasteurized milk can be hazardous to people allergic to penicillin.

In the book *Killers Within* the authors explain why antibiotics continue to be given in such high quantities to farm animals such as chickens, pigs, and cows: the reason is that antibiotics are in fact powerful *growth promoters*. This explains why dairy cows are usually so overdosed with antibiotics. [138]

> *Drinking a glass or two of milk each day may increase the risk of Parkinson's disease later in life. The risk of Parkinson's disease increases as the amount of milk consumed each day goes up. Heavy milk drinkers were 2.3-times more likely to develop Parkinson's disease than non-milk drinkers.*
> Source: Neurology, April 2005.

▶ **Growth Hormones.** The dairy industry is quick to say that they are not allowed by law to give *growth* hormones to dairy cows. But this is a misleading argument. Here are the facts:

Virtually all dairy cows get given between 50 and 60 types of hormones. The worst of these is a hormone called 'Insulin-like growth factor ONE' (IGF-1) which is very harmful to humans. IGF-1 *survives pasteurization and human digestion* and has been identified as the key factor in breast cancer growth.[5] IGF-1 from dairy milk is particularly harmful to humans because it has the same DNA composition as natural human growth hormone, and as a result growth hormones from cow's milk get fully assimilated into the human body. By drinking cow's milk, IGF-1 is delivered right into the body's cells.[3,4]

This in turn causes cancer. This is so because *all types* of cancer growth depend on our body's Insulin Growth Factor to take hold and grow. When IGF-1 from dairy milk is consumed this increases the risk of cancer by allowing cancers to grow and proliferate much more vigorously.

> *IGF-1 occurs in all kinds of dairy milk, in all countries, whether raw, pasteurized, organic, non-organic, homogenized, ultra-pasteurized, or whether made into yogurt, cheese, butter.*
> *If you consume dairy, you consume IGF-1*

Milk, whether human or dairy, is a hormonal delivery system designed to help the progeny grow quickly. **Dairy milk is specifically designed for rapid growth of calves.** When humans consume a cocktail of hormones designed for calf growth it plays havoc with the human body in many different and harmful ways.

Here are just a few of the many studies showing how IGF-1 in dairy milk causes illness:

IGF-1 is critically involved in the aberrant growth of human breast cancer cells. Journal of the National Institute of Health, 1991-3.

We manufacture IGF-1 in our bodies. We also consume IGF-1 in pasteurized, homogenized dairy milk. The tiny homogenized fat globules carry IGF-1 from milk through the stomach and gut into the bloodstream where they can circulate through the body to exert powerful growth effects. This IGF-1 allows cancers to grow.[60]

Estrogen regulation of IGF-1 in breast cancer cells would support the hypothesis that IGF-1 has a regulatory function in breast cancer. Molecular Cell Endocrinology, March, 99(2).

IGF-1 is a potent growth factor for cellular proliferation in the human breast carcinoma cell line. Journal of Cellular Physiology, January, 1994, 158(1).

IGF-1 plays a major role in breast cancer cell growth. European Journal of Cancer, 29A (16), 1993.

IGF-1 produces a 10-fold increase in RNA levels of cancer cells. IGF-1 appears to be a critical component in cellular proliferation. Experimental Cell Research, March, 1994, 211(1).

IGF-1 accelerates the growth of breast cancer cells. Science, Vol. 259, January 29, 1993.

A strong positive association was observed between IGF-1 levels and prostate cancer risk. Science, vol. 279, January 23, 1998.

IGF-1 can affect the proliferation of breast epithelial cells, and is thought to have a role in breast cancer. The Lancet, vol. 351, May 9, 1998.

IGF-1 strongly stimulates the proliferation of a variety of cancer cells, including those from lung cancer. Journal of the National Cancer Institute, vol. 91, no. 2, January 20, 1999.

IGF-1 is widely involved in human carcinogenesis. A significant association between IGF-1 and an increased risk of lung, colon, prostate, and pre-menopausal breast cancer has recently been reported. International Journal of Cancer, 2000 Aug. 87:4.

A raised level of IGF-1 has been associated with breast cancer for women and prostate cancer for men. Rosemary Hoskins, Food Fact no. 2, A Safe Alliance Publication, 1998.

By continuing to drink milk, one delivers the most powerful growth hormone in nature to his or her body (IGF-I). That hormone has been called the key factor in the growth of breast, prostate, and lung cancer. At the very best, or worst, this powerful growth hormone instructs all cells to grow. This might be the reason that Americans are so overweight. At the very worst, this hormone does not discriminate. When it finds an existing cancer, usually controlled by our immune systems, the message it delivers is: GROW! [60]

IGF-1 has been called "**plug and play cancer fuel**" by many. Here is what Dr. Sarfaraz K. Niazi (PhD pharmaceutical sciences, University of Illinois, USA) has to say regarding hormones in milk:

'Some dairy milk samples also show noticeable concentration of a growth hormone given to cows to promote their growth and increase milk production. Being fat-soluble, hormones are more concentrated in the cream. Hormones in milk are a serious threat to health because even at very low concentrations, they can cause severe imbalance of our physiologic system. They have also been implicated in many types of cancers and decreased resistance to infections and diseases. Though prohibited in some parts of the world, unscrupulous farmers continue to use hormones. Whatever a cow eats shows up in her udders. The grass, silage, straw, cereals, roots, tubers, legumes, oilseeds, oilcakes, and milk by-products, which contain a variety of chemical additives, make the diet of modern cow. The diet of cows is rife with pesticides, fertilizers, herbicides and traces of heavy metals along with chemicals from spoilage. With each glass of milk shoved down little Jane's or Johnny's throat, comes the increased chance of their developing atherosclerosis, cancer, autoimmune diseases, infections and a host of other diseases still unidentified, when they reach adulthood.'

Another little known fact about IGF-1 in dairy milk is that it accelerates early puberty in young boys and girls (the bovine growth factor accelerates the onset of puberty in humans). This makes you more prone to getting cancer later in life. Also, early puberty in girls causes depression, aggressiveness, social withdrawal, moodiness, behavioral problems, and a greater tendency to smoke and take drugs. Worse still, early puberty in a girl increases the risk of osteoporosis later in life (please see the chapter *Dairy Milk Effect on Young People* for a fuller explanation).

There are several reasons why dairy products raise a woman's hormone levels causing a variety of hormone-dependent problems from early onset of menstruation (menarche) to PMS and uterine fibroids - but one is unique to cow's milk. Cows are milked even while they are pregnant. As a result of the pregnancy, cows secrete high levels of estrogen into their milk. Source: Janowski T., *Mammary secretion of oestrogens in the cow*, Domest Anim Endocrinol. 2002 Jul; 23(1-2): 125-37.

Growth hormones occur naturally in *all milk* since hormones are present when cows lactate. But additionally, in the USA cows are regularly injected with the genetically engineered rBGH (**R**ecombitant **B**ovine **G**rowth **H**ormone). rBGH dramatically increases the amount of IGF-1 produced in dairy milk, and it is estimated that 90% of USA milk comes from rBGH cows!

This hormone (also known as rBST or Posilac) is given to cows to increase milk production by as much as 15 – 20%. The U.S. FDA approved the rBGH drug in 1993, but many countries are concerned about its safety on both human and animal health. Currently rBGH is allowed in the USA but its use in dairy cows is banned in the European Union, Canada, New Zealand, Australia and Japan, although many farmers flaunt the rules. Furthermore, there is no ban on the importation of milk into Europe that contains rBGH, and in fact some large coffee-shop chains do this. Also, many legally imported milk powders and dairy products contain rBGH. Therefore, if you consume dairy milk and dairy products it is difficult to escape rBGH wherever you live.

The dairy industry may argue that most rBGH is destroyed in pasteurization. But studies show that a large percentage does not get destroyed. Worse still, the harmful IGF-1 (a by-product of rBGH) does not get destroyed at all by pasteurization and passes into milk and dairy products. It is hoped that rBGH may one day be phased out of the dairy industry because of growing consumer resistance worldwide.

The vast majority of the USA's 1,500 dairy companies mix rBGH milk with non-rBGH milk during processing to such an extent that an estimated 80 to 90 percent of the U.S. dairy supply contains some percentage of rBGH. [123]

The rBGH hormone induces an abnormal level of insulin growth factor in dairy milk. Insulin growth factor is not destroyed during pasteurization and is not inactivated by digestion in the human gut. Insulin growth factor can be absorbed through the gut wall, particularly in infants, whose digestive tract is still developing. Insulin growth factor has been shown to abnormally increase body weight and increase liver weight. It also induces malignant transformation of normal human breast epithelial cells and stimulates the growth of the cancer cells. It has a similar association with colon cancer. Extract of letter from Samuel S. Epstein, M.D to David Kessler, head of the USA Food and Drug Administration.

Here is what Dr. Joseph Mercola (licensed Osteopathic physician and board-certified in family medicine, www.mercola.com) has to say regarding rBGH:

Recombinant Bovine Growth Hormone (rBGH) is a genetically engineered drug injected into cows, which increases the levels of cancer causing and other dangerous chemicals in milk. rBGH derived milk contains dramatically higher levels of IGF-1 (Insulin Growth Factor), a risk factor for breast and colon cancer. IGF-1 is not destroyed by pasteurization.

An article in "Cancer Research," June 1995, shows that high levels of IGF-1 are also linked to hypertension, premature growth stimulation in infants, gynecomastia in young children, glucose intolerance and juvenile diabetes. Dr. Samuel Epstein, professor of occupational and environmental medicine at the University of Illinois School of Public Health and chair of Cancer Prevention Coalition, Inc., reports that IGF-

1, which causes cells to divide, induces malignant transformation of normal breast epithelial cells, and is a growth factor for human breast cancer and colon cancer.*

Recombinant Bovine Growth Hormone is like "crack" for cows. Bi weekly shots "rev" up their system and force them to produce more milk for perhaps a few years, and then their milk production declines dramatically. rBGH also makes them sick. Their udders swell and develop painful, bloody lesions -- an infection known as "mastitis," which is "treated" by giving cows huge doses of antibiotics. [Mastitis creates pus in the milk]. *The cows suffer through shortened life spans and increased birth defects, rates of metabolic disease, infertility and stress.*

According to Dr. Michael Lam (USA), MD, MPH, ABAAM, CNCT, the widespread use of rBGH has been linked to the proliferation of breast, prostate, and colon cancer cells in humans. Selected studies have shown that men with an IGF-1 level of between 300-500 mg/dl have **more than four times the risk** of developing prostate cancer compared to those with a level between 100 to 185 mg/dl. This risk is even more pronounced in men over 60 years of age. The elevated IGF-1 levels were present several years before an actual diagnosis of prostate cancer (please see appendix five, *Dairy Milk and Prostate Cancer* for more information on this disease).

▶ **Bovine leukemia.** Bovine leukemia deserves a special mention: it is present in about half of dairy cows in Europe and America, and in other parts of the world the incidence is higher. There is increasing evidence that bovine leukemia is getting passed to humans through dairy milk, causing human leukemia and lymphoma (a kind of cancer). For example, dairy veterinarians and farmers have significantly elevated leukemia rates. Pasteurization does not always kill the bovine leukemia virus because very often, the pasteurization process is not carried out correctly or because of cross infection from raw milk to pasteurized milk (milk containers, equipment, etc). In tests to see whether other species of animals can catch bovine leukemia, virtually all tests proved positive.

▶ **Mucus.** Among dairy products, dairy milk is the worst because it causes more mucus in humans than any food you can eat. The casein in milk causes a thick dense mucus that clogs and irritates the body's entire respiratory system. This dense, gluey mucus coats the inside of the body and places an enormous burden on the eliminative faculties of the delicate mucus membranes. This in turn invites disease and prevents the immune system from keeping harmful viruses and bacteria at bay.

Eat casein and your body produces histamines, then mucous. This sludge congests your organs. Give up all milk and dairy products for just one week and an internal "fog" will lift from your body. [36]

This is what happens: The casein mucus congestion lines the epithelial cells in our airways and allows invading viruses to get past our defenses, causing infections such as colds and flu; plus many illnesses associated with the airways such as bronchitis, chest infections, coughs, aggravated asthma, and so on. Infections get past our defenses because the tiny hairs that line the mucus membranes in our airways get clogged up. Fig. 1 shows how each epithelial cell contributes a few hairs:

Fig. 1
Epithelial cells lining the airways

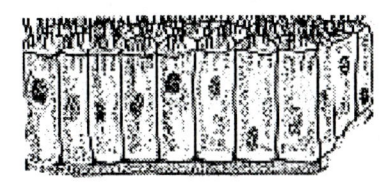

So when the hairs are clogged up with casein mucus they cannot catch and eject invading viruses, bacteria, dust and other debris. Healthy epithelial cells are able to undulate in a wave-like motion that carries debris out of the body. When the hairs are clogged with mucus, the undulating motion is ineffective.

As a result, immunity is lowered, and infections become more common. The mucus membranes of people who consume dairy milk on a daily basis are in a perpetual state of mucosal congestion. Few people note the ill effects because dairy milk tends to be consumed on a regular basis, providing a continuing state of mucosal congestion that is regarded as 'normal'.

'Eighty percent of milk protein is casein, a tenacious glue and allergenic protein. Eat casein and you produce histamines, then mucous. The reaction is often delayed, occurring 12-15 hours after consumption.... By eliminating all dairy milk for one week, most people note the difference which includes better sleep, more energy, better bowel movements, clarity of thought, muscle, bone, and back pain relief...and goodbye to nasal congestion.' [3]

▶ **Harmful fat.** Dairy milk contains saturated fat which is harmful to health. Whole milk is high in saturated fat which is known to cause obesity, heart disease, cancer and many other diseases in the human body.

Dairy milk also contains trans fats (trans fatty acids) a type of fat which is even more harmful than saturated fat. Trans fats are formed by heating unsaturated fat or by hydrogenation (mixing air into the fat). This changes the molecular structure. Such fats are harmful to health because they clog up arteries and veins and in so doing contribute to a multitude of diseases. Unlike saturated fat, trans fats penetrate more deeply into nooks and crannies of the body (including the brain) and are more difficult to get rid of.

All dairy milk contains trans fats, except non-fat milk. The level of trans fats in dairy milk varies, depending on animal feeds, grazing, and other factors. In the USA and some other countries, there is no requirement to state the level of trans fats on the label if the amount is not over 0.5g per 244g of fat. Consequently, no level of trans fats is shown on milk carton labels. But the 0.5g threshold is often breached because levels of trans fats vary considerably between 0.2g and 5.0g and random testing by the authorities, apart from being expensive and time consuming, is not enough to police the situation effectively.

> *'Trans fatty acid levels in dairy milk are quite high. Children should avoid trans fatty acids as a matter of family policy, otherwise you are doing them a considerable disservice* [at a critical time in their development]. *One should restrict foods that contain trans fatty acids'.*
> Source: Dr. Michael Schmidt, author of 'Brain-Building Nutrition' and a world authority on nutritional medicine.

What about lactose intolerance?

Dairy milk contains sugar (i.e. carbohydrate) in the form of lactose. This lactose is broken down by the digestive system and turned into blood sugar. The blood sugar (i.e. glucose) is then taken by the blood stream to the cells in your body where it is burnt to produce energy. Unfortunately, all humans are lactose intolerant, it's just a matter of degree.

When someone is said to be *lactose intolerant* it means the digestive system is not able to completely break down the lactose sugar in the milk. This inability results from a shortage of the enzyme *lactase*, which is produced by the cells that line the small intestine. As we get older, we produce less lactase, and therefore become more lactose intolerant. That is why the elderly instinctively shy away from dairy milk.

It is natural to lose the lactase activity in the gastrointestinal tract. It is a biological accompaniment of growing up. Most people do it. All animals do it. It reflects the fact that nature never intended lactose-containing foods, such as milk, to be consumed after the normal weaning period.[23]

Persons of all races are affected by lactose intolerance, with higher prevalence among Asian, African, and South American persons. In the USA the prevalence of lactose intolerance varies according to race. As many as 25% of the white population (prevalence in those from southern European roots) is estimated to have lactose intolerance, while among black, Native American, and Asian American populations, prevalence is estimated at 75-90%. Internationally, 75% of the world's population is estimated to be lactose intolerant. It is least common in races descended from northern Europe or from the northwestern Indian subcontinent

Males and females are affected equally. However, 44% of women who are lactose intolerant regain the ability to digest lactose during pregnancy. This is probably due to slow intestinal transit and bacterial adaptation during pregnancy.

Although lactose intolerance is a very common disorder that is present in many people, it is often ignored because it goes unrecognized. Symptoms of lactose intolerance include lose stools, abdominal bloating and pain, flatulence, nausea, and abdominal gurgling. To test yourself for lactose intolerance, see whether you get wind or a feeling of bloating within 5 - 30 minutes of consuming dairy milk.

A major problem is that people who suffer from lactose intolerance do not realize that it is being caused by dairy products (milk in particular is usually not suspected). Many times babies and toddlers suffer from wind and colic. However, the cause of all the pain, crying and distress on both the child and the parents may be the inability of the child to break down lactose. The fermentation of lactose in the bowels causes the formation of gases, including methane and carbon dioxide. These will cause the baby's intestines to inflate, causing pain and distress for all concerned. Unfortunately, doctors often find it difficult to pinpoint the presence of lactose intolerance and people with this condition are often wrongly classified as suffering from Irritable Bowel Syndrome (IBS).

We are, in fact, all lactose intolerant to a degree. Some people suffer badly from it, while others only get very mild symptoms of discomfort. This is so because people produce different amounts of lactase in the small intestine. For instance John may be producing just enough lactase to cope with a glass of milk in the morning before suffering any effects, while Jane is not even able to have a lick of ice-cream because it distresses her. The sad thing about lactose intolerance is that millions of people who consume dairy milk will suffer needlessly from its symptoms and make no association between the two, thus impairing their daily lives and well being. It should be noted that the non-dairy milks described in the recipes in this book contain no lactose, and therefore lactose intolerance is not an issue.

Does dairy milk provide any useful nutrients at all?

Talk to a milk producer an you will be told that dairy milk is loaded with vitamins, minerals, and other good nutrients. Indeed, a chemical analysis of dairy milk will look something like this:

Fig. 2
Typical nutritional analysis of dairy milk

Pasteurized whole milk (dairy milk)	Units	Value per 100 grams	Pasteurized whole milk (dairy milk)	Units	Value per 100 grams
Calories	kcal	60	Sodium (salt)	mg	40
Protein	g	3.22	Zinc	mg	0.40
Total Fat 3.25	g	Sat. 1.865 Mono. 0.812 Poly. 0.195 Other 0.378	Selenium	mcg	3.7
Lactose	g	5.26	Thiamin	mg	0.044
Calcium	mg	113	Riboflavin	mg	0.183
Iron	mg	0.03	Niacin	mg	0.107
Magnesium	mg	10	Pantothenic acid	mg	0.362
Phosphorus	mg	91	Vitamin B-6	mg	0.036
Potassium	mg	143	Folate	mcg	5

Extract from USDA National Nutrient Database for Standard Reference, Release 17 (2004)

Fig. 2 notes:

1. **Other kinds of dairy milk.** The figures in the above table will vary from country to country and also from milk type to milk type. Generally, the figures are similar for whole milk and the various low fat varieties except for the fat content.

On the face of it, you look at the table in Fig. 2 and you get the impression that dairy milk is full of healthy vitamins and minerals. The problem is twofold:

A. Poor absorption.

➢ People who consume dairy milk cannot absorb vitamins and minerals as efficiently as people who don't. When your internal membranes and organs are lined with and congested with thick casein mucus, the body simply cannot absorb nutrients efficiently, and only a fraction of the nutrients in the above table will actually get absorbed and used by the body. In particular, the kidneys get congested with casein and this in turn prevents certain vitamins and minerals from being absorbed into the body.

➢ In case you think this is an exaggeration, here is a scientific explanation: casein from dairy milk has a tendency to coat the digestive organs of the body with unwelcome mucus (including the kidneys). As a result, the kidneys do a poor job filtering the blood and keeping it clean. This in turn leads to poor cell functionality; in particular poorly cleaned blood affects oxygenation, and this prevents cells from fully absorbing the nutrients they need to stay healthy. When this happens, the cells do not communicate and work together properly (healthy cells are great team players!). The end result is disease, lethargy, and poor health.

➢ Milk curdles immediately upon entering the stomach, so if there is other food present the curds coagulate around other food particles and insulate them from exposure to gastric juices, delaying digestion long enough to permit the onset of putrefaction. Milk is made even more indigestible by the universal practice of pasteurization, which destroys its natural enzymes and alters its delicate proteins. The combination of putrefaction and indigestibility serves to prevent the absorption of vitamins and minerals in dairy milk.

B. Nutritional loss.

➢ **Indigestible protein.** The high content of indigestible animal protein in dairy milk will get excreted. What happens is that the protein gets broken down to an excess of amino acids that cannot be digested because of the highly acidic environment that is created. When this happens, the excess amino acids get flushed out of the body, mostly through urine and sweat. But on the way out, the amino acid molecules get stuck to molecules of magnesium, zinc, calcium and other nutrients, thus robbing the body of these valuable minerals. So even if some of the minerals in the above table get absorbed, most will 'turn around' and leave the body. This does not happen with amino acids from plant-based food, because the human body is able to use all the amino acids, with little or no excess.

➢ **Heat treatment.** All dairy milk must be pasteurized (i.e. heat treated) as it is mostly illegal to sell raw milk. The pasteurization process involves boiling milk to very high temperatures for half an hour or more, serving to destroy much of its vaunted nutritional benefits. The fact that the pasteurization-heating process kills all beneficial enzymes and many vitamins is not disputed, even by the milk industry.

Increasingly, dairy milk is being ultrapasteurized (sometimes known as UP or long-life milk). This involves higher temperatures and longer treatment times, making the milk even more indigestible and devoid of nutritional benefits. The industry says this is necessary because many micro-organisms have become heat resistant and now survive ordinary pasteurization.

Another reason for ultrapasteurization is that it gives the milk a longer shelf life — up to four weeks once opened and kept refrigerated. Milk producers are not advertising the fact that they are ultrapasteurizing the milk—the word is usually written in very small letters on cartons, and the milk is often sold in the refrigerator section as a marketing ploy (given its sterility it could be kept *unrefrigerated* until sold). In the USA virtually all national brands are ultrapasteurized.

➢ **Medication.** Dairy cows are heavily doped with hormones and antibiotics which get passed onto humans through the milk. Without medication, dairy cows would not be commercially viable. Antibiotics in particular have a dramatic effect on preventing vitamin absorption in the body. As a result, the antibiotics in pasteurized milk virtually cancel out many of the vitamins contained in the milk consumed. For example, research has shown that vitamin K in dairy milk hardly gets absorbed or used by the body because of antibiotics.

So we come back to the question: **Does dairy milk provide any nutritional benefits at all?** The answer is that although dairy milk contains some vitamins and minerals, they provide little nutritional benefit because they mostly do not get absorbed, and because dairy milk harms the body, including acting as a nutrient robber.

How is milk affected by pasteurization?

As mentioned, when dairy milk is pasteurized it is boiled several times to very high temperatures over 145°F which changes the molecular structure of milk. The purpose is to kill harmful pathogens, but in the process, it destroys most of the nutrients in milk.

Pasteurization destroys all valuable enzymes (lactase for the assimilation of lactose; galactase for the assimilation of galactose; phosphatase for the assimilation of calcium) and dozens of other precious enzymes. Without them, milk is very difficult to digest

In her book *Nurturing Traditions* (1999) Sally Fallon makes the following comment:

'Pasteurization is no guarantee of cleanliness. All outbreaks of contaminated milk in recent decades-- and there have been many--have occurred in pasteurized milk. This includes a 1984 outbreak in Illinois that struck 14, 216 people causing at least one death. The salmonella strain in that batch of pasteurized milk was found to be genetically resistant to both penicillin and tetracycline. Raw milk contains lactic-acid-producing bacteria which protect against pathogens. Pasteurization destroys these helpful organisms, leaving the finished product devoid of any protective mechanism should undesirable bacteria inadvertently contaminate the supply.

But that's not all that pasteurization does to milk. Heat alters milk's amino acids lysine and tyrosine, making the whole complex of proteins less available; it promotes rancidity of unsaturated fatty acids and causes vitamin loss. Pasteurization alters milk's mineral components such as calcium, chlorine, magnesium, phosphorus, potassium, sodium, and sulphur as well as many trace minerals, making them less available. There is some evidence that pasteurization alters lactase, making it more readily absorbable. This and the fact that pasteurized milk puts an unnecessary strain on the pancreas to produce digestive enzymes, may explain why milk consumption in civilized societies has been linked to diabetes.

Last, but not least, pasteurization destroys all enzymes in the milk--in fact, the test for successful pasteurization is absence of enzymes. These enzymes help the body assimilate all body-building factors, including calcium. After pasteurization, chemicals may be added to suppress odor and restore taste. Artificial vitamin D, shown to be toxic to arteries and kidneys, is added.'

The irony is that pasteurization kills just about everything that is good in milk, but does not kill everything that is bad. Virtually all the toxins and pollutants remain unaffected. Furthermore, some forms of harmful bacteria survive. During pasteurization milk is heated to 150-170 degrees Fahrenheit for thirty minutes to try to kill bacteria and to reduce chances of infectious diseases. However, it needs to reach 190 degrees to destroy b-coli, typhoid and tuberculosis. It doesn't kill streptococcus or salmonella in many cases. What it does destroy is the lactobacillus acidophilus that nature provides to keep harmful bacteria in check.

How is milk affected by homogenization?

Virtually all pasteurized milk *is also* homogenized. Homogenization is a mechanical process that forces the milk through thin nozzles to break down and disperse the fat globules into very small particles. This homogenization process keeps the fat evenly distributed throughout the milk and prevents it from floating up to the top of the milk bottle or carton.

Homogenization can cause health problems for three reasons:

1. **Increase in toxins.** The tiny homogenized fat globules that get through to the bloodstream act as an 'expressway' for harmful toxins, hormones, and proteins (lead, mercury, dioxins, IGF-1, etc) that may be present in the milk and food we consume. Normally, our body gets protected from the harmful elements of consumption: our digestive system and liver act to filter out harmful things in the food we eat. But when dairy milk is consumed, the tiny homogenized fat globules 'absorb' these harmful elements and carry them into the body, bypassing the liver.

   This homogenization process, referred to as *micronization of fat*, is so effective that some medications are encapsulated into micronized fat as a way of delivering them into the body orally instead of using injections.

The homogenized fat globules bind with pollutants and toxins in dairy milk and provide a perfect vehicle for delivering harmful substances straight into the bloodstream. Once there, the toxins get carried to our vital organs and other parts of the body where they get 'offloaded' when the micronized fat eventually dissolves, causing disease and illness. This is how harmful IGF-1 survives digestion and gets into all parts of the body.

Although the amount of toxins and heavy metals we consume may be very small, they accumulate in the body over a period of time. As heavy metals such as cadmium, mercury and lead are highly toxic, only small amounts are needed for serious illness to develop. Dairy milk provides more heavy metals than just about any other kind of food because of their presence in the milk, combined with a highly effective delivery system.

2. **Increase in harmful body fat.** Most of the homogenized fat globules that get through to the bloodstream do not get used as energy or as useful nutrition. Instead, they cause illness or get stored as surplus body fat. This occurs for four reasons:

- The homogenized fat globules are made of long chain saturated fatty acids (14, 16 and 18 chain carbon atoms). The 14 and 16 long chain fatty acids are known to increase the level of harmful (oxidized) cholesterol in the bloodstream, leading to arterial disease.

- Saturated animal fat consumed in the diet cannot be used by the body unless it is first converted into non-saturated fat. Since the body cannot easily convert 14 and 16 chain fatty acids into non-saturated fat, they get dumped by the bloodstream, i.e. stored as surplus body fat.

- The 14 and 16 chain homogenized fatty acids are more harmful than saturated fats (virtually on a par with trans fatty acids). This is so because, like trans fatty acids, they enter the body and become lodged within the cell membranes of various organs where they cause harm. They can do this because of their small size and because their molecular composition prevents them from being broken down and used by the body.

- Although the 14 and 16 chain homogenized fatty acids are technically classified as saturated fat they behave more like trans fatty acids inside the body. In pasteurized whole milk, most of the saturated fat is made up of 14 and 16 chain fatty acids (about 67%). This means that about two thirds of the saturated fat from dairy milk is not only fattening, but harmful on a par with trans fatty acids.

3. **Increase in allergy.** During homogenization there is a tremendous increase in the surface area on the fat globules (lots of small fat globules have a bigger total surface area than fewer bigger fat globules). This greater surface area makes the fat globules incorporate a much greater portion of casein and whey proteins.[13] This may account for the increased allergenicity of homogenized pasteurized milk.

Look at the label on a carton of pasteurized whole milk in the USA and you will see that it says it contains a zero amount of trans fatty acids (or it may not mention trans fatty acids at all). In reality, all milk contains trans fatty acids, but when the amount is below 0.5% per 100g of milk the authorities allow the labeling to show the amount as zero. This misrepresentation of trans fats is further compounded by the similarity of the tiny homogenized fat globules to trans fats, in terms of the harm they do to the body.

The case against homogenized milk is so overwhelming that virtually no health professional (unless allied to the milk industry) will say that it is good for you. Here are some extracts from some of the research:

Heart disease is proportional to the amount of homogenized milk consumed in a country. Finland has the highest consumption… and the highest heart disease rate followed by the US. Lowest consumption and lowest heart disease rates are found in France, Japan and Sweden. The Book Homogenized by Nicholas Samsidis, M.S.

Milk and milk products gave the highest correlation coefficient to heart disease. Survey of Mortality Rates and Food Consumption Statistics of 24 Countries, Medical Hypothesis, 7:907-918, 1981.

Milk consumption correlates positively with … coronary mortality. In comparisons between 17 countries, there is a good correlation between levels of mortality from heart disease. European Journal of Clinical Nutrition, 48, 1994.

Milk positively related to coronary heart disease for all 40 countries studied. Circulation, 1993; 88(6).

For heart disease milk was found to have the highest statistical association for males aged 35+ and females aged 65+. Alternative Medical Review, 1998 Aug, 3:4.

The fat in commercial milk is homogenized, subjecting it to rancidity. When milk is homogenized, small fat globules surround the xanthine oxidase and it is absorbed intact into your blood stream. There is some very compelling research demonstrating clear associations with this absorbed enzyme and increased risks of heart disease. Dr. Joseph Mercola (licensed Osteopathic physician and board-certified in family medicine, www.mercola.com).

As stated, almost all pasteurized milk *also* undergoes homogenization. This includes the various skim, low-fat, non-fat, and long-life varieties *(including organic dairy milk)*. As a result, millions of people all over the world are causing specific and life-long harm to their bodies as a result of consuming dairy milk.

***

Any dieticians and nutritionists who praise dairy milk as part of a well-balanced diet should hang their heads in shame. The same goes for school and hospital managers who allow dairy milk to be served to vulnerable children and adults. In the USA the USDA requires that every public school in the country serve milk. It's enough to make the angels weep when dairy milk is readily given to young children in schools in the belief that it is doing them good!

Dairy farmers and milk producers are urged to diversify or switch to non-dairy milk. The potential market for non-dairy milk (both raw materials and finished product) is huge and will grow exponentially as people turn away from dairy milk. Equally, restaurants and coffee shops are urged to offer non-dairy milk alternatives and take advantage of a growing market.

A ray of hope is on the horizon: an elementary school in Canada (Ecole Marie Poburan) has banned the sale of dairy milk in the school. The reason given was the serious risk to health caused by milk allergies. Jerry Zimmer, superintendent of the Catholic school, stated that '[some of] *the students have potentially fatal dairy allergies and the school board recommended stopping the milk program to protect them.*' Source: CBC News, May 30 2005.

And Palm Beach County schools, USA, announced that whole milk is being withdrawn from all its schools in favour of low fat milk because whole milk was making children obese and contributing to higher levels of harmful cholesterol. Source: www.sun-sentinel.com, 20 June 2005.

In a society where daily starvation (in the literal sense) is a thing of the past, **the consumption of dairy milk is worse than having no milk because it causes nothing but illness and poor health.** The late Dr. Benjamin Spock, America's leading authority on child care, spoke out against feeding dairy milk to children, saying it can cause anemia, allergies, and insulin-dependent diabetes and in the long term, will set kids up for obesity and heart disease, the number one cause of death in the First World.

This is what it comes down to: dairy milk is a substance designed for a calf, and as such is not fit for a human, whether raw or pasteurized. Pasteurized milk contains many harmful hormones, allergens and antibiotics, as well as saturated fats, oxidized cholesterol, toxins, blood, pus, feces, bacteria, viruses, PCB's, dioxins up to 200 times the safe level, heavy metals, and much more. Furthermore, pasteurized milk causes specific harm to the arteries and heart arising from calcification, as explained later in this book.

There are dioxins in milk and other dairy products. The higher up you go in the food chain, the more concentrated are these terrible man-made chemicals in an animal's flesh and body fluids. There are a lot of things in milk that you don't want in your body. Every sip of milk has virus, pus, bacteria, powerful growth hormones, proteins, allergens, antibiotics, pesticides, fat, oxidized cholesterol and dioxins.[36]

Dioxins are the most deadly substances ever assembled by man... 170,000 times as deadly as cyanide.[37]

The largest contributors to daily intake of chlorinated insecticides are dairy products.[38]

Milk is filled with dead cells, loaded with pus from cows that have mastitis which is treated with antibiotics, it is chock-full of pesticides, and it contains [harmful] bacteria. Milk contains a "one-two" punch of fat and cholesterol, and has IGF-1, a hormone that allows cancer to grow in humans.[60]

Numerous studies are continually revealing the harm caused by dairy milk, covering a multitude of diseases. For example, several studies show a link between dairy milk and ***ovarian cancer***:

- A major study of more than 60,000 women carried out over 13 years found a direct link between dairy milk consumption and ovarian cancer. It found that drinking more than one glass of milk a day may double the risk of ovarian cancer! The study found that lactose in milk (rather than fat) was to blame.[28] Lactose increases the absorption of calcium, which in turn increases the harmful calcium yo-yo effect explained in appendix four. And this in turn increases the risk of micro-calcification in the ovaries, leading to ovarian cancer.

- A study compared ovarian cancer incidence with per capita milk consumption in 27 countries. *'A significant positive correlation was found between ovarian cancer and milk consumption.'* The study concluded that this was due to lactose in milk.[131]

- A study of consumption of dairy foods among women found *'a highly significant trend for increasing ovarian cancer risk.'* The Study concluded that this was due to lactose consumption in milk.[132]

- Regular milk consumption doubles the risk of ovarian cancer and failure to consume vegetables regularly nearly quadruples the risk.[153]

- *Poor absorption of lactose* [from dairy milk] *may more than double the risk of ovarian cancer in women.* American. Journal of Epidemiology, 1999;150

- *IGF-I* [in dairy milk] *can stimulate normally slow-growing cancers (like breast, ovarian, and prostate) to grow very quickly, causing them to appear in a decade or two or even less.* Delicious 12/95.

- *Galactose* [in dairy milk] *is linked both to ovarian cancer and infertility...women who consume dairy products on a regular basis, have triple the risk of ovarian cancer than other women.* The Lancet 1989; 2.

- *IGF-I* [in dairy milk] *reacts in a synergistic manner with estrogen, and plays a role in the growth and proliferation of ovarian cancer.* J-Clin-Endocrinol-Metab, Feb. 1994, 78(2).

***

Try the following test: stay off dairy milk for just five days and see how you feel. By switching from dairy to non-dairy milk you won't miss it.

People who stop consuming dairy milk for a week report that they begin to feel less bloated, more energetic, clear-headed, and healthier. The change will be gradual, but after about four weeks the improvement in health can be dramatic, particularly for asthmatics and people with congested airways.

The imperative here is to switch from dairy milk to non-dairy milk and enjoy a dramatic improvement in your health. By using the recipes in this book you can now replace dairy milk with super-healthy home-made milk and continue to enjoy the same drinks, breakfast cereals and other foods that previously 'required' dairy milk. Also, by consuming home-made milk, you will be getting lots of valuable vitamins, minerals, and other nutrients that can be safely assimilated and used by the human body. But best of all you can say goodbye to dairy milk!

And if you're concerned about surplus body weight, home-made milk provides an ideal source of nutrition as part of a well-balanced diet.

***

Dairy Milk Effect on Osteoporosis

Does regular consumption of dairy milk cause osteoporosis?

Many factors can contribute towards osteoporosis such as smoking, heavy alcohol consumption, early menopause in women; even certain medical conditions can precipitate osteoporosis. However, the evidence strongly suggests that dairy milk is the biggest *dietary* cause of osteoporosis. Furthermore, diet is one of the main factors affecting osteoporosis. New and exciting discoveries explain why dairy milk promotes osteoporosis, and this is fully presented in this chapter.

Do other dairy products also cause osteoporosis?

It depends on how much cheese, yogurt, quark and other dairy milk products you consume. A high regular consumption of these products will contribute to osteoporosis, but for special reasons dairy milk is by far the biggest dietary cause of the disease.

What exactly is osteoporosis?

A typical dictionary definition goes like this: **It is a disease in which the bones become extremely porous, are subject to fracture, and heal slowly.**

Here is a medical definition: *'Osteoporosis is a disease of bone in which the amount of bone is decreased according to the bone mineral density (BMD) as measured by DEXA: a BMD of 2.5 standard deviations below the peak bone mass (20 year old person standard) is considered osteoporosis.'*

In fact, the main form of osteoporosis (responsible for the vast majority of cases) is nothing more than the premature aging of the bones. Every human being will get osteoporosis if they live long enough. Problems arise when you get osteoporosis before you reach the end of your life. People as young as thirty can get osteoporosis, and for those afflicted it is a terrible and painful disease.

As explained in the introduction to this book, it used to be thought that osteoporosis was a ***calcium deficiency disease*** and this was generally put forth by those who favoured dairy milk. On the other side of the fence, those opposed to dairy milk have generally proclaimed it to be a ***disease of excessive calcium loss***. The battle between these two sides still rages and even some doctors and nutritionists don't know what to think because there are health professionals on both sides of the fence.

The conundrum that we have is this: Calcium in dairy milk has been shown to increase bone density in regular consumers, yet the highest incidence of osteoporosis is also found in regular dairy milk consumers. The close correlation between osteoporosis and dairy milk consumption is examined in this chapter, and the explanation to this conundrum is revealed.

To finish answering the question: osteoporosis is nothing more than the premature aging of bone-making cells. These bone-making cells are responsible for making new bone material to replace old bone material which is always in a process of decomposition. If we have enough bone-making cells to do the job we don't get osteoporosis. But when the number of bone-making cells dwindles, we begin to get osteoporosis because the rate of making new bone does not keep up with the rate of decomposition of old bone. So when we talk about the 'aging' of bone-making cells, we are talking about the erosion of the total population of bone-making cells.

The traditional approach to combating osteoporosis has been to use medications that increase BMD (bone mineral density) or reduce bone decomposition. Both these approaches have largely failed as evidenced by the growing epidemic of osteoporosis worldwide. Also, some health professionals exhort patients to take more exercise and consume high calcium food or supplements in an effort to increase BMD. But as we shall see this kind of advice is mistaken. Osteoporosis is not a disease of low BMD. If that were the case osteoporosis could be easily cured by increasing BMD. Quite simply, osteoporosis is a disease caused by a lack of bone-making cells. For a full explanation, please see **Appendix Two, The Root Cause of Osteoporosis** and then come back to this page.

Isn't calcium in dairy milk good for the bones?

It is often said that dairy milk provides a good source of calcium for healthy bones and teeth. Ask most people the question: **why is milk good for you?** and the reply will usually be '*Because it has calcium.*' The belief that dairy milk is good for bones is strongly ingrained in society because for generations we have been taught this at school, and this is what our parents and teachers have told us. Also, this belief is strongly reinforced by a vast dairy industry that spends millions of dollars a year on advertising and sponsorship. It's easy to be seduced into thinking dairy milk is good for health when you see good-looking celebrities and healthy athletes advertising dairy products.

Is it any wonder that when it comes to giving up milk we hesitate? If so many people believe that milk is good for the bones, surely they cannot all be wrong? The whole subject of milk and calcium is further confounded by a fundamental truth: **calcium in dairy milk actually causes osteoporosis!** It is ironic that dairy milk's strongest selling point is the goodness of its calcium, when the exact opposite is true: as explained later, the calcium in dairy milk is among the biggest causes of osteoporosis in the world today!

> *Countries with the highest rates of osteoporosis, such as the USA, England, and Sweden, consume the most milk.*[34]
>
> ***
>
> *Women consuming greater amounts of calcium from dairy foods had significantly increased risks of hip fractures.*[35]
>
> ***
>
> *There's really no good evidence that increasing milk consumption by adults will reduce their risk of fractures.* Source: Harvard Professor Walter Willett, one of the top health researchers in the USA.

If osteoporosis is about the aging of the bones, how does this happen?

As explained in *Appendix Two*, our bone-making cells are responsible for making new bone material to replace old bone material that is continually in a process of melting away. When new bone can be made quickly enough to keep up with old bone decomposition, we avoid weakening of the bones, and osteoporosis is kept at bay.

If we have enough bone-making cells to do the job there is no problem. But as we get older, we gradually lose bone-making cells and when their number dwindles, bones begin to weaken, i.e. they get more porous and more likely to fracture. So to slow down the aging of bones we have to slow down the rate at which we lose bone-making cells. Bone aging is the same as erosion of bone-making cells.

You may wonder why the body does not replace bone-making cells as they are lost? The answer is that the body does indeed do this, but as we get older less and less bone-making cells can be replaced (please see appendix two for a full explanation).

You may also wonder why we lose bone-making cells? The answer is that every time the bones receive the raw materials for making new bone (namely calcium) some of the bone-making cells get used up in the bone-making process. Harm is caused when calcium is made to go into and out of the bones (a kind of calcium yo-yo-effect), as this uses up more bone-making cells than otherwise. This in turn leads to osteoporosis.

The process of aging is, in general, simply the process of losing body cells. Our body muscles shrink with age as muscle cells are lost. Our skin gets wrinkled and 'old looking' because it contains less body cells to keep it firm. And our bones become porous and weaker as we lose bone-making cells.

Using the skin again as an example, if the skin is over-exposed to the sun on a regular basis it ages more quickly. This happens because when the sunlight 'burns' the skin it kills the cells on the surface of the skin, forcing the cells to renew themselves again and again. This in turn erodes the total population of skin cells. Then, as skin cells dwindle, they leave microscopic holes in the skin, making the skin loser, more wrinkled, and blotchier, i.e. the skin has aged.

When dairy milk is consumed excess calcium is absorbed into the bloodstream and then into the bones. This happens because when the bloodstream receives the calcium from the digestive system, the bloodstream has to get rid of it. It does this by dumping some of the calcium into the bones, some into nooks and crannies of the body causing harmful calcification, and some gets excreted in the urine. The bloodstream is compelled to do this as it tries to restore its 'default' level of nutrients. This default level is a particular mix of nutrients that blood always likes to keep as it travels around the body.

Why is dairy milk singled out as a major cause of osteoporosis?

Weight-for-weight, some food products contain more calcium than dairy milk, but they are never consumed in the same quantity or frequency, and they are not as acidic. Dairy milk is singled out as the biggest *dietary* cause of osteoporosis for five reasons: **excess calcium, high acidity, lactose absorption, frequency of consumption, and added vitamin D.** Let's look at each of these five factors as together, they galvanize milk into the harmful calcium yo-yo effect that erodes bone-making cells as explained in see appendix four.

1. **Excess calcium.** Dairy milk provides by far the **biggest source of excess calcium in the human diet** – it has the highest concentration per serving of highly absorbable calcium. And since dairy milk, in all its guises, is consumed in much higher quantities than any other high-calcium product, it contributes much more **excess calcium** than any other kind of food.

I would call milk perhaps the most unhealthful vehicle for calcium that one could possibly imagine, which is the only thing people really drink it for, but whenever you challenge existing dogma...people are resistant. Source: Neal Barnard, M.D., Director of the *Physician's Committee for Responsible Medicine.* www.pcrm.org.

Mark Hegsted, retired professor of nutrition at Harvard University, USA, believes we get too much calcium. In an article in the *Journal of Nutrition* he writes: *'Hip fractures are more frequent in populations where dairy products are commonly consumed and calcium intakes are relatively high. Is there any possibility that this is a causal relationship? It will be embarrassing enough if the current calcium hype* [to consume more dairy milk] *is simply useless; it will be immeasurably worse if the recommendations* [to consume dairy milk] *are actually detrimental to health.'*

Professor Hegsted considers that high calcium consumers permanently damage their ability to effectively use dietary calcium or even to conserve calcium in the bones later in life, and that this explains why high dairy milk consumers so often end up with rampant bone loss.

It has been argued that the poor ratio of calcium and magnesium in dairy milk prevents calcium from the milk being absorbed into the bloodstream or bones. This is not so for the following reasons:

- Dairy milk has a ratio of about ten parts calcium to one part of magnesium. This same ratio exists in human milk. However, human milk gives the baby excellent strong bones, therefore the ratio in dairy milk cannot be faulted as a poor ratio.

- Mother's milk certainly does not enhance osteoporosis in suckling. On the contrary, mother's milk enables infants to grow stronger bones very rapidly. This means the calcium/magnesium ratio is correct for good assimilation of calcium. As dairy milk has a similar calcium/magnesium ratio the calcium in dairy milk ***does*** get assimilated into human bones, but in so doing it weakens bones and promotes osteoporosis by eroding bone cells.

- There is no natural or 'correct' ratio based on two parts of calcium to one part of magnesium (a 2:1 ratio). Such a ratio is arbitrary and has never been proved as a necessary ratio for calcium assimilation into bone. Further proof of this is the fact that ratios of calcium and magnesium vary wildly in all types of human food with no underlying pattern of a 2:1 ratio.

- Milk consumers also eat other foods that may contain magnesium. The human body is able to store magnesium in a pool of nutrients for use as required. Hence, even the argument that dairy milk contains too little magnesium for bone assimilation does not hold true.

- There is evidence of an association between high magnesium intake and hip fracture risk.[116] A high ratio of 2:1 for calcium/magnesium may therefore not be good for health. The implication here is that magnesium encourages the assimilation of calcium into bone, thus adding to the harmful calcium yo-yo effect.

- Many studies, usually quoted by the dairy industry, show that calcium in dairy milk is indeed absorbed into bones in spite of low magnesium. Ironically, by proving that calcium is assimilated (and bone density is increasaed) these same studies provide evidence that dairy milk erodes bone cells and causes osteoporosis.

2. High acidity. The body chemistry is very sensitive to what is called pH. The pH level measures the acidity and alkalinity in the body from 1 to 14. So water at 7 pH is neutral, and the blood is on average 7.365 pH. Different areas of the body have different ideal pH levels. Over-acidification of body fluids and tissues underlies all disease. It also weakens the immunity, making infection more likely and more severe. In terms of the diet, no food is completely alkaline or completely acidic. But the body loves high alkaline food and hates high acidic food. The more alkaline food and less acidic food you eat, the healthier you will be. [84]

The body's chemistry cannot work unless the pH balance is maintained within very strict limits. What this means is that if what you eat is acidic, the body rigorously neutralizes the blood to keep the pH balance where it is wanted. Now it is the protein in our diet that causes acidity. A high protein diet means a high acid diet. We have all heard that protein is made up of amino acids. The problem is that proteins from *animal* sources (such as dairy milk) are particularly high in acid, specifically sulphur amino acid which converts to sulfate and makes the blood acidic. During the process of neutralizing this acid, calcium which is alkaline is pulled from the bones.

So as dairy milk is very acidic because of the high content of animal protein, when it is consumed it makes the digestive system very acidic. This in turn makes the bloodstream acidic and compels the body to defend itself by trying to become more alkaline. Many studies corroborate this:

'When you eat acidic foods, the body tries to return to its alkaline state the only way it can – by withdrawing calcium from your bones...osteoporosis is a calcium-robbing problem, not a calcium –deficiency problem. Dairy milk is highly acid-forming. It can increase cancer risk. The idea that dairy products are healthy is pure hype – a cultural myth. Milk is full of components of no use to us, and they must either be converted to use (wasting our body's resources in the process) or eliminated as toxins.' [84]

'You should avoid too much protein. Getting too much protein can leach calcium from your bones. As your body digests protein, it releases acids into the bloodstream, which the body neutralizes by drawing calcium from the bones. Animal protein seems to cause more of this calcium leaching than vegetable protein does.' [130]

So the source of calcium to neutralize the acidity caused by dairy milk *comes from the bones*. You may be wondering why the body cannot use the calcium in the milk to neutralize the acidity instead of pulling calcium from the bones. The answer is that the calcium in the milk is still in the process of being absorbed from the digestive system and there is insufficient to neutralize the high acidity that was caused as soon as the milk was consumed.

As the acidity in the blood is gradually neutralized and reduced, the bloodstream will now have too much calcium (a combination of calcium coming from the milk and coming from the bones, although some of the calcium will have been lost in the process of neutralizing the acidity).

The bloodstream now acts to get rid of the excess calcium, and it does this by putting some back into the bones, some is excreted through the kidneys, and some is dumped as calcification in different parts of the body. This is how the harmful calcium yo-yo effect is started off – see appendix four.

3. Lactose absorption. The calcium in dairy milk gets readily absorbed into the bloodstream with help from lactose. This powerful milk sugar enhances the permeability of the intestinal mucus, which in turn increases absorption of calcium into the bloodstream.[159]

Many studies confirm this:

The protective effect of lactose against reduced bone calcium accretion may be due to increased calcium absorption. [160]

These results suggest that lactose or its component sugars enhance jejunal calcium absorption in proportion to their effect on fluid absorption.[161]

Milk calcium may be absorbed in distal intestine in the absence of vitamin D, under the influence of lactose. Dairy products do not contain anything likely to inhibit the intestinal absorption of calcium like phytates, oxalates, uronic acids or the polyphenols of certain plant foods. [162]

It is now generally agreed that lactose, at least in high doses, increases the passive absorption of calcium in the absence of vitamin D and, consequently, decreases intestinal calcium concentration and active transport of calcium. [163]

When you examine the research on this subject confusion arises between absorption and assimilation. Numerous studies show that lactose dramatically increases absorption of dairy milk calcium into the bloodstream. Other studies say that lactose has little or no effect on calcium absorption, but here the studies are referring to the *assimilation of calcium into the bones* rather than into the blood.

By enhancing absorption of calcium into the bloodstream, the lactose in dairy milk increases the harmful calcium yo-yo effect described in appendix four – point two. This in turn erodes bone-making cells.

4. Frequency of consumption. Dairy milk is usually consumed on a daily basis. Additionally, the total consumption when added up is typically two to three cups daily. In the USA, average daily consumption is over three cups daily (remember that 2 cups equals 1 pint, and 4 cups equals 1 US quart).

Other dairy products such as cheese contain more calcium than dairy milk (weight for weight) but are never consumed in the same kind of volume.

Many people may not drink dairy milk on its own, but when consumed with tea, coffee, breakfast cereals, desserts, sauces, as yogurt, ice-cream, flavoured drinks, and many other guises, the total amount soon adds up. This, plus the regularity of consumption is what causes the harmful calcium yo-yo effect and erosion of bone-making cells.

5. Added vitamin D. As explained later in this chapter, and in appendix four, the high amount of vitamin D3 added to US and Canadian milk causes calcium to be pulled from the bones yet again, adding to the harmful *calcium yo-yo effect* that erodes bone-making cells.

So coming back to the question 'why is dairy milk singled out as a major cause of osteoporosis?' the answer is because it offers a unique cocktail of factors that is tailor-made for promoting osteoporosis. The high calcium, high acidity, effect of lactose, and regularity of consumption all serve to pull and push calcium in and out of the bones (the *calcium yo-yo effect*), and this erodes bone-making cells, leading to osteoporosis. And in some countries such as the USA and Canada, the high amount of vitamin D3 added to dairy milk further exacerbates the harmful calcium yo-yo effect. *No other human food has this particular combination of factors that make it so harmful for bones.*

Does that mean calcium in the food we eat is harmful?

As mentioned, when the bloodstream receives excess calcium from the diet it parks some of the excess in the bones. It does this in response to hormones that compel the bloodstream to get rid of excess calcium in a kind of 'knee jerk reaction'. As a result, the blood stream will later run low on calcium so it pulls the parked calcium back into the bloodstream. Then later, when further excess calcium is received from the diet, the cycle is repeated, setting up a 'yo-yo' effect of calcium going into and out of the bones. This is what causes osteoporosis because bone cells wear out much more quickly than otherwise. Children brought up on dairy milk will have less bone-making cells in later-life, increasing the risk of osteoporosis.

The phenomenon of calcium going in and out of bones is well known to bone scientists (referred to as 'bone tunrover'), and medical textbooks refer to the calcium in bone as being either 'stable bone' or 'exchangeable bone' although in reality there are no two separate bone areas as such. The purpose of exchangeable bone is to provide a 'calcium warehouse' for the bloodstream to call upon whenever it needs calcium. However, the less often this calcium warehouse is used the better, as bone-making cell erosion is then minimized.

When dairy milk is avoided and a nutritious varied diet is consumed the bloodstream gently feeds the calcium it receives from the food into the bones in a one-way street. This does also wear out bone-making cells *but at a much lower rate* that avoids osteoporosis in old age. Also, this avoids harmful calcification because the bloodstream is never forced to get rid of excess calcium – it virtually all goes into the bones and stays there.

> *'Osteoporosis affects an estimated 10 million Americans, and each year, about 1.5 million suffer a fracture as a result. Another 34 million Americans have less severe bone-thinning but enough to still risk a fracture. Half of all Americans older than 50 will be at risk of fractures from too-thin bones by 2020.'*
> Source: Announcement from the US Surgeon General, 18 March 2005.

At what age should I start to care for my bones?

There is a misconception that once your bones have stopped growing they are set for life. This misconception may arise from confusion between *bone mass* and *bone density*.

Bone mass refers to bone volume, i.e. the *outside* dimensions of the bone. This can be measured using special computerized equipment. Alternatively, a bone can be immersed into a bucket of water so as to gauge the amount of water dispersed.

Bone density refers to the amount of calcium and minerals *inside* the bone, i.e. the bone content. This can be measured using bone density measuring equipment.

The Merck Manual of Geriatrics says: *'The increase in bone mass during growth results from an increase in bone size, not bone density (bone mass per unit volume). After growth stops, the bones continue to increase slowly in girth (except the mandible, which gets smaller). However, between ages 40 and 50, bone density begins to progressively decrease. Bone density does not tend to result from decreased bone production; bone remodeling can actually increase with aging.'*

Unfortunately, medical literature often refers to 'bone mass' when in fact it is referring to 'bone density'.

To put this simply: *bone mass* (size of bones) stays about the same throughout life whatever your lifestyle. *Bone density* gradually decreases with age, but is constantly changing throughout life, depending on lifestyle. Osteoporosis relates to bone density, not bone mass. Doctors refer to 'peak bone mass' as meaning the maximum amount of bone (in size and density) that is reached when the bones stop developing by about age 30.

It is critical to develop maximum 'peak bone mass' while the body is growing as you only get one chance. Once you are grown up it is too late to increase bone mass. Good bone mass provides the framework (literally) for a strong and healthy body. Good nutrition and a healthy lifestyle during childhood and adolescence will ensure good bone mass for life.

To understand peak bone mass in another way, think of your skeleton as a retirement bank account. From birth until age 30 or so, you continually make deposits into your account. When you retire at age 30, the deposits stop and you have to start making withdrawals for the rest of your life. Thus, the size of your bank account at age-30-retirement is analogous to your peak bone mass. This is the bone you will have to work with for the rest of your life. [128]

Our larger long bones, such as our arm bones and leg bones, are very dense, and they are completely replaced about every 10-12 years. Our less dense bones, such as our spine and the ends of our long bones, turn over every 2-3 years. Thus, as you can see, we always have the opportunity to be creating better bone for ourselves. However, although we can gradually improve the quality of our bones once grown up, it is a very gradual process. The size of bones cannot be significantly influenced, once grown up, because when new bone is made, it replaces old bone *as it melts away*, and so the overall size and shape of bones is maintained.

So throughout life new bone is being created and old bone is being decomposed. Up until your teen years more bone is created than is lost (hence bones get bigger). During your twenties and thirties, bone created and lost is about even (hence bone size and density stay about the same). Then gradually, from your forties onwards more bone is lost than created (hence bone density, and to a small extent bone size, is reduced).

The danger here is the belief that consuming calcium-rich foods such as dairy milk is the best way to protect bones in children and adults. As we shall see, we need very little calcium in our diet, and **the less calcium we consume the more we will protect our bones** by virtue of protecting the 'shelf life' of bone-making cells.

So, to answer the question, *yes*, we should always be looking after our bones, and one of the best ways of doing this is to avoid dairy milk.

Avoiding osteoporosis is not about assimilating more calcium into bones, it's about not consuming too much calcium. The secret to strong healthy bones is a low calcium diet!

To summarize, it is vitally important to look after your bones as early as possible in life for two reasons:

1. You want to develop good bone *mass* while growing up because you only get one chance in life to influence the *size* of your bones. Once your bones stop growing in your mid-twenties, that's it. They will basically stay like that for the rest of your life. Also, good bone mass goes hand in hand with a strong healthy body.

2. At any age, young or old, you want to maintain good bone *density* so that your bones are strong enough for normal everyday activities. You do not want to develop *high* bone density as the greater the bone density the greater you erode bone-making cells. Achieving exactly the right amount of bone density is *easy and automatic* when you consume a nutritious varied diet because the body uses hormones to make sure that only the exact right amount of calcium is assimilated into bones. But when you consume dairy milk this hormonal control goes haywire with the consequence that you increase bone density to a harmful level. It is harmful in the sense that bone-making cells get eroded as a result of the calcium yo-yo effect (see appendix four), thus increasing the risk of osteoporosis.

How is calcium used by the body?

Every cell in the body needs calcium. The body uses the calcium as physical bridges between cells over which they communicate (cells talk to each constantly, using a chemical code language). They need to talk all the time so that they can 'vote' on when to die, when to divide, and so on.

Since cells are in a 'permanent state' of dying and being renewed (e.g. through cell division), the calcium communication bridges between cells need constant renewal. The body also needs calcium for many other functions. Consequently, the bloodstream is permanently carrying calcium all over the body to places where it is needed. The bloodstream gets its calcium from the food we eat or from the body's *calcium warehouse*.

This 'warehouse' is located in the hip and thigh bones, the biggest bones in the body (and to a lesser extent in the lower vertebrae, the tibia, and fibula). This is where the body 'stores' calcium for servicing the whole body.

Technically, what happens is that the calcium gets put into the fluid around osteoblast cells in the hip and thigh bones and new bone matrix is formed by osteoblast secretion. In the process, 50% to 70% of the osteoblasts 'sacrifice their lives' and get trapped inside their newly created bone material and cease to be osteoblasts. In this way new bone material gets manufactured to help keep the bones dense and strong.

Whenever the blood gets low on calcium, it gets replenished from the hip and thigh bones if no calcium is forthcoming from the digestive system. In this event hormones pull calcium from the bones, thus wasting the efforts (and lives) of bone-making cells – the calcium yo-yo effect.

Adequate calcium in the blood is so vital to a wide variety of body functions that our internal biochemistry will not tolerate a deficiency even for short periods. Consequently, the bloodstream can never be without calcium (and many other minerals) that are being carried around the body all the time. As the calcium is carried around in the bloodstream it gets fed to the millions of cells that make up our body.

So as calcium in the bloodstream gets depleted, it gets replenished with fresh calcium, either from the food we eat or from the calcium warehouse. But whenever the bloodstream has **more than enough calcium** problems arise: as fully explained in appendix four, some of the excess calcium is 'parked' in the warehouse thus adding to the harmful calcium yo-yo effect that erodes bone cells, and some of it ends up being excreted or getting dumped in the body in the form of harmful calcification.

Osteoporosis develops because old bone is constantly being decomposed regardless of anything else, and if new bone formation is not keeping up, microscopic holes develop in the bones, making them weaker and weaker.

To summarize: As explained in *Appendix Two*, each time calcium is assimilated into bones, either permanently or temporarily, bone-making cells get used up. When excess calcium is consumed on a regular basis, as in the case of dairy milk, bone density is increased, but at a price that erodes bone-making cells more quickly than otherwise.

Therefore, the less frequent the movement of calcium in and out of bones the better, as this minimizes erosion of bone-making cells and reduces the risk of osteoporosis. Once osteoporosis develops, consuming more calcium will not increase bone density because there will not be enough bone-making cells to process the calcium. If anything, the increased consumption of calcium will only serve to make matters worse as it will further erode precious bone-making cells.

What is meant by 'excess calcium'?

We have seen how bones age more quickly when we consume *excess calcium*. The key then is to consume enough calcium for good health, and avoid *excess calcium*. Most of the harm occurs when **too much** calcium is absorbed into the bloodstream, because this sets up the calcium yo-yo effect that erodes bone-making cells more quickly (see *Appendix Four, The Calcium Yo-Yo Effect*). As with all minerals, the body normally absorbs just as much calcium from our food as it needs. Only about 200 mg is absorbed into the blood, on the average, whether we consume 300 mg or 700 mg calcium daily, or sometimes even when we consume up to 1200 mg supplementary calcium daily. In order to absorb the right amount of calcium, absorption rate decreases when we consume more calcium.

But when we consume *excess calcium*, the absorption rate cannot be sufficiently decreased; about 5% of dietary calcium on top of 1500 mg a day is additionally absorbed into the blood. For example, consuming 5 times more calcium than before, a group of girls did, in fact, absorb twice as much calcium (as before) into the blood. [106]

Why is excess calcium assimilated into the bones?

This is to prevent the blood-calcium level from rising too much. Muscles can only function if calcium from inside the muscle cells can be moved to the outside of the muscle cells. Every time you move your arm you are moving calcium in or out of muscle cells in your arm. If the blood-calcium level were too high, this wouldn't be possible; it would be lethal since breathing requires muscle-action. To keep you alive excessive dietary calcium is temporarily stored in the bones, prior to excretion. Normally the blood contains a total of 500 mg calcium. The difference between highest and lowest blood-calcium level is only 26%, thanks to the three different hormones that prevent our blood from containing too much (or too little) calcium. After the *excess calcium* has been metaphorically parked in the bones two of these hormones pull the calcium back from the bones (thus wasting the efforts and sacrifices of bone-making cells), and the third one stimulates the dumping or the excretion of the pulled calcium.

Why don't the bones hold on to that excess calcium?

It used to be thought that we can prevent osteoporosis by stacking more calcium into the bones, and many doctors and nutritionists still believe this: *'The more calcium your bones contain, the longer it will take before they are empty.'*

This would be a simple solution if the bones did indeed hold on to that extra calcium, but our bones are built according to a plan - and the amount of calcium in the bones has to be according to that plan. Just as piling up bricks in your bedroom does not make your house better or stronger, stacking extra calcium into the bones is not an improvement either. To be able to go to bed or live in your house properly, you chuck the bricks out.

The redundant calcium in your bones is always chucked out eventually. The amount and speed at which calcium is created into *stable* new bone cannot be forced – the body has to be allowed to do this task at its own good pace. To keep redundant calcium in your bones, you have to keep on consuming excess calcium daily. But no matter how much milk you drink, or supplementary calcium you take (or don't take), your bones always end up with less calcium at the age of 70 than at the age of, say, 30.

Redundant calcium in reality refers to an exchange of calcium, i.e. calcium goes into the bones and later that same day (or same hour) other calcium comes out of the bones. As there has been no significant net gain of calcium, it is referred to as 'redundant calcium' or 'excess calcium.' When dairy milk is consumed it triggers a movement of calcium in and out of the bones several times a day, depending on the frequency of consumption (see appendix four). This in and out movement of calcium (the yo-yo effect) is what erodes valuable bone-making cells, increasing the risk of osteoporosis.

To clarify further, when dairy milk is consumed this is what typically happens to the calcium:

1. About a third of the calcium in dairy milk gets absorbed into the bloodstream and the rest is excreted. [122]

2. Of that one-third-calcium, some of it gets assimilated into the bones to increase or maintain bone density, and some of it is redundant calcium that comes out again (the calcium yo-yo effect).

3. The redundant calcium is eventually excreted or dumped in the body to cause calcification.

So some of the calcium from dairy milk does indeed stay in the bones and some does not. This is why milk consumers have dense (but over-aging) bones. But increased bone density happens at a terrible price: The daily calcium yo-yo effect wears out bone-making cells, speeding up the onset of osteoporosis. If, for example, you have been absorbing 400 mg instead of 200 mg dietary calcium into the blood daily since childhood, these cells have had to process 2.9 million mg *more* calcium during, say, 40 years.

Virtually all physicians know that blacks consume **much less** milk than whites; the most common reason given is that many blacks are lactose intolerant.[155] Yet it is well documented that black Americans have a much lower incidence of osteoporosis compared to white Americans:

- *Black women had a 30% to 40% lower risk of fracture, compared to white women, no matter what their bone mineral density levels were.*[156]
- *Osteoporosis is twice as common in white men as in black men.*[157]

In a major *University of Pittsburgh* study in May 2005 [156] osteoporosis incidence between white and black American women was compared to see why the disease was so much lower among black women. The study was led by Stephen Honig, M.D. (Director, Osteoporosis Center, Hospital for Joint Diseases, New York City). Dr. Honig said '*the study suggests the reasons that black women have lower rates of fractures may be related to **lower bone turnover**, racial differences in hip axis length or bone size differences.*' 'Bone turnover' refers to the amount of bone material made and then lost (the calcium yo-yo effect described in appendix four). ***This and other research shows a strong correlation between low milk consumption and low osteoporosis due to a reduced calcium yo-yo effect.***

To avoid osteoporosis you want to minimize the calcium yo-yo effect. It cannot be completely avoided, but ideally you want a one-way street of calcium going into the bones. And you only want enough calcium going in to keep the bones normally healthy, because every time calcium goes in bone-making cells get used up. Above all, you want to reduce as much as possible the very harmful yo-yo effect.

This is best achieved by eating a nutritious and varied diet devoid of dairy milk because that way you 'drip-feed' small amounts of calcium and supporting minerals into the bloodstream. In this scenario, the calcium gets well assimilated into the bones. Little or no calcium is pulled out again because the bloodstream will be receiving a small, steady amount of calcium and supporting minerals from the digestive system. This minimizes the calcium yo-yo effect and the wearing out (i.e. the aging) of bone-making cells. The end result is that you do not get osteoporosis.

> **Getting exactly the right amount of calcium (and supporting minerals) in the diet for healthy bones is very easy: just eat a nutritious and varied diet – the body will then automatically take exactly what it needs for healthy bones, thus minimizing the risk of osteoporosis**

A *dairy milk* consumer may have high BMD (bone mineral density) should he/she be tested. But this would be a 'fool's paradise' because it would not reveal the dwindling population of bone-making cells. It would not show the looming osteoporosis that may be just around the corner. The regular consumption of dairy milk creates a hidden ticking bomb inside your body. The ticking bomb is osteoporosis, and it is well hidden for two reasons:

1. No medical bone test can reveal how many bone-making cells have been used up and how many are left. This means osteoporosis could be imminent or still some time away.

2. A bone test showing high BMD gives the dairy milk consumer a false sense of security and further convinces him/her to continue consuming dairy milk thus ignoring the ticking bomb.

Should I increase my bone mineral density by consuming calcium-rich food?

If less calcium is consumed, the bone-making cells age slower: a low calcium intake throughout adolescence has been shown to beneficially retard *and prolong* longitudinal bone growth in rats. [107]

It is not being suggested that anybody deliberately adopt a low calcium diet – too little calcium in the diet is of course bad for bones because a truly poor BMD (bone mineral density) can eventually promote osteoporosis. This is so because very low BMD makes bones porous and weak, and likely to fracture. It can take many years to recover from chronically poor BMD even if you have no shortage of bone-making cells. And if you're already approaching old age, you cannot afford the recovery time – you in effect have osteoporosis. This scenario is a possibility in cases of chronic starvation, but would be very rare in developed countries.

To truly eat a diet that contains *insufficient* calcium would be a hard thing to do because almost all food contains calcium in varying degrees, and you only need to absorb less than half a gram a day for optimum bone health.

What is being suggested is that you eat a nutritious and varied diet that contains a mix of foods, some of which will be high in calcium and some low, but without dairy milk and little or no dairy products. Also, eat all foods in moderation – never eat any particular food to excess. By doing this you avoid harmful excess calcium; instead, you get enough calcium and nutrients for the body to take exactly what it needs and keep your bones normally strong and healthy (and minimize bone-making cell erosion).

It's easy to construct a dairy-free diet that delivers sufficient calcium. By relying on [food from] ***plants rather than cows to provide your calcium needs, you also avoid cholesterol, saturated fat, somatic (pus) cells, potential risks arising from rBGH injections, and a number of other undesirable elements that come in every glass of milk.*** Source: Physicians Committee for Responsible Medicine, USA.

Society has been so conditioned to equate high assimilation of calcium with good bone health that we have to make a conscious effort to change our mind-set. We have to realize that high calcium intake *causes* osteoporosis and low calcium intake *prevents* osteoporosis. We have to literally turn our preconceptions on their head! It is infinitely preferable to have low BMD and more bone-making-cell potential than high BMD and less bone-making-cell potential. Having a low BMD does not mean that your bones are weak, it means that your bones are strong and healthy for normal everyday living. Think of low BMD as being normal and natural, and high BMD as being abnormal and harmful.

Coming back to the question '*Should I increase bone mineral density by consuming calcium-rich food?*' The answer is NO. If you do increase your BMD (bone mineral density) as a result of consuming calcium rich foods such as dairy products, you will exhaust your bone-making cells sooner. A high BMD means stronger bones, but not *healthier* bones. Just as bodybuilders have stronger muscles but not *healthier* muscles – most body builders experience muscle problems in later life because, like bone-making cells, their muscle cells age prematurely. The more the bone-cell aging is accelerated, the sooner the bone building capacity will be exhausted. This is why, in those countries where the average BMD is highest, the hip-fracture incidence is highest too.

Does this mean that low BMD protects against osteoporosis?

If BMD is 'low' because you consistently consume a diet that avoids calcium supplements and high-calcium dairy food, then the answer is **yes** although I prefer to use the word 'normal' rather than 'low'. Having a normal BMD is the best way to prevent osteoporosis and maintain strong bones. If calcium intake is very low, there will still not be a lack of calcium for healthy bones. [108] On the contrary the bones will not age prematurely by virtue of a low calcium yo-yo effect. But if the BMD is low as the result of exhausted bone-making cells then you have osteoporosis, and in this scenario a low BMD will get worse and cannot be reversed.

BMD is low in osteoporosis due to the lack of new bone-matrix. Holes develop that do not contain calcium. So BMD can be low in good healthy bones **and** it can be low in weakened osteoporotic bones, which is what makes it so confusing for so many scientists and nutritionists!

I often see women in their forties who bring in the results of a "baseline" bone density measurement test and are shocked to find that they have osteopenia (mild low bone mass) or even osteoporosis (more severe low bone mass). They ask me why they are losing bone so rapidly. In the vast majority of cases, these women are not rapidly losing bone and in fact, have perfectly healthy, normal bone tissue, just less of it. They wonder why, then, if their bones are healthy, they have less bone than the "average" woman's. I explain that, ten to twenty years ago, they probably achieved a lower peak bone mass than the "average" woman, probably due to genetic factors. Some women just have smaller and thinner bones than other women. [128].

In another study it was found that people who avoid dairy milk because of their lactose intolerance had a more healthy bone mineral density that their milk-drinking peers: *In African American premenopausal women, lactose tolerance facilitates the dietary intake of calcium when compared with their lactose intolerant counterparts. Low calcium intake is associated with higher bone mineral density.*[158]

A healthy person who is avoiding dairy milk and consuming a mixed diet of nutritious food will have a 'low' (i.e. **normal)** BMD and healthy bones. This protects the bones against any future osteoporosis because even in old age enough bone-making cells will still be available for making new bone at a rate that more or less keeps up with bone decomposition.

If I avoid dairy milk, should I be eating calcium-rich foods?

The short answer is ***no***, you should not be eating calcium-rich foods. Nor should you deliberately try to eat a very low calcium diet – **let the body work out how much calcium it needs.** The key to avoiding osteoporosis is not the amount of calcium you eat, but how quickly you wear out bone-making cells.

Building a strong skeleton during childhood is essential for combating bone-loss and fractures in later life, but you don't do this by consuming dairy milk, taking calcium supplements, or eating calcium-rich foods. You do it by eating a well-balanced diet that avoids dairy products (particularly dairy milk). Such a diet should be nutritious with a good variety of fruit, vegetables, salads, nuts, seeds, and pulses. It is best to have three or four small meals over the day rather than one or two big meals. This is important because it reduces the number of times the body has to borrow calcium from bone to maintain adequate levels of calcium in the bloodstream (i.e. it reduces the harmful calcium yo-yo effect that ages bones). When at work, try to eat a healthy snack mid morning or mid afternoon, e.g. a piece of fruit, some nuts/seeds & raisins, a salad sandwich, or carrot and celery sticks. You can even take non-dairy milk to work, using a screw-top beaker.

If you are not vegetarian or vegan, keep meat consumption to a minimum by giving preference to unpolluted cold-water sea food. Cooked meat protein is more acidic (and less nutritious) than cooked fish protein A well-balanced diet that avoids dairy milk products will provide all the calcium and supporting minerals that you need for good bone assimilation while minimizing erosion of bone-making cells.

There is no need to plan how much calcium you are eating or which foods to combine – by simply eating a healthy varied diet that **avoids dairy milk products** you will automatically get exactly the right amount of calcium needed to protect bones. This is so for two reasons:

1. Once the bloodstream has absorbed enough calcium from the diet, hormones are triggered to stop further absorption. This prevents excess calcium being absorbed into the bloodstream and consequent erosion of bone-making cells. The calcium-hormones function like a fire brigade: when little calcium is being consumed, they are not activated that much, which is good: no fire. When too much calcium is consumed, the calcium-hormones are very active, stimulating absorption of calcium into the bones, and subsequently expelling the calcium from the body (the calcium yo-yo effect). The more this process is accelerated, the more the bone cells erode.

2. We only need a tiny amount of calcium to develop and maintain strong bones (less than half a gram a day). Nutritionists cannot agree how much calcium we need each day because several factors can affect how calcium is absorbed. This is what is generally recommended:

The RNI (Reference Nutrient Intake) is a daily amount that is enough or more than enough for 97% of people. The RNI (similar to the *Recommended Daily Allowance/Intake*) is as follows:

UNITED KINGDOM	
Age	Calcium requirement (mg/day)
0-12 months (non breast fed infants only)	525mg
1-3 years	350mg
4-6 years	450mg
7-10 years	550mg
11-18 years	(boys)1000mg, (girls) 800mg
19+ years	700mg
Pregnant women	700mg
Breastfeeding women	700+550mg

The table below shows the amounts recommended by the Osteoporosis Society of Canada and by the US Institute of Medicine:

CANADA		USA	
Age	Calcium requirement (mg/day)	Age	Calcium requirement (mg/day)
Not given	Not given	0–6 months	210
Not given	Not given	7–12 months	270
Not given	Not given	1–3 years	500
4-8	800	4–8 years	800
9-18	1300	9–18 years	1,300
19-50	1000	19–50 years	1,000
50+	1500	51–70+ years	1,200
Pregnant/nursing women	18+: 1000	Pregnant/nursing women	<19: 1,300 >19: 1,000

Generally then, official sources vary but on the whole they recommend a minimum of 1 gram a day, because it is known that only about a third of a gram of calcium gets absorbed from dairy products (which is more than enough for the bones). The high acidity of dairy milk ensures that about two thirds of the calcium in milk gets excreted without being absorbed into the bloodstream or bones.

Weight for weight, plant-based foods contain less calcium than dairy milk, but a higher percentage of the calcium gets assimilated calmly into the bones without causing the harmful calcium yo-yo effect. Hence, achieving enough calcium for optimum health *without dairy milk* is easily accomplished by eating a nutritious and varied diet of fruit, vegetables, salads, nuts, seeds, and pulses.

Restrict consumption of grains to occasional helpings of whole grain foods. Avoid processed and cooked foods as much as you can – the fresher and more natural the food the better. Eat plenty of fresh fruit and make sure you get enough omega 3 and DHA oil in your diet. It does not matter if some days you eat less or more than one gram of calcium. Also, it does not matter if some days you eat less fruit or less nuts, or miss a meal. The body is surprisingly flexible and adaptable. To get strong bones and avoid osteoporosis it is best to be focused on a good *variety of quality food* rather than on the amount of calcium you eat.

According to the United States Department of Agriculture the average American consumes about 29 ounces of dairy milk per day (that's at least three cupfuls per day). That means the average American is consuming about 1.087g of calcium a day just from milk. When you add other calcium-rich foods that are typically consumed (pizzas, yogurt, ice-cream, etc.) you can see that most people consume far too much calcium for their own good.

In Canada, Australia and New Zealand milk consumption is similar to the USA. In Northern Europe the consumption of dairy milk is about 20% higher than the USA, and in Southern Europe, 20% lower. In South America consumption is about 50% lower, and in Eastern Europe it is 50% *higher* than the USA! In Asia, consumption is 70% lower compared the USA, and in China there is virtually no dairy milk consumption.

Are calcium and vitamin D supplements good or bad for bones?

Calcium supplementation causes excess calcium which in turn wears out bone-making cells in the same way that dairy milk does. We have to remember that whenever calcium is assimilated into bones (even small amounts of 'healthy' calcium) this kills 50% to 70% of the osteoblasts attending to the newly arrived calcium. The best and only way to combat osteoporosis is to minimize the amount of calcium that goes into bones, as this minimizes erosion of bone-making cells.

However, calcium supplements that are formulated with magnesium, manganese, and boron (and ideally vitamin K) can be required for bones *in extreme cases* of nutritional deficiency – circumstances which are rarely seen in developed countries. The combination of these four nutrients ensures good assimilation into bone, **but the price you pay is a higher rate of bone cell erosion.** It could be that in cases of literal starvation or serious malnutrition, calcium supplementation is preferable, even if this means a higher erosion of bone-making cells.

Note that vitamin D in dairy milk does not help the body absorb calcium until the vitamin D has first been absorbed into the bloodstream. *The vitamin D necessary to absorb calcium moving down the intestine must already have been in the bloodstream for a while – what is present with that calcium (in milk) is useless at that stage.*[46]

This means that by the time the vitamin D in milk arrives at the bloodstream and is ready for action, there is an absence of calcium from milk in the intestines (unless a person is continually consuming milk). In the absence of calcium waiting to be absorbed from the intestines into the bloodstream, the vitamin D acts to pull calcium from the bones. For this reason, dairy milk with added vitamin D is particularly harmful, because it contributes to the calcium yo-yo effect (see ***Appendix Four***).

European Union countries only add a trace amount of synthetic vitamin D2 to dairy milk. Most tropical and sunny countries add no vitamin D. Many other countries, such as the USA and Canada, add vitamin D3 to dairy milk. Vitamin D3 can only be obtained from animal sources, typically from pig skins, sheep skins, raw fish livers, and pig brains, and then used as a milk additive. (**Note:** the dairy industry euphemistically refer to these animal sources as 'lanolins'). Clearly, the use of animal derived additives in milk can conflict with many cultures, religions, and diets.

Vitamin D3 is the vitamin our bodies make in response to sunlight and it is about nine times more powerful than the synthetic vitamin D2.

Sunlight and dairy milk don't mix

If you drink milk with added vitamin D and if on that same day your skin receives sunlight, it can be unhealthy.

Some people may scoff at the suggestion that vitamin D from sunlight can be unhealthy, but this would be a misrepresentation. It is only unhealthy when the human body being presented to the sun is a dairy milk consumer. As mentioned, the body stops converting sunlight into vitamin D when it has enough, but the body has no way of knowing that an additional wave of vitamin D will be coming from dairy milk or supplements.

Thus, a North American dairy milk consumer is likely to have vitamin D3 from milk in the digestive system but not yet absorbed into the blood. If in parallel with this, it is being generated from sunlight, there will come a point later in the day when there is an excess of D3 in the body, causing calcium to be pulled from the bones. This scenario is played out almost daily by millions of Americans and Canadians, adding fuel to the harmful calcium yo-yo effect. People who take vitamin D supplements run the same risk.

Another danger is that in the absence of calcium waiting to be absorbed from the intestines, the vitamin D provided by dairy milk may cause harm by increasing absorption of heavy metals. *Vitamin D increases intestinal calcium and phosphate absorption. Not so well known, however, is that vitamin D stimulates the co-absorption of other essential minerals like magnesium, iron, and zinc; toxic metals including lead, cadmium, aluminum, and cobalt; and radioactive isotopes such as strontium and cesium. Vitamin D may contribute to the pathologies induced by toxic metals by increasing their absorption and retention.*[47]

The high amount of added vitamin D3 increases health risks for US and Canadian milk consumers

Getting vitamin D from sunlight is much safer than getting it from dairy milk, because as mentioned the body stops making vitamin D from sunlight when it has made enough. The presence of vitamin D in dairy milk is yet another risk to health.

The solution then is to get your vitamin D from sunlight and avoid vitamin D supplements. You cannot overdose on vitamin D from sunlight (although you might get sunburn!) because the body stops making vitamin D as soon as it has enough for the task in hand. That way, vitamin D from sunlight is always beneficial.

Incidentally, sunlight does not actually give you vitamin D – it triggers the body into making the vitamin D that it needs. To get enough vitamin D from sunlight white people need to expose their limbs (or arms and head) to direct sunlight for at least 10 minutes daily. Alternatively, exposing yourself to bright daylight (sun shining through clouds not thick enough to obscure the contour of the sun) for at least 30 minutes can be just as good. Dark skinned people require up to ten times more exposure time than white people, depending on skin pigmentation. If you live in parts of the world above or below 40 degrees latitude the UV sunlight is not so strong, and more sun exposure is required. Always be careful to not get sunburn.

If you have children, make sure they get the same kind of exposure as adults. Note that attempting to acquire vitamin D from sunlight through window glass is not very successful. This is because some of the UV spectrum (required for vitamin D) gets filtered out as sunlight passes through glass. For example sunlight passing through clear 4mm glass loses about a third of its UV light spectrum. Thicker glass or double glazing will be much less effective for this purpose.

Getting enough sunlight should become an important daily routine in your life. Vitamin D is essential for good health and for life itself because its main function is to make sure the bloodstream always has a set level of calcium for feeding to millions of cells all over the body. However, your health/bones will not suffer if you get no vitamin D for several days or even a week or so, providing this does not happen very often.

Vitamin D foods for non-vegetarians include cod liver oil, egg yolks, and oily fish. For vegetarians/vegans sources include fortified breakfast cereals, margarines, and other non-animal foods fortified with vitamin D.

To summarize: unless you rarely venture into sunlight, or unless prescribed by a health professional, it is generally best to avoid calcium and vitamin D supplements altogether. This is because vitamin D greatly increases the amount of calcium absorbed from the diet (or re-absorbed back from the bones). This in turn can cause the harmful **calcium yo-yo effect** that erodes bone-making cells. If you feel you cannot get enough vitamin D from the diet or from sunlight/daylight, then a *small* vitamin D supplement may be justified. If supplementing with vitamin D on its own take it during or after a meal. If you take it on an empty stomach, the vitamin D will pull calcium form the bones, adding to the harmful calcium yo-yo effect.

There have been hundreds of scientific papers showing the damaging effects of added vitamin D [to milk]; among these effects are kidney stones and urinary calculi, hypercholesterolemia, and damage to the eyes. [53]

Consumption of dairy milk may not provide a consistent and reliable source of vitamin D in the diet. Samplings of milk have found significant variation in vitamin D content, with some samplings having had as much as 500 times the indicated level, while others had little or none at all. [133, 134]

Too much vitamin D can be toxic and may result in excess calcium levels in the blood and urine, increased aluminum absorption in the body, and calcium deposits in soft tissue. [64]

Note: if considering giving calcium or vitamin D supplements to an infant under two please see the chapter '**Dairy Milk and Young People: Is dairy milk good for growing bones and teeth?**'

Where is the proof that a low calcium diet is best for bones?

This question will be answered under three headings:

Country comparisons	Calcium intake	Effect of estrogen

Country comparisons

Many scientific studies have looked at the incidence of osteoporosis and hip-fractures in different countries. The analysis shows a strong and irrefutable correlation between high milk consumption and the incidence of osteoporosis.

For example in Hong Kong in 1989 twice as much dairy products were consumed as in 1966 and osteoporosis incidence tripled in the same period. Today their milk consumption level is almost "European", and so is osteoporosis incidence. This shows that osteoporosis is not genetic, since their brothers in nearby China, who consume very little milk, have very low rates of osteoporosis.

In Greece the average milk consumption doubled from 1961 to 1977 (and was even higher in 1985), and during the period 1977 - 1985 the age adjusted osteoporosis incidence almost doubled too.

Like Australians and New Zealanders, Americans consume three times more milk than the Japanese, and hip-fracture incidence in Americans is therefore 2½ times higher. Among those within America that consume less milk, such as the Mexican-Americans and Black Americans, osteoporosis incidence is two times lower than in white Americans.

The highest milk consuming countries in the world (per capita) include Ireland, Austria, The Netherlands, Romania, Sweden, Finland, and the USA. In these countries the incidence of hip-fractures and osteoporosis has sky rocketed.

A specific study carried out in the Eighties compared rates of hip-fractures in the US, Finland, Sweden and Switzerland where three times more milk was consumed comapred to Venezuela and Chile. The results showed that the per capita hip-fracture incidence in Venezuela and Chile was more than three times lower. [111]

Later, in 2001 Merck & Co, USA, reported that *'hip fracture rates increased with age and were higher in women than men. Age-adjusted hip fracture rates were highest in Finland, the USA, and Sweden for men; and in Switzerland, the USA, and Scotland for women'* (Jack Guralnik, The statistical characteristics of human populations). These same countries are among the top 15 milk-consuming countries in the world.

Chinese people consume very little milk (8 kilos per year) and hip-fracture incidence, therefore, is among the lowest in the world. Hip-fracture incidence in Chinese women is 6 times lower than in the USA (the average American consumes 254 kilos per year).

In other countries such as Gabon, Guinea, and Togo very little milk is consumed and osteoporosis is extremely rare. In the Democratic Republic of the Congo, Liberia, Ghana, Laos and Cambodia even less milk is consumed (average person: 1 to 3 kg a *year*), and age-related hip-fracture is too rare to quantify.

It is very simple: where the most milk is consumed (and hence most calcium), the osteoporosis incidence is highest. The less milk consumed, the lower is the osteoporosis rate. [112]

There are many studies that show why dairy milk is bad for bones:

Consumption of dairy products, particularly at age 20 years, were associated with an increased risk of hip fractures...metabolism of dietary protein causes increased urinary excretion of calcium. [166]

Countries with the highest rates of osteoporosis, such as the USA, England, and Sweden, consume the most milk. [34]

Women consuming greater amounts of calcium from dairy foods had significantly increased risks of hip-fractures. [35]

Women who ate most of their protein from animal sources [i.e. consumed dairy products/meat] *had three times the rate of bone loss and 3.7 times the rate of hip-fractures of women who ate most of their protein from vegetable sources. An increase in vegetable protein intake and a decrease in animal protein intake may decrease bone loss and the risk of hip-fracture.* [99]

Several studies show dairy milk is bad for children and this was reinforced by a major US study in March 2005: it was found that milk and dairy products do not promote healthy bones in children and young adults. The *'Physicians Committee for Responsible Medicine'* found that after analyzing 58 studies, a clear majority of these studies found no positive relationship between calcium intake from dairy products and bone health. Also, previous studies that showed a relationship between milk and bone health were confounded [invalidated] because of the statistical distortion caused by the addition of vitamin D into milk. The study also pointed out that Americans are some of the world's highest consumers of dairy products, and US rates of osteoporosis and bone fracture are also among the world's highest. [22]

Calcium intake

We have seen how excess calcium such as that provided by dairy milk or supplements can harm bone-making cells by making them age more quickly and hasten osteoporosis. Clearly, one can increase BMD (bone mineral density) by high-calcium intake. But equally, one can increase BMD by low-calcium intake. [109,110] The former is harmful, the latter is not.

Consumption of excess calcium causes high but unhealthy bone mineral density. It is unhealthy because it is based on a dwindling population of bone-making cells.

Consumption of moderate amounts of calcium causes healthy normal bone mineral density. It is healthy because it is based on a long-lasting population of bone-making cells.

Excess calcium, as provided by dairy milk, causes bone-making cell erosion because of its high calcium and high acidity content.

Compared to other foods, only dairy products (or calcium supplements) are capable of greatly increasing calcium intake. This is proven by the fact that average BMD is highest in those countries where the most dairy milk is traditionally consumed.

In a large study carried out by Aberdeen and York Universities [115] it was concluded that taking vitamin D and calcium supplements does not prevent fractures. The study looked at a total of 8,614 elderly people carried out over several years. The objective was to see if taking calcium and vitamin D supplements helps prevent or heal fractures. Control groups and dummy pills were used as part of the research. The studies examined the effect of taking calcium and vitamin D on people who had already had a fracture, and were taking no other medication. Professor Adrian Grant, who led the research, said older frailer people were more likely to have vitamin D deficiency and therefore more likely to benefit from supplements. But the research proved otherwise. Professor Grant said their study *'indicates that routine supplementation with calcium and vitamin D, either alone or in combination, is not effective in the prevention of further fractures.'*

Commenting on the 'Aberdeen study' Jackie Parrington, deputy chief executive of the UK National Osteoporosis Society, said: *'The results show that the benefits of calcium and vitamin D as a treatment option to prevent further fractures are uncertain....older people should consider eating a healthy, well mixed diet to ensure they get the full range of vitamins and minerals.'*

The *Aberdeen study* shows that elderly people with signs of osteoporosis do not benefit from calcium and vitamin D supplements. If osteoporosis were a disease caused by insufficient calcium in the bones it is reasonable and likely that calcium and vitamin D supplements would help. Why didn't they? The answer is that osteoporosis is not a disease of calcium insufficiency in the diet or in bones – it is a disease of *bone-making cell* insufficiency. As already stated, when osteoporosis begins to develop it means you no longer have enough bone-making cells to keep pace with the melting away of old bone. No amount of calcium and vitamin D can generate more bone-making cells. In fact, throwing calcium at the problem is counter-productive because it further erodes bone-making cells, making the onset of osteoporosis even worse!

Other studies have come to similar conclusions: high calcium intake does not lower risk. The *Harvard School of Public Health,* USA, says: *'Long-term studies cast doubt on the value of consuming large amounts of calcium: In particular, these studies suggest that high calcium intake doesn't actually appear to lower a person's risk for osteoporosis. For example, in the large Harvard studies of male health professionals and female nurses, individuals who drank one glass of milk (or less) per week were at no greater risk of breaking a hip or forearm than were those who drank two or more glasses per week. Other studies have found similar results.'*

The very extensive Harvard studies into osteoporosis clearly show that consuming more calcium does not reduce hip fractures. This adds further weight to the growing evidence that osteoporosis is not about calcium insufficiency, or even calcium loss, it is about the premature aging of bone cells.

Here are brief details of some other studies showing that a higher calcium intake does not protect bones:

- A study of 65,000 Swedish women (pub.1995) found that high calcium intake did not protect against hip fracture. [116]

- A study of 43,063 men (pub.1997) looked at adult calcium intake and the risk of bone fractures in Health Professionals. It concluded that there was no relation between calcium intake and the incidence of forearm or hip fractures in men. [129]

- In a major 12-year study among 77,761 women (pub.1997) scientists examined whether higher intakes of dairy milk and other calcium-rich foods during adult years can reduce the risk of osteoporotic fractures. It was found conclusively that higher consumption of milk or other food sources of calcium by adult women does not protect against hip or forearm fractures. [130]

Further evidence that osteoporosis is not caused by insufficient calcium is to be found inside the human body itself. It is a medical fact that the bloodstream always has to maintain a minimum level of calcium. This has been proven by examining the calcium blood levels of osteoporosis patients – they are no different to healthy individuals or to postmenopausal women. *Everybody* has the same minimum level of calcium circulating in the blood at all times.

The bloodstream is always compelled to maintain a 'default level' of calcium for feeding to body cells everywhere, including bone cells. When it runs low, it re-stocks on calcium from the digestive system or by pulling calcium from the bones. This means everybody, including those with osteoporosis, have always been 'fed' the minimum amount of calcium needed for strong bones. It is very difficult to not get enough calcium in your diet for the body's requirements. Even a junk-food diet high in coffee, sodas, alcohol, and little or no fresh fruit and vegetables, will have plenty of calcium. The only way to not get enough calcium is to deliberately avoid foods with calcium or to live in conditions of literal famine.

Effect of estrogen

Appendix three explains how estrogen protects bones. It does this by reducing the harmful calcium yo-yo effect that erodes bone-making cells. Proof that estrogen acts to protect bones from becoming weak can be found in any medical textbook or by consulting the numerous research papers on the subject. The fact that estrogen protects bones is universally accepted by medical scientists.

Estrogen is a hormone made by the body and is present in both women and men. In women the natural estrogen produced by their own body protects the bones and has other important functions relating to femininity. In men a non-feminizing version of estrogen is made from testosterone, and just as in women, it protects the bones.

The role played by estrogen proves that a low calcium diet is best for bones. This is so because estrogen protects the bones by **reducing** the amount of calcium assimilated into the bones. ***In other words, it reduces the harmful calcium yo-yo effect.*** It does this by stopping osteoblasts from accepting more calcium and making new bone material. By slowing down the rate at which osteoblasts process calcium into new bone, osteoblasts suffer less erosion (they are made to work less hard, thus minimising the erosion of bone-making cells).

So estrogen keeps osteoporosis at bay by ***reducing the amount of calcium*** that goes into bones and protecting the precious population of bone-making cells. For a fuller explanation please see appendix three, **How Estrogen Protects Bones**.

When postmenopausal women no longer have as much estrogen as they need for strong bones, several things can be done to protect bones as summarized at the end of this chapter. It is unfortunate that some doctors who prescribe estrogen to postmenopausal women *also* prescribe calcium supplements. In such situations women should consider seeking a second opinion from a bone specialist, as taking calcium supplements can be counter-productive and may even hasten the onset of osteoporosis.

> **Estrogen and calcium do not act in concert, they fight each other. Calcium supplements reduce the effectiveness of estrogen by preventing estrogen from shielding bone cells from further erosion.**

What does the milk industry say about osteoporosis?

When confronted with evidence of a strong correlation between dairy milk consumption and the incidence of hip-fractures and osteoporosis how does the milk industry respond? A typical response is likely to go like this:

> *Hip-fracture incidence varies worldwide, with numerous factors, among them age, gender, reproductive history, hormonal status, race,*

institutionalization, medical comorbidities, hip geometry, medications, bone density, body habitus, diet, smoking, alcohol, fluoridation of water supplies, environment, climate, and osteopenia, all influencing risk. The incidence of hip-fractures is therefore not related to dairy milk consumption, it is due to many factors.

This kind of response is an attempt at obfuscation. Every disease in the world can be attributed to a variety of factors, and naturally different factors can indeed affect osteoporosis. The point here is that dairy milk is the biggest *dietary cause* of osteoporosis, and diet is known to be one of the biggest factors affecting osteoporosis. Clearly, some factors, such as smoking, may indeed affect how calcium (and anything else!) is absorbed and hence how healthy the bones remain, **but it does not follow** that the incidence of hip-fractures is therefore not related to dairy milk consumption.

As mentioned, there is an irrefutable and strong correlation between high milk-consuming countries and osteoporosis. For example, look at any set of statistics that include Denmark, Norway, Australia, New Zealand, Canada, USA, Netherlands, Austria, Finland, and Ireland. These ten countries are among the highest milk-consuming countries in the world on a per capita basis. These same ten countries are also among the highest for hip-fractures and osteoporosis on a per capita basis.

Alternatively, just look at Eastern Europe, the highest milk-consuming region in the world. Eastern Europe has more per capita osteoporosis, heart disease, and cancer than any other region of the world. Northern Europe and America are not far behind.

When it comes to preventing osteoporosis people with a vested interest in dairy milk typically use generalizations like this:

'Adequate calcium and vitamin D consumption contributes to the achievement of optimum bone mass and life-long protection against osteoporosis.'

Another generalization often quoted goes like this:

'Dairy milk provides an important source of calcium as part of a balanced diet.'

Generalizations like these are meaningless and misleading. What is meant by 'Adequate calcium and vitamin D consumption?' Does this include or exclude dairy milk? What about calcium and vitamin D supplements? What is meant by 'optimum bone mass' – does this refer to bone size, or to mineral density caused by a high calcium diet or a low calcium diet? What is meant by 'balanced diet'? If this means eating a varied and nutritios diet, this is a given, but it does not follow that dairy milk is an important source of calcium! Anyhow, the last thing we need is a rich source of calcium.

Bland generalizations are often used when you don't know the answer or when you want to defend the indefensible.

Interestingly, osteoporosis, heart disease and other milk-related illnesses are higher in cold climate countries and lower in hot regions of the world. The explanation is that you lose excess calcium in your sweat.[145] Hence, the harmful calcium yo-yo effect (appendix four) is somewhat ameliorated in hot climates that make you sweat more. The dairy industry is quick to say that higher rates of osteoporosis are due to poor (cold) climatic conditions and not related to milk consumption. However, the correct explanation is that **milk consumption is very much to blame**, it's more a matter of how much you sweat. It does not follow that dairy milk does not increase the risk of osteoporosis.

Here is a more specific argument put forward in favour of dairy milk. The text that follows is taken from a major dairy milk website: *Calcium, which is important for healthy bones and teeth, is abundant in dairy milk. So is protein. Although it's possible to get ample calcium without milk, it does take some careful planning. But in dairy milk the calcium is well absorbed by the digestive tract because the vitamin D and lactose found in milk facilitate calcium absorption. Therefore, dairy milk provides a good source of calcium and protein.*

Let's briefly dissect the above statement:

1. '*Calcium, which is important for healthy bones and teeth, is abundant in dairy milk. So is protein.*'

Yes, calcium is abundant in dairy milk and this is the problem! It causes excess calcium in the bloodstream, and over time this wears out valuable bone-making cells.

Regarding teeth, far from building up strong teeth, dairy milk actually does the opposite. Firstly, regular dairy milk consumption speeds up the onset of osteoporosis, and osteoporosis will dramatically weaken the teeth. This is so because teeth are entirely dependent on a strong bone structure in the jaw. Secondly, the lactose in milk, which is a form of sugar, coats the teeth with acidity. This strips the delicate enamel coating and causes tooth decay. If dairy milk must be consumed, it should be done only at mealtimes so as to minimize the acidic effects.

> **'Milk may cause cavities'** *Canadian Dental Association*

The habit of giving a child a bottle or drink of milk before bedtime is one of the biggest causes of childhood tooth decay because, unless the teeth are cleaned *very thoroughly*, the lack of saliva during sleep will allow the plaque to proliferate and cause harm. *Human* milk does not do this because

(i) the lactose content is different, (ii) it has anti-infective properties, and (iii) by the time the baby has teeth it will hardly be consuming human milk.

The indigestible protein in dairy milk serves to acidify the digestive system, inhibit digestion of nutrients, rob the body of valuable minerals, and promote cancer arising from the putrefaction of the protein in the digestive tract. Above all, the acidity caused by indigestible protein acts to pull calcium from the bones, exacerbating the harmful calcium yo-yo effect.

2. *'Although it's possible to get ample calcium without milk, it does take some careful planning.'*

We only need a very small amount of calcium for good health. When the bloodstream is presented with small amounts of calcium it triggers a hormone called 'calcitonin'. This hormone acts to help the newly arrived calcium get assimilated. When a large amount of calcium is presented to the bloodstream (as in the case of dairy milk), production of calcitonin is inhibited but not enough to stop some of the excess calcium getting through to the bones. Then other hormones are triggered to pull calcium out of the bones. This cycle of calcium movement in and out of the bones is repeated several times daily in people who consume dairy products. This in turn leads to erosion of osteoblasts and the onset of osteoporosis.

Regarding 'careful planning' the strongest and biggest-boned animals on earth do not plan what they eat and their diets are entirely based on plant foods. There is no need for any kind of 'planning' or food combining because virtually all foods contain calcium in varying degrees.

3. *'But in dairy milk the calcium is well absorbed by the digestive tract because the vitamin D and lactose found in milk facilitate calcium absorption. Therefore, dairy milk provides a good source of calcium and protein.'*

Two thirds of the calcium does not get absorbed because of the acidity in milk, and because the calcium binds with casein and leaves the body. About a third of the calcium does indeed get absorbed into the bloodstream with help from the vitamin D and lactose found in milk. But that is where the problem lies because, as stated, it causes excess calcium in the bloodstream, ultimately speeding up the onset of osteoporosis. Also, some of this excess calcium causes harmful calcification and serious illness.

> **A major study carried out with Harvard nurses *(American Journal of Public Health 1997;87:992-7)* concluded that dairy milk consumption does not protect against bone fractures. The study of 77,761 women over a 12-year period showed that fractures were higher in women who drank more milk, and lower in those who drank less milk.**

The imperative here is to protect healthy bones and teeth by *avoiding* dairy milk. If you continue to consume dairy milk it becomes *even more important* to take measures to protect bones.

Why do osteoporosis organizations recommend dairy milk as a good source of calcium?

This is a good question. Osteoporosis is so widespread throughout the world that many countries have organizations set up to fight both osteoporosis and arthritis as they have much in common. Some of these organizations recommend dairy milk (among other foods) as a good source of calcium, and hence as a way of fighting osteoporosis.

Why do they do this? Is it out of ignorance or because they have not kept up to date with the latest research? This is puzzling, since they are bound to take advice from qualified doctors and nutritionists.

The answer is likely to be a combination of three factors:

1. **Dairy sponsorship:** It is a fact that many osteoporosis organizations receive ongoing lobbying and funding from the milk and dairy industries. This funding can be in the form of direct cash payments, or in the form of sponsorship for 'charitable' events, exhibitions, seminars, and the like.

2. **Out of date knowledge:** Sometimes new research and discoveries can take a long time to percolate down and change pre-conceived ideas about a particular disease. In the case of osteoporosis, there is a perverse (yet erroneous) logic that goes like this:

- *You get osteoporosis when bone density becomes too weak, making bones more likely to fracture.*
- *The best way to combat osteoporosis is to prevent bone density from becoming too weak, and one way to do this is to consume calcium rich foods. We know that absorbing more calcium into bones increases bone density and makes bones stronger.*
- *Since dairy milk is rich in calcium, it has to be good for the bones, particularly as research shows that drinking milk increases bone density.*

This perverse logic, however false and out of date, is nevertheless strongly ingrained in society and in the minds of some health professionals. As a result, such advice is still issued by many osteoporosis organizations.

3. **Misguided advice:** Some osteoporosis organizations may have people on their boards who have financial interests in the milk and dairy industries. It is not at all unusual for osteoporosis organizations to take advice from health professionals associated with the dairy industry. Such people may quite openly receive funding or sponsorship from the dairy industry. No doubt such advice is given in good faith, however misguided and erroneous.

For example the *National Osteoporosis Society* in the UK readily admits they receive funding from the National Dairy Council, and (at the time of writing) this is stated on their website. In the USA the *National Osteoporosis Foundation* has received donations from *Dairy Farmers Inc*. Both these organizations mention dairy milk as a food source for calcium.

This is not to say that osteoporosis organizations do not provide a valuable service, but it does mean that some of their comments about milk and dairy products may not be wholly impartial. Osteoporosis organizations everywhere are urged to review their policy regarding dairy milk and fully honour their commitment to helping people fight osteoporosis.

> **The U.S. FDA takes the view that *dairy milk* accounts for 1% to 1.5% in skeletal loss per year**

Why is osteoporosis more prevalent in women?

Statistics show that women are about two to three times more likely to get osteoporosis compared to men. Why is this so? The answer lies with estrogen. It is well known that estrogen helps protect bones, and this is due to a slowdown in the calcium yo-yo effect which in turn slows down the aging of bone cells (please see **Appendix Three: Estrogen Myth** for a technical explanation).

All bone-scientists acknowledge that if the female body has sufficient estrogen at its disposal all the time, osteoporosis risk is far lower. That is why for women the osteoporosis risk is higher than for men: in women the estrogen level is far lower every 4th week, and the bones are less protected at that time. And in postmenopausal women, estrogen level is permanently decreased.

Women and men both lose bone at the rate of about 0.5% to 1% per year. It's a very slow rate of bone loss. But after menopause, some women can lose 2% to 5% of their bone per year, which is a tremendous amount of bone loss. [That's 5 to 10 times more bone loss per year after the menopause].[76]

Remember that somebody with a higher BMD (bone mineral density) can be closer to getting osteoporosis than somebody with a lower BMD – what counts is the remaining bone-making-cell potential left in the body. A postmenopausal woman can have a bone test that shows 'low' BMD and yet still have perfectly healthy bones with no prospect of osteoporosis. Another postmenopausal woman can have a bone test that shows high BMD and yet be much closer to getting osteoporosis. There are no known tests that can determine the state of health of bone-making cells.

Furthermore, bone testing machines are notoriously unreliable and inaccurate, and it is a myth that the diagnosis of osteoporosis, as a measure of low bone density, is accurate, valid, and reliable. [136]

Telling postmenopausal women to increase calcium consumption, take calcium/vitamin D supplements, or increase their exercise is not the solution as this is likely to make matters worse! [121]

> *92% of American women over 45 do not know that collapsing bones in the spine, called compression fractures, are the most common consequence of osteoporosis. Yearly, 300,000 American women suffer a hip-fracture caused by osteoporosis and within a year one fifth will die. Half of the survivors never fully recover and require long term nursing care. Osteoporosis is not something you should ignore.*

The prospect of osteoporosis for menopausal women is not inevitable. Many women live into their 90's and even become centenarians while still maintaining good bones. How do they do this? They do it by combining several factors: avoiding dairy milk (and consuming few, if any, dairy products) throughout their lives, eating a healthy diet, walking a lot, and getting daily sunlight. Other factors may also play a part such as not smoking or drinking, being physically active, avoiding stress, and having a menopause late in life. All these factors help reduce the rate at which bone-making cells are worn out, thus allowing new bone to be made at a rate that more or less keeps up with bone decomposition.

What should a postmenopausal woman do to prevent osteoporosis?

Here is a check list:

- *Avoid dairy products* and follow the advice given in this chapter.

- *Avoid calcium and vitamin D supplements* unless prescribed by a trusted health professional on medical grounds.

- *Eat a wide variety of good nutritious food*. This will ensure the right amount of calcium and supporting nutrients are assimilated in a healthy manner while minimising erosion of bone-making cells.

- *Eat boron rich foods*. This mineral acts to slow down or stop more calcium and magnesium going out of the bones than is coming in (thus reducing the calcium yo-yo effect). This in turn helps to slow down or prevent osteoporosis. Boron may mimic the action of estrogen. In one report, postmenopausal women lost calcium and magnesium from their bodies when they were made boron deficient, and retained those minerals on a boron-supplemented diet; they also manufactured more estrogen and testosterone when on boron supplementation. In another study, vitamin D status improved in boron-deficient women after they received boron.[21]

Boron food sources

Virtually all vegetables, particularly potatoes, avocados, and green leafy vegetables. Most nuts, including peanuts. Most fruit and fruit juices, particularly apples, pears, plums, grapes, prunes, and all types of dried fruit. Also chocolate, coffee, beer, dried beans, peanut butter, raisin granola/bran cereals, and wine. Most non-dairy milks are high in boron, particularly those made from nuts or soybeans. Meat, fish, and dairy products contain no boron or very little.

- *Consider taking estrogen supplements* under the guidance of a health professional. This does not necessarily mean taking 'full-blown HRT' – a low-dose estrogen supplement can be a viable alternative. However, be aware that in some circumstances estrogen supplements my increase the risk of breast cancer.

- *Consider taking DHEA supplements* as this stimulates the body into making estrogen, which in turn protects bones. For some women this may be a good alternative to taking estrogen supplements or HRT. However, DHEA is a powerful hormone, and it should be taken sparingly, under medical supervision. To get more information on DHEA go to www.lef.org and enter 'DHEA' in the search box, then scroll down fully to see all the results. (Note: DHEA can be equally effective for men.)

- *Take the right kind of exercise* that best combats osteoporosis (see chapter titled *Dairy Milk Effect on Physical Fitness*). Taking the wrong kind of exercise can increase the risk or severity of osteoporosis.

- *Stay informed.* Keep up to date with medical developments relating to osteoporosis and the menopause. Do this by keeping up to date with health news, by consulting health professionals, and by researching information on Internet. For example, be aware that (as explained in this chapter) a low bone-density test does not necessarily indicate that you are on the road to osteoporosis.

- *Should you already have osteoporosis,* know that there are several kinds of treatments and medications available. If prescribed drugs to combat osteoporosis, check them out on Internet and seek a second opinion – such drugs may be counter-productive or ineffective. Never take medication without understanding all the consequences.

In a nutshell, what is the best way to avoid osteoporosis?

The acronym **S.P.E.N.D.** summarizes five key points to remember:

Sunlight is good. Get daily sunlight or bright daylight for vitamin D. This ensures the right amount of calcium is made available to the body.

Pills for supplementing calcium and/or vitamin D should be *avoided* (unless prescribed by a health professional) because they can cause calcium excess and erosion of bone-making cells.

Exercise the right way. Know which kind of exercise helps bones. Some kinds of physical activity actually weaken bones. (See chapter *Dairy Milk Effect on Physical Fitness*).

No dairy milk. Avoid all kinds of dairy milk, and minimize consumption of cheese, yogurt and other high calcium dairy products.

Diet: variety is best. Eat a good mix of fruit, vegetables, salads, nuts, seeds, and pulses. This gives the body an optimum amount of calcium and supporting nutrients for strong, healthy bones and teeth.

> Osteoporosis is not about calcium insufficiency or calcium loss, it's about the premature aging of bone-making cells

Healthy Bones Quiz

The following *Healthy Bones Quiz* helps identify things you can do straight away to reduce your risk of osteoporosis. It is not intended as a checklist of all risk factors, such as age, gender, etc. as these are beyond your control. Also, realize that the *Healthy Bones Quiz* does not address certain medical conditions which can promote osteoporosis.

Answer YES, NO, or SOMETIMES for each question. For the sake of your health you must be completely truthful in your answers.

YES = 2 points
SOMETIMES = 1 point
NO = 0 points

1. Do you get at least 15 minutes sunlight (or 45 minutes bright daylight) on your skin every day? YES/SOMETIMES/NO

2. Do you avoid calcium supplements (formulated with or without vitamin D)? YES/SOMETIMES/NO

3. Do you avoid vitamin D supplements (formulated with or without calcium)? YES/SOMETIMES/NO

4. Do you walk or move around on your legs for at least 60 minutes a day (or at least 120 minutes every other day)? YES/SOMETIMES/NO

5. Do you avoid all kinds of dairy milk? YES/SOMETIMES/NO

6. Do you avoid high-calcium dairy products (e.g. cheese, yogurt, quark) more than 3 days a week? YES/SOMETIMES/NO

7. Do you eat at least three of the following six food categories every day: fruit, vegetables, salads, nuts, seeds, pulses?
YES/SOMETIMES/NO

8. Do you avoid cigarettes? YES/SOMETIMES/NO

9. Do you avoid weight-loss supplements and drugs that affect the natural hormonal balance of your body? YES/SOMETIMES/NO

10. Do you avoid excessive alcohol consumption?
YES/SOMETIMES/NO

Score 15 to 20 points = Very good. Focus on any questions not answered YES and take remedial action.

Score 10 to 15 points = Not so good. You need to carefully evaluate questions not answered YES and take corrective action as soon as possible.

Score under 10 points = You may be at risk of osteoporosis even if a test shows you have high bone mineral density. Re-evaluate your priorities and consider a change in lifestyle for the sake of your health. If you cannot make the necessary changes in your life so as to bring your score up to at least 15, consult an osteoporosis health professional.

What about bone density scans?

A bone density scan uses low-dose X rays (typically DEXA equipment) that measures the mineral density of bones. According to a DEXA test, number 1 is the baseline measurement for normal bone density. So a score above 1 indicates high bone density. Between 1 and -1 is regarded as 'borderline' bone density. Between -1 and -2.5 is regarded as low bone density. And below -2.5 means you have osteoporosis.

As already explained in this chapter, a low BMD (bone mineral density) of, say, -1 does not necessarily mean unhealthy bones. On the contrary, it could mean that the bones are perfectly healthy. What counts is whether your bone-making cells are getting depleted, and this is not reflected in bone density scans.

If you have a bone scan that shows *low* bone density you have to ask your self the following question: *Is my DEXA result low because my bone-making cells are getting depleted or because, in the process of preserving my bone-making cells, the bone density is low but healthy?*

If you have a bone scan that shows **high** bone density you have to ask yourself a similar question, but with greater urgency: *Does my **high** DEXA result reflect depletion of bone-making cells, thus increasing the risk of osteoporosis? Or does it mean I have high bone density without depletion of bone-making cells?* The higher the score the more likely the answer is YES to the first part of this question and NO to the second part.

Hence, whether low or high, the question that really matters is whether bone-making cells are being depleted. Since current technology cannot answer this question you need to examine lifestyle factors to find ways of slowing down the erosion of bone-making cells.

In the above **Healthy Bones Quiz** if your score is below 15, and if this reflects a life-long score, then it is more likely that your bone-making cells are being depleted. This can be the case whether your DEXA result is low or high.

Note that you can now use the above **Healthy Bones Quiz** to answer the question: *Why does person XYZ have a low bone density reading?* For example, if Mrs. Jones has a low bone density reading of -1.2 and her result of the **Healthy Bones Quiz** is 14, a study of the quiz answers will reveal what she can do about it. If her quiz result is, say, 19, she can be more confident that her bones are healthy in spite of the negative bone scan reading. If the bone scan reading is above 1, taking the **Healthy Bones Quiz** becomes more critical because a person with a high bone scan reading is more likely to get osteoporosis than a person with a low reading!

Whatever the result of your bone density scan, you should take action to protect your bones (it is never too late). Do this by studying the above **Healthy Bones Quiz** and take action to convert all answers to a YES answer. Clearly, you should also follow any advice given by a bone health professional. Should the advice be in conflict with the advice given in this chapter (some health professionals are not up to date with the latest research) seek a second opinion or refer the health professional to this book.

Dairy Milk Effect on Calcification

More people die of heart disease and cancer than any other kind of illness. These diseases affect men and women of all ages, races, and in all countries. There are many risk factors that cause these diseases such as poor diet, smoking, pollution, insufficient exercise, and so on. Many of these risk factors are common to both heart disease and cancer.

But new research is revealing an extraordinary story: *calcification* is emerging as the underlying cause of heart disease and cancer, and dairy milk is a major player in this unfolding story. Increasingly, scientists are realizing that harmful calcification is at the root of a multitude of diseases. That in fact, calcification is responsible for more deaths through illness than anything else.

Diseases caused by calcification

Here is a list of some of the diseases caused by calcification: [17]

- Aging skin
- Alzheimer's
- Arthritis
- Bone spurs
- Breast implant calcification
- Bursitis
- Cancer (bone, brain, breast, colon, prostate, and ovarian)
- Cataracts
- Diabetes (type 2 in adults)
- Gallstones
- Glaucoma
- Heart disease
- Kidney stones
- Liver cysts
- Macular degeneration
- Multiple sclerosis
- Prostatitis
- Psoriasis
- Salivary gland stones
- Scleroderma
- Stroke
- Tendinitis

A dictionary definition of **calcification** refers to a '*Deposit of calcium salts in the tissues that produce hard, inelastic nodules.*' So here we are **not** talking about the healthy assimilation of calcium into the bones or the body cells – we are talking about the harmful accumulation of calcium into parts of the body where it causes serious disease.

Calcification is a rock-hard mix of calcium and phosphorus. Normally this mix is essential for building bones and teeth. But as we age, and sometimes when we are still young, some of it goes haywire, stiffening arteries, roughing up skin, destroying teeth, blocking kidneys and salting cancers. The arithmetic is frighteningly easy. Calcification doubles in the body about every three or four years. We can have it as teenagers and not notice, although it mysteriously accelerates in some athletes. Then as we age and also live longer, it becomes so endemic that most people over seventy have it. Calcification contributes to most diseases that kill us, including heart disease, diabetes and cancer. The numbers are staggering. For the 60 million Americans who have heart disease, most have calcification. Of the millions of women who develop breast or ovarian cancer or who have breast implants, calcification is a warning. Men with prostate disease often have it, as do kidney-stone sufferers. Athletes with stress injuries like bone spurs and tendonitis get it frequently. Most of us don't know the pervasiveness of calcification because it has a different name in many diseases, and here are just a few: dental pulp stones, hardening of the arteries, kidney stones, pitcher's elbow, bone spurs, microcalcification in breast cancer and "brain sand". Many doctors are unaware of new studies that show calcification is toxic, causing acute inflammation, rapid cell division and joint destruction. In June 2005 British researchers published proof in the leading medical journal Circulation Research *that calcification causes inflammation in the arteries. If true, the British discovery would force a re-evaluation of the whole medical approach, not only to inflammation but also to the foundations of heart disease, looking at calcification as a prime culprit.* Source: Edited extract from Douglas Mulhall's comments (co-author of *The Calcium Bomb*), Nexus Magazine, Volume 12, Number 5 (Aug- Sep. 2005).

Factors affecting calcification

Calcification occurs when several factors come into play as follows:

1. The bloodstream always carries phosphorus and calcium around the body for feeding to body cells to keep them healthy. But sometimes these two minerals get dumped into nooks and crannies around the body. This leads to harmful calcification in places where nanobacteria are lurking. The existence of nanobacteria, only discovered a few years ago, is now widely accepted by scientists. Nanobacteria are difficult to study because they are 1000 times smaller than bacteria, and because they take days rather than hours to multiply.

2. The nooks and crannies where calcification occurs can be just about anywhere: the arteries and veins, the brain, organs of the body, the eyes, even the sex organs! And when calcification occurs, it acts as an anchor point for further calcification to build up over time.

3. Nanobacteria use calcium and phosphorus from the bloodstream as their food or raw materials to produce calcium phosphate. This calcium phosphate acts as a kind of cement that creates and develops the harmful calcification deposits in our body.

4. There is increasing evidence that dairy milk is a major contributor to calcification because it provides nanobacteria with the raw materials (calcium and phosphorus) that it needs for calcification to develop.

Examples of calcification

Example 1: The elbow.

The photographs show and example of calcification of the elbow joint:

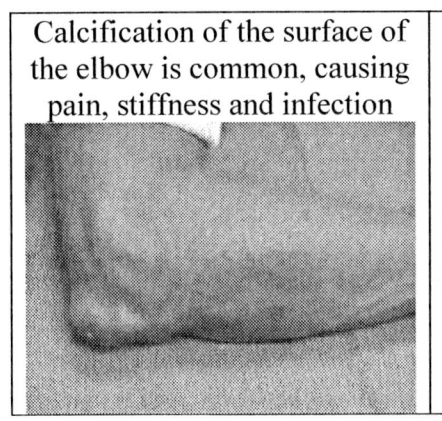

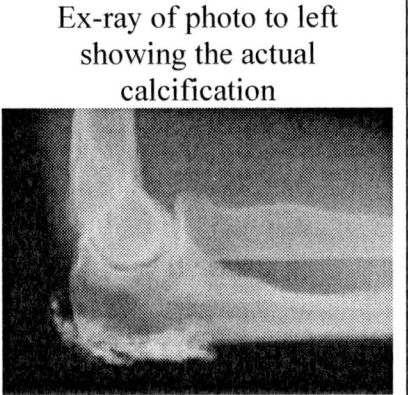

Calcification of the surface of the elbow is common, causing pain, stiffness and infection	Ex-ray of photo to left showing the actual calcification

Example 2: Prostate cancer.

Several studies show that high dairy milk consumption increases the risk of prostate cancer, but the culprit is *calcium* rather than fat. Calcification caused by dairy milk acts to prevent the prostrate from functioning efficiently, leading to cancer. A major Harvard study confirms this:

A strong case can be made that higher calcium intake is associated with an increased rather than a decreased risk of prostate cancer. Several case-control and prospective cohort studies have found positive associations between calcium intake and prostate cancer risk. Most prospective cohort studies, but not all, support an association between **higher intake of milk** *or dairy products and risk of prostate cancer. In addition, countries with* **greater per capita consumption of milk have higher prostate cancer** *mortality rates. Dairy fat was not associated with risk of prostate cancer.* [Several studies] *also reported an association* [of prostate cancer] *with calcium, independent of dairy fat. It is thus of concern that three recent prospective studies all found an increased risk of prostate cancer associated with high calcium intake.* [140]

(Please see appendix five, **Dairy Milk and Prostate Cancer** for more evidence on this subject).

Example three: Breast cancer.

As mentioned in another part of this book, dairy milk increases the risk of breast cancer in women by suppressing the natural production of progesterone (and by promoting cancerous cellular growth through bovine IGF-1). This happens because bovine sex hormones interfere with a woman's body chemistry. That is not to say that the genes you inherit do not play a part. The latest research shows that you can inherit a predisposition to breast cancer. But whether or not you inherit this predisposition, life-style factors such as the consumption of dairy milk can make breast cancer more likely.

When dairy milk is consumed regularly, an environment is created in the arteries of the breast that allows breast cancer to develop. More specifically, breast cancer occurs when micro-calcification in breast arteries cause cells to become more vulnerable to mutation and uncontrolled growth. This micro-calcification is caused by nanobacteria that get 'fed' with calcium and phosphorus in the bloodstream. The greater the calcium yo-yo effect (see appendix four) the greater the risk of micro-calcification in breast arteries.

The incidence of hypercalcemia (medical term for high calcium in the blood that leads to harmful calcification) is highest in lung cancer, and second highest in breast cancer.[152] The fact that calcification can cause cancer is well known to medical science. Many authoritative studies show how the tiny particles that make up calcified deposits can trigger inflammation and changes in cellular growth.

The incidence of breast cancer is higher in postmenopausal women because they lack estrogen. When the female body is low in estrogen the harmful calcium yo-yo effect is more pronounced (estrogen acts to slow down the calcium yo-yo effect as explained in appendix two, and dairy milk acts to increase the calcium yo-yo effect).

*The correlation with breast cancer was particularly strong in postmenopausal women. Positive correlations between foods and cancer mortality rates were particularly strong in the case of meats and **milk** for breast cancer.* [141]

Cholesterol is not the culprit

Coming back to heart disease for a moment, it is now realized that it is not caused by cholesterol. In fact, cholesterol is the body's best friend and vital to life. We need it to digest food, to make use of vitamins, to produce hormones, to protect the body against heart disease and cancer, and many other vital functions.

The latest research is clearly showing that dictary cholesterol is not a major cause of high blood cholesterol levels. We now know that it's the saturated fat in our diet that adversely affects our blood cholesterol level rather than the cholesterol that we eat.

Dietary cholesterol is not the same as blood cholesterol. Dietary cholesterol, when consumed from foods such as eggs, does not have a major effect on the overall amount of cholesterol in the blood of most people. It is now widely accepted that reducing *saturated fat* intake (including milk fat) is the most important dietary factor in reducing blood cholesterol levels. Milk is very high in myristic acid (a kind of saturated fat) which is known to raise LDL (bad) cholesterol levels leading to illness.

This does not mean that the cholesterol contained in the food we eat is good for you. It means there is no apparent need for cholesterol in the diet and there is no evidence of any beneficial effects of dietary cholesterol. The human body is perfectly capable of making as much cholesterol as it needs for good health.

Note however, that when food containing cholesterol is cooked/pasteurized, this oxidizes the cholesterol and this is bad for health. Oxidized cholesterol causes cancer, interferes with the body's capacity to make use of polyunsaturated fats, and promotes harmful arterial plaque. [103-105]

The point here is three-fold: (i) dairy milk contains oxidized cholesterol which provides raw material for arterial plaque, (ii) dairy milk provides saturated fat which in turn raises levels of bad (LDL) cholesterol and consequent heart disease, and (iii) dairy milk feeds calcium and phosphorus to nanobacteria which leads to arterial *calcification* and heart disease.

Excessive milk consumption may adversely affect the [blood] *circulation on account of the high calcium content of milk and because lactose promotes the intestinal absorption of calcium. Excessive calcium intake may cause calcification and rigidification of the large elastic arteries, which could be an important factor in causing heart disease.*[61]

How arteries get clogged up

The sequence of events leading up to clogged arteries goes like this:

1. The artery walls contain living cells. Sometimes something causes these cells to mutate, forcing them to duplicate at an extraordinary rate eventually creating a bulge inside the arterial wall. Why do cells mutate and multiply in this way? It is thought the answer is multi-faceted and related to poor diet, pollution, smoking, alcohol, defective genes, and stress.

2. The bulges created by the uncontrolled growth of cells are usually benign tumors called "*atheromas*". They can grow so large that they cause the inner lining of the artery to rupture, causing a lesion which acts as an anchor point for plaque to 'get a hold'.

3. Nanobacteria in the bloodstream get stuck to the lesions caused by the atheromas and other 'anchor' points in arteries and veins. Also, the bloodstream always carries around a certain level of 'home made' cholesterol (a mix of LDL/bad and HDL/good cholesterol). LDL cholesterol is sticky and therefore some of it sticks to the inside walls of arteries at the mentioned anchor points along with nanobacteria. Other passing debris from the bloodstream (including dairy milk fatty acids) gets stuck to the LDL cholesterol and the plaque begins to grow.

4. The *calcification* process begins when the bloodstream 'unintentionally' feeds phosphorus and calcium to the nanobacteria in the plaque. (In effect, nanobacteria suck calcium and phosphorus from the bloodstream). Over time, the plaque grows with a mix of LDL cholesterol, fatty acids, phosphorus, calcium, and other debris. The plaque gradually hardens as the nanobacteria secrete calcium phosphate in and around the plaque.

It is a safe bet that nanobacteria get the calcium and phosphorus from the blood. [137]

5. Similar calcification may also occur around the heart's four valves, narrowing the valves and leading to conditions such as *calcific aortic valve stenosis*.

This is what the renowned *Mayo Clinic* says on the matter:

Nanobacterium sanguineum is recognized as an emerging infectious disease. Nanobacteria have been shown to cause the calcification in coronary artery disease and vascular disease atherosclerotic plaque.[51]

Coronary heart disease continues to be a major cause of death and disability in developed nations, and projections from health authorities indicate that with continued inroads of antimicrobial therapies into underdeveloped regions, cardiovascular diseases may overtake infection as the primary cause of morbidity and mortality worldwide.

Calcium mineral deposits frequently form in atherosclerotic plaque. Calcification is a common and early feature of atheroma that almost invariably indicates the presence of plaque when found in the coronary arteries. Because calcium deposits are a surrogate measure of coronary atherosclerosis, clinical interest has focused on the utility of noninvasive detection of calcium as a coronary risk–stratification tool.[52]

Some doctors may disagree with this saying that not all plaque is calcified, and not all calcification is a sign of narrowed arteries. That may be; nevertheless, nearly all the research is saying that *most arterial plaque* is formed with the aid of calcification. Without calcification, the plaque is unable to grow and solidify.

Further evidence of the role that nanobacteria play in causing calcification and disease was provided in May 2005 by Dr Olavi Kajander, a pioneer in nanobacteria research:

Nanobacteria have the ability to replicate or propagate, and to create calcium phosphate coated vesicles or shells around themselves. These bony like particles ultimately accumulate and become calcified plaques. More specifically, a nanobacteria has a core phospholipid vesicle, surrounded by a calcium phosphate layer that binds proteins from its surroundings. These proteins involve blood clotting proteins, inflammation promoters and regulators, and many other proteins that are implicated in many diseases. Nanobacteria or calcified nano-particles are like ticking time bombs. The particles carry many of the known proteins implicated in coronary artery disease and many other diseases associated with pathological calcification or plaque. Therefore, the particles are capable of activating multiple disease pathways. This leads us to believe that many diseases such as kidney stones, atherosclerosis, prostatitis, arthritis and psoriasis are local manifestations of a systemic disease.[154]

The table that follows shows the strong correlation between high milk consumption and circulatory disease, by country.

Fig. 3
Top ten milk consuming countries (per capita)

Highest dairy milk consumers	Highest circulatory deaths
1. Ireland	1. Poland
2. Austria	2. Romania
3. Romania	3. Ireland
4. Sweden	4. Austria
5. Finland	5. Germany
6. Poland	6. Finland
7. United Kingdom	7. United States
8. New Zealand (12)*	8. United Kingdom
9. Denmark (11)*	9. Sweden
10. Netherlands (13)*	10. Norway

Source: Amalgamation of data from the OECD health data (www.nationmaster.com), the United States Department of Agriculture, (www.usda.gov), and *The Demographic Yearbook 2003.*

*Given that there are hundreds of countries in the world, the correlation in the above table is extraordinary. The table shows that all the biggest milk consuming countries *also have* the highest rates of circulatory deaths, *and in a similar ranking.* In fact, only New Zealand, Denmark and The Netherlands are not shown in the second column, but they are not far behind. The figures in brackets in the first column show what their ranking would be in the second column.

Whichever way you look at the statistics there is a striking correlation between high milk-consuming countries and the incidence of circulatory disease, i.e. disease related to clogged arteries and the circulation of blood.

What causes calcification?

Traditionally, doctors have said that fatty deposits trigger calcification and this is why plaque builds up in arteries. But this does not explain why calcification occurs in parts of the body where there are no fatty deposits, such as cataracts in the eyes. In the ground-breaking book *'The Calcium Bomb'*[17] the authors Mulhall and Hansen postulate that harmful calcification of the body is caused by nanobacteria. More specifically, the process of calcification goes like this:

(Summarized extract from 'The Calcium Bomb')

1. Nanobacteria enter the bloodstream directly or through the digestive system, from a variety of sources (pollution, contaminated water, the diet, and other possible sources).

2. Some nanobacteria get excreted harmlessly, while others get carried by the blood to locations where they get stuck in arteries and veins where blood flow is reduced at a splitting, a bend, or narrowing in capillary beds of tissue or at a site of injury or tumor growth.

3. These nanobacteria get fed by the bloodstream and are able to multiply and form a colony. Using calcium and phosphorus from the bloodstream the nanobacteria create calcium phosphate crystals which lead to harmful calcification. This harmful process occurs in arteries, organs, the eyes, the brain, and many other parts of the body where nanobacteria get a hold.

4. The calcification process caused by nanobacteria occurs whether the level of calcium in the blood is high or not high.

How does dairy milk come into this?

As mentioned, dairy milk appears to provide the raw materials for nanobacteria to grow and multiply by feeding them with phosphorus and calcium. To explain this further this is what happens when dairy milk is consumed:

1. **The calcium yo-yo effect.** Dairy milk consumption leads to a harmful *calcium yo-yo effect* (see appendix four). This in turn raises levels of calcium and phosphorus in the blood to an excessive level. This triggers PTH (parathyroid hormone) which compels the level of calcium in the blood to be lowered. When this happens, the bloodstream gets rid of excess calcium and phosphorus by putting some of it into bone, some of it is

excreted or lost through sweat, and some it gets dumped in arteries, veins, and other parts of the body causing harmful calcification. Hence, when the bloodstream dumps excess calcium and phosphorus it gets fed (inadvertently) to nanobacteria. ***Calcium and phosphorus are the raw materials that nanobacteria need to grow and flourish.***

The incidence of osteoporosis is likely to go hand in hand with the incidence of harmful calcification because osteoporosis is a reflection of the calcium yo-yo effect, and the calcium yo-yo effect is a major instigator of harmful calcification.

2. **Other foods.** Some other foods besides dairy milk are also high in calcium, or high in phosphorus, but they do not act to feed nanobacteria. This is so because dairy milk is unique in having a combination of four factors: high calcium, high phosphorus, high acidity, and high daily consumption. (Most milk consumers consume it on a daily basis).

3. **Healthy assimilation.** When dairy milk products are avoided in place of a healthy varied diet of fruit, vegetables, salads, nuts, seeds, & pulses, the calcium and phosphorus from the diet gets assimilated into the bones instead of causing harmful calcification. This happens because the body is able to control exactly how much calcium and phosphorus gets absorbed into the blood and hence into the bones. When this happens there is little or no *calcium yo-yo effect*, and consequently there is little or no dumping of calcium and phosphorus in places where nanobacteria lurk. With a dairy milk consumer, the *calcium yo-yo effect* makes the bloodstream dump calcium and phosphorus into calcified areas several times a day, depending on how often dairy milk is consumed.

Further evidence

Harmful calcification arises as a result of several factors coming together (as with most diseases there is no single cause). These factors are:

> Factor 1: Existence of nanobacteria.
> Factor 2: Existence of calcification.
> Factor 3: Existence of food source for nanobacteria.

Factor 1: Existence of nanobacteria.

The existence of nanobacteria inside the human body is no longer disputed as there is plenty of evidence to prove this. Consider the following:

➢ Livestock are known to harbour nanobacteria in abundance and that is why livestock serum is the 'industry standard' used for laboratory cultures of nanobacteria.

➢ It is well known that a lactating mammal such as a cow excretes toxins through her milk. This includes pesticides, chemicals, hormones, antibiotics, and bacteria (and there is no reason to think that nanobacteria are exempt from this process). These toxins and bacteria bind with the fat in milk, which serves to 'protect' and carry the toxins into the body when consumed. The propensity for toxins to bind with fat when fatty food is consumed is well documented. This is how toxins get stored inside surplus-body-fat. Normally, the body does quite a good job filtering out the toxins we consume so that they do not get into the bloodstream to cause harm. But in the case of dairy milk, all of which is homogenized, this does not happen:

Homogenizing milk involves the breaking down of fat particles to such a small size that the milk looks nice and smooth with no chunks of cream, but these smaller fat particles can permeate the intestines and end up in your blood stream. On the other hand, fresh unhomogenized milk... is natural and not a harmful form of fat. The larger fat molecules pass through the digestive system and nutrients are properly absorbed without fat entering the bloodstream. [97]

What happens is that the tiny homogenized fat globules act to carry toxins (and nanobacteria) into the bloodstream, bypassing the body's defenses. Once in the bloodstream, the toxins and nanobacteria get deposited almost anywhere in the body!

➢ *Because nanobacteria are in livestock, this suggests that they come from an environmental source. Many people eat red meat, and because calcium-encased nanobacteria may not be eradicated by cooking, they might enter [the body] that way.* [17]

➢ *How are humans exposed to nanobacteria? 'Cows seem to be hosts to nanobacteria, and biopharmaceutical cell culture (fetal bovine serum used as a supplement) are occasionally contaminated with nanobacteria.* [57]

➢ *Nanobacteria in clouds could play a crucial role in the spread of disease and in the formation of rain drops.* [56]

➢ *Experiments have shown that nanobacteria are excreted from the body in urine and their dispersal from the ground into the atmosphere and stratosphere appears to be inevitable.* [93]

➢ Nanobacteria are likely to be all around us, in nature, in rain, on grass pastures, and inside our bodies. People who are HIV positive have particularly large counts of nanobacteria. In 2004, researchers reported finding nanobacteria in everything from heart disease to cancer and kidney stones. [168]

➢ The issue is not whether we have nanobacteria in our bodies (we most likely do) – the issue is *what can we do* to starve nanobacteria and prevent them from proliferating inside the body causing calcification.

Factor 2: Existence of calcification.

➢ Nanobacteria cause calcification by secreting calcium phosphate. But they can only do this if fed calcium and phosphorus from the bloodstream. Therefore, it is likely that ***any dietary source*** that causes the bloodstream to dump calcium and phosphorus in the body will promote nanobacteria calcification. Dairy milk is tailor made for being this principal source.

➢ Doctors have known for a long time about the many diseases caused by harmful calcification. The fact that calcification occurs and is rampant throughout the world is not disputed. What is new is the role that nanobacteria play in the calcification process, and further research in this area can be expected.

As mentioned, there is mounting evidence that nanobacteria exist in the environment generally, all around us. Also, there is little doubt that nanobacteria feed on the calcium and phosphorus in the bloodstream, causing them to multiply and cause calcification. Without nanobacteria, calcification would not occur and the components of arterial plaque would most likely be excreted or stored inside body fat instead of clogging arteries.

Further evidence of a correlation between calcification and dairy milk can be found in the fact that the incidence of osteoporosis is much higher in people with heart disease. Dairy milk is the common link between osteoporosis and heart disease, as explained in appendix seven.

Factor 3: Existence of food source for nanobacteria.

➢ Dairy milk is increasingly being shown as the major piece of the calcification jigsaw puzzle – a kind of 'missing link' that adds light to the calcification process. Put simply, calcification occurs because ***nanobacteria get fed*** rather than because ***nanobacteria are present*** in the body.

In effect, dairy milk provides an ideal mix of ingredients for the formation of harmful calcification, whether it be arterial plaque or calcified concretions in different parts of the body. Virtually no other food product has the effect of dumping calcium and phosphorus into the tissues of the body to serve as food for nanobacteria. Dairy milk, with its unique combination of high acidity, high calcium & phosphorus, and high regularity of consumption all serve to complete the jigsaw puzzle that forms harmful calcification.

➢ *An increasingly vast set of data is linking the process of vascular **calcification** to the metabolism [consumption] of calcium and phosphorus...a case could be made to recommend restriction of* [**milk** and milk derivatives]. Source" Nunes JP, Med Hypotheses. 2005 May 16.

➢ *The calcium excess resulting from **milk** consumption tends to **calcify** the aorta, deteriorating its elasticity, resulting in lower diastolic pressure. When that becomes inadequate, the heart dies of ischaemia. The human* *habit of consuming the* **milk** *of another species invalidates the natural expedient for ensuring calcium intake according to needs. The lactose of cow's milk causes the absorption of its calcium content whether it is needed or not. Briefly, the intake of excess calcium in old age results in the hardening of the arteries, hence its connection with mortality from coronary heart disease.* Source: Dr. S Seely, The connection between milk and mortality from coronary heart disease, *Journal of Epidemiology and Community Health* 2002;56:958.

➢ *Excessive [dairy]* **milk** *consumption may adversely affect the circulation on account of the high calcium content of* **milk** *and because lactose promotes the intestinal absorption of calcium. Excessive calcium intake may cause* **calcification** *and rigidification of the large elastic arteries, which could be an important factor in causing myocardial ischaemia.* Source: Dr. Seely S, Possible connection between milk and coronary heart disease: the calcium hypothesis, Med Hypotheses. 2000 May;54(5):701-3.

➢ *The potential hazard of a high intake [of dairy* **milk** *calcium] is that a small fraction finds its way into soft tissues. The aorta is notably prone to* **calcification**...*The best cure would be prevention: the reduction of intake of calcium in prosperous countries.* Source: Seely S, Is calcium excess in western diet a major cause of arterial disease? Int J Cardiol. 1991 Nov;33(2):191-8.

➢ *A multi-country statistical approach involving 32 countries is used to find dietary links to ischemic heart disease (IHD) and coronary heart disease (CHD). For IHD,* **milk** *carbohydrates were found to have the highest statistical association for males aged 35+ and females aged 65+...In the case of CHD,* **non-fat milk** *was found to have the highest association for males aged 45+ and females aged 75... Lactose and calcium in conjunction with homocysteine from consumption of* **non-fat milk** *may also contribute to* **calcification** *of the arteries.* Source: Grant WB, **Milk** and other dietary influences on coronary heart disease, Altern Med Rev. 1998 Aug;3(4):281-94.

To summarize, the above research shows that dairy milk causes calcification, but until now the reasons were not clear. With recent discoveries in the world of nanobacteria a clearer picture is emerging.

A combination of three factors is showing a strong and direct association between dairy milk consumption and harmful calcification. These are:

Factor 1: Existence of nanobacteria in the human body.
Factor 2: Existence of calcification caused by nanobacteria.
Factor 3: Existence of food source for nanobacteria provided by dairy milk.

Anybody who consumes dairy milk will get the right mix of ingredients for calcification to develop (whether you are overweight or slim). In the book *The Calcium Bomb* [17] the authors state that a healthy lifestyle is unlikely to get rid of harmful calcification once formed, and that antibiotics are required for eradication. This may be so. However, by avoiding dairy milk, further calcification is likely to be greatly reduced or avoided altogether (and who knows, it may even reduce existing calcification). Also, if you have little or no harmful calcification in your body to start with, the avoidance of dairy milk is likely to go a long way to preventing the onset of calcification.

Some may argue that nanobacteria will suck calcium and phosphorus from the bloodstream whatever the level of these minerals in the blood. That therefore dairy milk is irrelevant, since nanobacteria get fed regardless of what is consumed. This argument has little merit for the following reasons:

1. There is no evidence that nanobacteria get fed calcium and phosphorus from the bloodstream when the level of these minerals in the blood is mostly low (i.e. at default level). The blood is compelled to always carry a minimum default level of these two minerals (plus a host of other nutrients). The National Cancer Institute, USA, states: *Normal blood calcium levels are maintained within narrow and constant limits.*

Good health is synonymous with a default level of nutrients in the blood as this reflects the fact that the body is being allowed to function properly. If nanobacteria could thrive even when the *default* level of calcium and phosphorus applied, this would mean that nanobacteria could thrive even in a perfectly healthy person. There is no evidence for this.

2. There is overwhelming evidence that high levels of calcium in the bloodstream (known medically as hypercalcemia) cause harmful calcification. There is no evidence that default levels of calcium in the bloodstream can lead to calcification.

3. There is increasing evidence that dairy milk causes excess levels of calcium in the bloodstream and consequent calcification (see evidence in this chapter). Since calcification is caused by nanobacteria, it is very likely that the high blood levels of calcium and phosphorus provided by dairy milk are to blame.

4. No other food source is known to raise levels of calcium and phosphorus in the blood to the extent or frequency accomplished by a regular consumption of pasteurized dairy milk. Several studies show unequivocally that when hypercalcemia occurs, the bloodstream is compelled to get rid of the excess calcium, resulting in harmful calcification. Given that dairy milk causes hypercalcemia (see above mentioned studies and appendix four), it is unrealistic to argue that dairy milk consumption has no impact on the incidence of harmful calcification.

The imperative here is to avoid dairy milk as there is increasing evidence that regular consumption leads to calcification, a ticking bomb in the form of serious disease, a poor quality of life, premature ageing, and early death.

Dairy Milk Effect on Protein

The average American or European consumes three to five times as much protein as necessary. Most of this is excess protein from dairy and animal sources which is not digested properly and is hazardous to health.

Outdated education has left most people badly misinformed about our body's protein needs. Several generations of school children and doctors were taught incorrectly that we need meat, dairy food and eggs for protein. The meat, dairy food and egg industries have funded this 'nutritional education' over generations and it has become official doctrine in many countries.

In the last twenty years or so experts in the field of nutrition and medical science have drastically changed their thinking about human protein needs but this updated knowledge has been very slow to reach the public.

The medical and nutritional establishment has been slow to accept evidence that is contrary to the status quo of self-serving 'nutritional education', sponsored by the meat and dairy industries. Increasingly though, doctors and nutritionists are steering people away from animal foodstuffs in favour of more fresh fruit and vegetables.

These enlightened professionals are saying that **modern research has shown that medical problems are caused by consuming too much protein, rather than not getting enough.** Protein is an extremely important nutrient, but when we get too much protein it causes problems. In the book *Your Health, Your Choice,* Dr. Ted Morter, Jr. warns, '*In our society, one of the principal sources of physiological toxins is too much protein.*'

Excess protein causes cancer

It may come as quite a shock to people trying to consume as much protein as possible to read in major medical journals and scientific reports that excess protein has been found to promote the growth of cancer cells and can cause liver and kidney disorders, digestive problems, gout, arthritis, calcium deficiencies (including osteoporosis) and other harmful mineral imbalances.

It has been known for decades that populations consuming high-protein dairy diets have higher cancer rates and lower life-spans (averaging as low as 30 to 40 years), compared to cultures subsisting on low-protein vegetarian diets (with average life-spans as high as 90 to 100 years).[6]

Numerous studies have found that humans on high-protein diets (and animals subjected to high-protein diets) have consistently developed higher rates of cancer. T. Colin Campbell, a Professor of Nutritional Sciences at Cornell University and the senior science advisor to the American Institute for Cancer Research, says there is '*a strong correlation between dietary protein intake and cancer of the breast, prostate, pancreas and colon.'* Likewise, Myron Winick, Director of Columbia University's Institute of Human Nutrition, has found strong evidence of *'a relationship between high-protein diets and cancer of the colon.'*

In *Your Health, Your Choice,* Dr. Morter writes, *'The paradox of protein is that it is not only essential but also potentially health-destroying. Adequate amounts are vital to keeping body cells healthy but regular consumption of excess dietary protein congests your cells and forces the pH of your life-sustaining fluids down to cell-stifling, disease-producing levels. Cells overburdened with protein become toxic.'*

Writing in the Sept. 3, 1982 issue of the *New England Journal of Medicine,* Dr. Barry Branner and Timothy Meyer state that *'undigested protein must be eliminated by the kidneys. This unnecessary work stresses out the kidneys so much that gradually lesions are developed and tissues begin to harden.'* In the colon, this excess protein waste putrefies into toxic substances, some of which are absorbed into the bloodstream. Dr. Willard Visek at the University of Illinois Medical School, warns: *'A high protein diet also breaks down the pancreas and lowers resistance to cancer as well as contributing to the development of diabetes.'*

In another Study in the *New England Journal of Medicine* evidence was presented that showed dairy milk as the cause of diabetes in **every one of 142 diabetic children** in the study. Each child produced antibodies in response to milk proteins. These antibodies (triggered fight invading milk proteins) turned on the children's own insulin-producing beta cells located in the pancreas. [125]

Protein in dairy milk weakens bones

There are numerous studies linking osteoporosis with high consumption of both protein and calcium, as found in dairy milk.[7]

For example, the March 1983, the *Journal of Clinical Nutrition* found that by age 65, the measurable bone loss of milk and meat-eaters was five to six times worse than of vegetarians. The Aug. 22, 1984 issue of the *Medical Tribune* also found that vegetarians have 'significantly stronger bones.'

For every gram of protein that you eat, you lose 1 to 2 mg of calcium in your urine.[90] African Bantu women average only 350 mg. of calcium per day (far below the National Dairy Council recommendation of 1,200 mg.), but seldom break a bone, and osteoporosis is practically non-existent, because they have a low-protein diet.

At the other extreme, Eskimos (the Inuit) have the highest calcium intake in the world (more than 2,000 mg. a day), and they suffer from one of the highest rates of osteoporosis because their diet is also the highest in protein.

The explanation for these findings is that dairy milk products leave an acidic residue, and a diet of acid-forming foods requires the body to balance its pH by withdrawing calcium (an alkaline mineral) from the bones. When this happens the bloodstream gets overburdened with calcium coming from two directions: the bones and the digestive system. This then triggers the harmful *calcium yo-yo effect* described in appendix four.

Dr. John McDougall reports on one long-term study, finding that even with calcium intakes as high as 1,400 mgs. a day, if the subjects consumed 75 grams of protein daily, there was more calcium lost in their urine than absorbed into their body.

In another study nutritional researcher Robert P. Heaney found that as consumption of protein increases, so does the amount of calcium lost in the urine (*Journal of the American Dietetic Association*, 1993): '*This effect has been documented in several different study designs for more than 70 years*' he writes, adding, '*the net effect is such that if protein intake is doubled without changing intake of other nutrients, urinary calcium content increases* [i.e. calcium is lost] *by about 50 percent.*'

Less protein is better for health

The human species has evolved as a mammal that thrives on low protein and gets sick on high protein. Millions of years ago our brains got bigger and made a quantum leap from ape to human because we ate a diet high in **unsaturated** fats, not because we ate meat, bone marrow, protein, or saturated fat.

Most recent research worldwide, both scientific and empirical, shows convincingly that our past beliefs in high protein requirements are incorrect, and that the actual daily need for protein in human nutrition is far below that which has long been considered necessary. Researchers working independently in many parts of the world arrived at the conclusion that our actual daily need for protein is only 25 to 35 grams (less than one ounce!).[7]

In his 1976 book, **How to Get Well**, Dr. Paavo Airola, Ph.D., N.D says: '***The metabolism of proteins consumed in excess of the actual need leaves toxic residues of metabolic waste in tissues, causes autotoxemia, overacidity and nutritional deficiencies, accumulation of uric acid and purines in the tissues, intestinal putrefaction, and contributes to the development of many of our most common and serious diseases, such as arthritis, kidney damage, pyorrhea, schizophrenia, osteoporosis, arteriosclerosis, heart disease, and cancer. A high protein diet also causes premature aging and lowers life expectancy.***'

It is easier to meet our minimum daily protein requirements than most people imagine since most fruit and vegetables contain protein in varying degrees. Because much of what experts once believed about protein has been proven incorrect, U.S. government recommendations on daily protein consumption were reduced from 118 grams to 56 grams in the 1980's.

Today the RDA for protein is based on body weight and is set at 0.8 grams per kilogram of body weight (that's 0.36 grams per lb. of body weight). Many nutritionists now feel that 20 grams of protein a day is more than enough, and warn about the potential dangers of consistently consuming much more than this amount. The average American consumes a little over 100 grams of protein per day!

Drastically reduced recommendations for protein consumption are an obvious indication that official information about protein taught to everyone from school children to doctors was incorrect, but there has been no major effort to inform the public that what we were taught has been proven wrong. So there are large numbers of people with medical problems caused by eating more than four or five times as much protein as necessary, yet their misguided obsession is still to ensure that they get enough protein.

Nutritionists now generally agree that it is very easy for a vegetarian to get sufficient protein. There are two reasons why we have such low protein requirements: (i) the human body recycles 70 percent of its proteinaceous waste, and (ii) our body loses only about 23 grams of protein a day.

The 'complete protein' myth

The need to consume meals containing 'complete protein' is based on an erroneous myth. Another fallacy is that 'food combining' is necessary to obtain 'complete protein' from vegetables. Both of these theories have been completely disproved, because we now know that people can completely satisfy their protein needs and all other nutritional requirements from fresh fruit, nuts, seeds and vegetables without worrying about food combining or adding protein supplements or animal products to their diet.

In fact, the whole theory behind the need to consume 'complete protein' (a belief once accepted as fact by medical and nutritional experts) is now disregarded. For example, Dr. Alfred Harper, of the US National Research Council, and Chairman of Nutritional Sciences at the University of Wisconsin states: *'One of the biggest fallacies ever perpetuated is that there is any need for so-called complete protein.'*

Protein is composed of amino acids, and these amino acids are literally the building blocks of all protein. Our body needs a total of 23 amino acids to make the protein that it needs for optimum health. Eight of these 23 amino acids are termed *'essential amino acids'* because our bodies cannot make them. But all eight essential amino acids are abundant in fresh fruit and vegetables. The other 15 amino acids are easily and comfortably made by the body. In this way, the body makes exactly the amount of protein that it needs for good health, without any harmful excess.

Best way to get protein

There are many vegetables and some fruits that contain *all eight essential amino acids*, including carrots, brussels sprouts, cabbage, cauliflower, corn, cucumbers, eggplant, kale, okra, peas, potatoes, summer squash, sweet potatoes, tomatoes and bananas.

But the reason we do not need all eight essential amino acids from one food or from one meal is that our body stores amino acids for future use. From the digestion of food and from recycling of proteinaceous wastes, our body maintains an amino acid pool, which is circulated to cells throughout the body by our blood and lymph systems. These cells (and our liver) are constantly making deposits and withdrawals from this pool, based on the supply and demand of specific amino acids.

It is known that protein gets destroyed at temperatures over 145 F. At this temperature the chemical bond and structure of protein is 'denatured' and once this happens, there is nothing we can do to 'un-de-nature' protein. Dairy milk is pasteurized at 145 F for 30 minutes, then 161 F for 15 seconds, and then at other higher temperatures going up to 212 F.

So when we consume the cooked protein in dairy milk it is denatured and only a very small portion actually gets assimilated. The excess **indigestible protein** acts to rob the body of valuable minerals in the process of travelling through the intestines. Worse still, this excess protein putrefies in the intestines causing illness and carcinogens which can eventually lead to cancer. When animal protein in dairy milk is cooked with pasteurization, this creates mutagens. These are chemicals that can alter the DNA in the nucleus of a living cell and increase the risk of the cell becoming cancerous.

As stated, humans do not need much protein for good health. The protein content of *human milk* is about 0.9%, the lowest among mammals. When you get your protein from plant based sources you physically cannot eat an excess of protein – you always get exactly what your body needs. With dairy milk and animal foodstuffs, you always get an excess of protein because the human body cannot break down and use all the amino acids in the protein – these excess amino acids are bad for health, causing numerous illnesses including osteoporosis and cancer.

As the animal-based protein travels along the human gut, it putrefies causing carcinogens and other unhealthy agents inside the body. Only carnivorous animals manage to break down and use up animal protein with complete efficiency – they can do this because their gut length is short and the animal protein passes through their body before putrefaction takes place. The human intestines share characteristics common to both omnivores and carnivores, so some of the animal protein does get digested but not with complete efficiency compared to carnivores.

Furthermore, once consumed, the protein in dairy milk has a tendency to putrefy more quickly than protein in meat because of the highly acidic environment created by the milk. The human intestines require an alkaline environment for efficient digestion – the acidic and 'cooked' protein in pasteurized milk is not only indigestible, it creates a bad acidic environment for the digestion of *all other food.*

Protein, when properly assimilated, helps the body to develop and grow, but you don't need much protein to grow a strong and healthy body. After all, the strongest animals on earth (think of gorillas, horses, elephants) eat a very low protein diet, yet they are strong and full of energy and stamina. Protein is for building body cells. Fuel for providing our cells with energy comes from the glucose and carbohydrates of fruit and vegetables.

Dairy milk protein bad for children

For infants and children, the indigestible protein in dairy milk does not promote healthy body growth. On the contrary, it promotes poor body growth (and ill health) arising from the harmful calcium yo-yo affect explained in appendix four. Also, dairy milk affects body growth by robbing the body of valuable minerals, from a loss of energy, and from a loss of appetite for more nutritious foods such as fruit and vegetables.

As pointed out by John Robbins in *Diet for a New America,* many studies have shown that protein consumption is no higher during hard work and exercise than during rest. Robbins writes, '*True, we need protein to replace enzymes, rebuild blood cells, grow hair, produce antibodies, and to fulfill certain other specific tasks. But study after study has found that protein combustion is no higher during exercise than under resting conditions. The popular idea that we need extra protein if we are working hard turns out to be simply another part of the whole mythology of protein, the 'beef gives us strength' conditioning foisted upon us by those who profit from our meat habit.*' To demonstrate how well-founded this position is in current scientific knowledge, Robbins quotes the National Academy of Science as saying, '*There is little evidence that muscular activity increases the need for protein.*'

Protein requires more energy to digest than any other type of food. In '*Your Health, Your Choice*' Dr. Ted Morter, Jr. writes: '*Protein is a negative energy food. Protein is credited with being an energy-producer. However, energy is used to digest it, and energy is needed to neutralize the excess acid ash it leaves. Protein uses more energy than it generates. It is a negative energy source.*'

> *'You need protein to build muscle but too much can lead to long-term side effects, like putting the kidney under too much pressure. The body can only store a certain amount of protein, too much can damage the kidney.'*
> Source: Claire MacEvilly, Tufts University, USA, and nutrition scientist for the British Nutrition Foundation.

Professional athletes are now being told that protein saps energy from working muscles and that too much protein is actually toxic. Phrases like 'protein power,' 'protein for energy,' 'protein pills for the training athlete' are now known to be false and misleading. If you are a meat eater, avoiding dairy milk protein is even more critical for good health.

The biggest harm caused by dairy milk when it comes to body growth is IGF-1. As explained in the chapter **Dairy Milk effect on Health**, IGF-1 from cow's milk is a growth hormone that plays havoc with the human body. It does this by over stimulating harmful cell growth setting up markers for a higher risk of cancer later in life. *'IGF-1 has been called the key factor in the growth and proliferation of cancer in humans by more than one microbiologist and cancer researcher.'* [60]

In summary, we don't need as much protein as we have been taught and consuming too much protein, as provided by dairy milk, is unhealthy. We don't need to eat 'complete protein.' Our body does need protein but only in small amounts. By eating a varied diet of fruit, vegetables, salads, nuts, seeds, and pulses we will get all the protein the body needs. Many of the milk recipes in this book provide easily digested protein because they are plant based and because very little or no cooking is involved.

When assimilated, protein provides the building blocks for our living cells. The highly cooked protein in *pasteurized* dairy milk gets poorly digested, robs the body of valuable minerals, depletes your energy, and causes mutagens which can develop into cancer. Worse still dairy milk protein promotes the harmful **calcium yo-yo effect** described in appendix four, and this in turn can lead to osteoporosis and to a multitude of diseases caused by calcification. Hence, there is a direct link between dairy protein and harmful calcification.

The imperative then is to avoid the indigestible protein provided by dairy milk. You will then begin to feel more energetic, and as your health gradually improves you will feel better and lose surplus body fat.

Dairy Milk Effect on Young People

Many parents have been brought up on the notion that dairy milk is an important source of nutrition for infants and children. We are told many times throughout our lives that children need dairy milk for good health. In many countries we see that dairy milk is dispensed freely to school children and this further reinforces the sanctity of dairy milk.

When you have your child's best interest at heart, and when you have spent a whole life-time being told that dairy milk is good for children, it is only natural to question the wisdom of depriving a growing child from consuming dairy milk. To deal with such concerns we will address three questions:

1. **Is dairy milk good for body growth?**
2. **Is dairy milk good for brain development?**
3. **Is dairy milk good for strong bones and teeth?**

At the end of this chapter infant milk-feeding is examined, from breast-feeding to weaning.

Is dairy milk good for body growth?

The simple answer is that dairy milk provides ***poor body growth*** rather than good body growth. Better body growth is obtained by avoiding dairy milk. This is so because the protein in dairy milk gets poorly digested, because the homogenized saturated fat in the milk is bad for health, and because the consumption of dairy milk fills you up, making you less likely to consume more nutritious growth-promoting food.

The protein in dairy milk gets poorly digested because the pasteurization process destroys enzymes needed for milk-protein digestion. Another reason is that humans lack rennin, an enzyme required for efficient digestion of milk protein.

At least 50% of all children in the USA are allergic to milk. Dairy products are the leading cause of food allergy, often revealed by constipation, diarrhea, and fatigue. Many cases of asthma and sinus infections are reported to be relieved and even eliminated by cutting out dairy. [23]

Humans have evolved to thrive on a low protein diet, and hence a high protein diet leads to illness and *poor body growth*. We need very little protein for optimum health (about 1 ounce daily), and we can easily get this from a variety of fruit, vegetables, salads, nuts, seeds, and pulses. At this point the reader is urged to review the chapter ***Dairy Milk Effect on Protein*** before continuing with this chapter.

> *Asthma, rhinitis, dermatitis, and gastrointestinal manifestations are common diseases of infants and children, and cow's milk appears to be the most common offending food.*[24]
>
> Does your child have coughs, colds, and ear infections? *Remove dairy products from a child's diet and watch what happens. After an initial period during which nose and ear problems persist (as the body clears out the residue mucus), the runny nose and ear problems go away and stay away.* [40]

Excess protein

Body growth occurs as a result of *hormonal activity* (instigated by the pituitary gland and liver) which affects bone and muscle growth. The *rate* of body growth is not dependent on the amount of protein that you eat. For example, if John eats more protein than George it does not mean this will make John grow better than George. In fact, any excess protein eaten by John could cause bad health, and provided George is not eating too little protein, he will grow a strong and healthy body. Protein is simply one of the many nutrients needed for good body growth.

Clearly, good body-growing nutrition is critical at a time in life when a child is growing up. The problem is that the highly cooked indigestible protein in pasteurized milk does not get used by the body for growth and nutrition. As the indigestible protein travels through the intestines it sticks to valuable minerals and carries them out of the body. This robs a child of nutrients at a critical time in life when maximum nutrition is needed for body growth.

Another problem is that as the protein travels along the intestines it quickly putrefies causing carcinogens which may lead to cancer in later life. This occurs because of the acidic environment created by the dairy milk and because the undigested protein stays in the intestines long enough to putrefy.

Homogenized saturated fat

As mentioned in previous chapters, the tiny fat molecules created in the milk by homogenization act to carry toxins (including heavy metals) into all parts of the body. This in turn affects healthy body growth. The harmful effects of homogenization are greatly underrated and not well publicized by the health industry.

Iron deficiency

Iron is needed for good bone marrow formation and therefore has a direct effect on body growth. During the first 6 months of life, babies are usually protected against developing iron deficiency due to the stores of iron built up in their bodies before they are born. However, when over six months old, as infants continue to undergo significant growth, they usually do not take in enough iron through breast milk alone.

If consuming dairy milk, iron deficiency is exacerbated for three reasons:

1. Dairy milk contains virtually no iron and therefore contributes nothing towards the prevention of anemia. The trace amount of iron that dairy milk contains (less than one milligram per quart) gets poorly absorbed: the indigestible protein in milk binds with the iron and leaves the body without being absorbed into the bloodstream.

2. Dairy milk makes an infant less interested in eating other foods that are good for body growth and that provide better sources of iron. This is so because dairy milk is filling, thus satiating feelings of hunger for more nutritious food.

3. Dairy milk causes some infants to lose iron from their intestines through intestinal bleeding (the harsh casein in milk irritates the delicate lining of the baby's intestines). This bleeding is pervasive and usually not sufficiently severe to be noticed in stools, but enough to cause anemia. It is estimated that half the iron-deficiency in infants in the USA is from cow-milk induced intestinal bleeding! Many studies have been carried out that show how dairy milk causes intestinal bleeding. Here are extracts from some of these studies:

Milk consumption has been shown to cause intestinal bleeding, resulting in low hemoglobin count. The result: weakness, depression, irritability.[3]

Babies who are fed whole cow's milk during the second six months of life may experience a 30% increase in intestinal blood loss and a significant loss of iron in their stools.[12]

Children with iron deficiency had a higher intake of cow's milk compared to those with sufficient iron. Intake of cow's milk is significantly higher in children with iron deficiency.[13]

Cow's milk-induced intestinal bleeding is a well-recognized cause of rectal bleeding in infancy. In all cases, bleeding resolved completely after instituting a cow's milk-free diet.[14]

Significant rectal bleeding is the most common symptom in cow's milk allergy.[15]

Cow's milk has been linked to a variety of health problems, including hemoglobin loss, mood swings, depression, and irritability.[16]

The association with anemia and acute intestinal bleeding in infants is known to all physicians.[60]

Early puberty

As mentioned in the chapter **Dairy Milk Effect on Health** the growth factor IGF-1 in dairy milk accelerates early puberty in boys and girls. This promotes behavioral problems and sets up markers for cancer later in life. Additionally, in the case of women, early puberty increases the risk of osteoporosis.

For example, let's say a girl reaches puberty at age 10 instead of 14 (not unusual), and reaches the menopause at 50. In this situation, her bones have processed 4 extra years of calcium by age 50. This means 4 extra years of depletion of valuable bone-making cells, making the onset of osteoporosis that much closer than otherwise.

An increase in calcium utilization is associated with the earliest physical signs of puberty. We conclude that longitudinal data demonstrate a change in bone mineral metabolism during early puberty associated with maturation of the hypothalamic-pituitary axis and physical changes of breast development. These changes lead to increases in multiple aspects of calcium metabolism during early puberty. Source: Stevan A, et al, *Calcium Absorption, Bone Mass Accumulation, and Kinetics Increase during Early Pubertal Development in Girls*, The Journal of Clinical Endocrinology & Metabolism Vol. 85, No. 5 1805-1809.

Acne

Although not related to body growth, here's a good way to convince teenagers to give up dairy milk: it causes acne! What happens is that steroids (androgens) in dairy milk stimulate the glands of hair follicles, making them secrete more sebum than usual. If you consume dairy milk the indigestible protein causes the skin to retain more water than normal. This in turn 'pinches' the sebum canal and prevents the free-flow of sebum to the skin. The result: acne. Giving up dairy milk will make your skin look and feel much better because less water will be retained in skin cells, freeing skin pores and allowing natural oils to keep your skin smoother and healthier.

IGF [in milk] *contributes to the increase in sebum production during puberty.*[49]

About 80% of [dairy] *cows are... throwing off hormones continuously...* [milk is] *implicated as a factor in the development of acne... teenage acne patients improved as soon as milk drinking stopped.*[50]

About 80% of cows that are giving milk are pregnant and are throwing off hormones continuously, including progesterone. This breaks down into androgens, which have been implicated as a factor in the development of acne. Adolescence is a time when milk consumption tends to be high, with many teenagers priding themselves on drinking 3-4 quarts daily. Dr. Jerome has found that acne improved as soon as the teenagers stopped drinking milk. [139]

Combination of factors

If your child is consuming dairy milk on a regular basis the sooner you switch the child to non-dairy milk the better. Failing this, you need to take extra care to ensure he/she gets adequate nutrition. Good body growth comes from good overall nutrition. Since we only need a small amount of protein for good body growth, and since virtually all foods contain protein in the form of amino acids, this should not be a concern.

When you eat well for optimum nutrition, you feel better, you have more energy, you suffer less stress, you think more clearly, and all these factors are necessary and inter-related for good body growth.

> *Myth:* **Children born to vegetarians and vegans are smaller than children born to meat eaters.**
>
> *Reality:* **Birth weights of infants born to well nourished vegetarian and vegan women have been shown to be similar to birth-weight norms and to birth weights of infants of non vegetarians.**
> Source: Pediatrics. 1989;84

Dairy milk makes you feel under-par, less energetic, less healthy, and hence more stressed. For a child or teenager, these factors combine together to inhibit good body growth and create markers for ill health later on in life. The biggest and strongest animals on earth do not eat animal protein (think of gorillas, elephants, buffaloes, horses, and rhinoceros). Bones get big and strong from the assimilation of *minerals* rather than protein. Therefore, healthy body growth is best achieved by giving more attention to eating a wide variety of fruit, vegetables, salads, nuts, seeds and pulses (as this will automatically provides an optimum level of vitamins, minerals and protein), rather than being concerned with the actual amount of protein consumed.

Protein misconceptions

There is a misconception that we need a little protein every day for good health. As explained in the chapter **Dairy Milk Effect on Protein** it does not matter if, on some days, you consume no protein. This is so because the body keeps a pool of amino acids, and it makes the amount of protein it needs, as and when needed. The most important thing for body growth is to get a wide variety of nutrients from the diet (and avoid the indigestible protein provided by dairy milk!). The many non-dairy milk recipes in this book provide a wide variety of nutrients, including easy-to-digest protein, providing an ideal source of nutrition for a growing body.

Another misconception is that we should not combine protein food with carbohydrate food as this can lead to poor digestion – research has proven this to be false.

Also, there is a misconception that humans require some degree of saturated fat in their diet for good health or body growth. In fact, **no amount of saturated fat (from the diet) is required for good health** because the body can easily and comfortably make any saturated fat that it may need.

This does not mean that eating foods with saturated fat is necessarily bad for health – some are bad (e.g. dairy milk), and some are not bad (e.g. coconuts).

Harmful fats in dairy milk

When it comes to dairy milk, the saturated fat breaks down as follows:

Saturated fat type	Percentage of total saturated fat
Myristic	16%
Palmitic	45%
Stearic	19%
Other saturated fats	20%

Two thirds of the fat in whole milk is saturated. As you can see in the above table most of the saturated fat is made up of myristic, palmitic, and stearic fat.

None of these three fats are good for health when obtained from homogenized pasteurized milk because they mostly get stored as body fat rather than being used for energy or nutritional purposes.

It is difficult to label any particular fat as being either good or bad as so much depends on the context (the nature of the food, how cooked, how much and what else eaten, etc).

However, some studies have shown that myristic acid & palmitic acid can promote harmful LDL cholesterol, heart disease, obesity and illness in humans. Here are some examples from such studies:

• *Myristic and palmitic acids may have a negative effect on cardiovascular health.*[27]

• *A large number of human and animal experiments subsequently confirmed that saturated fatty acids with chain lengths of 12 to 16 carbon atoms (lauric, myristic, and palmitic acids) were the most active in raising serum* cholesterol concentrations, whereas fatty acids with chain lengths of 10 or fewer carbon atoms or 18 carbon atoms (stearic acid) had no effect.[55]

It used to be thought that dietary cholesterol and total fat were the major causes of harmful cholesterol. Later on it became clear this was not so. That in fact, certain fatty acids are responsible for promoting harmful cholesterol. It was found that saturated fatty acids with 12–16 carbon atoms [the fats most prominent in dairy milk] *were the most important determinants of harmful cholesterol in the blood. These fatty acids have a strong cholesterol elevating effect and are strongly related to long-term heart disease mortality.*[87]

It is appreciated that some plant-based foods also contain saturated fat, particularly some kinds of nuts and seeds, e.g. coconuts. But these saturated fats are mostly *medium chain fats* and as such they more readily convert into energy or into *unsaturated* fats, once consumed. The body can then use these unsaturated fats for many important tasks, including making any *saturated* fat it might need for body growth and health.

Infants, and indeed children up to the age of 12, need to get about fifty percent of their calories from fat. Within this there must be a substantial amount of unsaturated fatty acids. If fat intake is restricted during childhood you may arrest development of the brain and other organs, with possible life-long consequences. Unfortunately, many infants consume large amounts of dairy milk, which is high in harmful saturated fat and low in good unsaturated fats.

Some parents have attempted to provide a low fat diet to their infants by feeding them low fat or skim milk. But giving low fat dairy milk to infants and children causes harm because the protein to fat ratio is too high.

In the highly acclaimed book *'Brain-Building Nutrition'* the author explains that the saturated fats found in milk and dairy products are, on the whole, not healthy because they are high in Omega-6 fats, low in Omega-3 fats, and milk has no DHA, the most important fat required for good brain development. Here are some extracts from the book:[25]

- *From age one to age two, the fat requirement of a child is still higher than that of an adult, so cutting out fat is dangerous, and cutting out unsaturated fatty acids can be disastrous.*

- *Saturated fat* [of the kind that breaks down to unsaturated fat once consumed] *is good for rapid body growth but poor for rapid brain growth. Unsaturated fatty acids* [from the diet] *have a less dramatic effect on body growth, but are critical for brain growth. Saturated fatty acids can easily be made by the body from simple raw materials.*

- *Prior to 2001 infant formulas contained no DHA and many formulas were derived from cow's milk which is high in saturated fat. This may account for the fact that formula fed infants tended to do worse on various types of visual, attention and intelligence tests. Most formula manufacturers will eventually rectify this problem.*

- *Unfortunately, the trend among many adolescents is toward high-saturated fat food that is rich in trans-fatty acids. On the other side of the coin are children who restrict their diets in various ways…gymnasts restrict calories to remain fit, runners load up on carbohydrates and restrict fat with the mistaken belief that this improves endurance, body-builders load up on high-protein foods and saturated fat, consuming very low amounts of unsaturated fatty acids.*

- *The results [of studies into the effects of dietary saturated fats] were pretty clear. Animals who were fed the high-saturated-fat diets had the lowest performance on memory tests. Those fed the diets lowest in saturated fat did the best.*

These extracts point towards the importance of giving children and teenagers a diet low in animal saturated fat, and high in *unsaturated* fats. For good body growth a child needs plenty of good unsaturated fat in the diet, the kind of fat you don't get from dairy milk. The human body can easily make **the right kind and the right amount of saturated fat** that it needs, and it does this best by using unsaturated fats, i.e. the kind of fats you get from plant-based foods.

The dairy industry goes to extraordinary lengths to promote milk in schools through sponsorship, advertising, and even by subsidizing school-milk costs ('Get them hooked on milk while they're still young'). Typically, the promotional literature states:

'Milk is an exceptional drink. It can make an important contribution to the diets of children and teenagers. Dairy milk during school recess stops children feeling hungry, helps them to concentrate, and provides almost every vitamin and mineral needed for a healthy diet.'

Hunger in school children can easily be assuaged by giving them *non-dairy* milk. Commercially produced non-dairy milk such as soy or rice milk is widely available in a variety of convenient carton sizes (with or without straws). Alternatively, school chefs can easily make non-dairy milk in bulk, using the recipes in this book. Giving dairy milk to school children does not help them to concentrate – *assuaging their hunger* (from any food source) is what helps them to concentrate. Dairy milk does not provide 'almost every vitamin and mineral' needed for a healthy diet – this is completely untrue. Most of the vitamins and minerals in dairy milk fail to get absorbed and get excreted: the indigestible protein in milk prevents absorption of most vitamins and minerals by causing mucosal congestion and high acidity. Furthermore, dairy milk provides no fibre, no brain-development fats, no health-promoting enzymes, and no energy for daily activities. However, dairy-milk does provide school children with a cocktail of harmful saturated fat, cancer-causing bovine hormones, and a multitude of chemicals that cause ling-term illness. By promoting ill-health, dairy milk actually holds children back from doing well at school.

***

Is dairy milk good for brain development?

We have seen why the *saturated* fat in dairy milk is bad for health. Now let's look at *unsaturated* fat.

The consumption of foods with unsaturated fat is essential to life. In fact, the human species was able to evolve a big brain and make a quantum leap from the animal kingdom *only because we started to eat foods with unsaturated fat.* These unsaturated fats came from flowering seed plants, nuts, grubs, insects, and sea food. Other mammals who ate meat and lived away from the coast-line failed to evolve a large brain.

The dairy industry would argue that milk does provide valuable unsaturated fatty acids like LA (linoleic acid), GLA (gamma linoleic acid), and oleic acid. Dairy milk also contains unsaturated fat called AA (arachidonic acid). Let's look at each of these:

1. **LA** is an Omega-6 fatty acid which is present in dairy milk, only in small, *trace amounts*. This fat is widely available from many vegetable oils, and from seeds, nuts, corn, grains, sea vegetables, and green leafy vegetables. The body needs LA to make important brain fats.

2. **GLA** is also an Omega-6 fatty acid which is present in dairy milk, only in small, *trace amounts*. This fat is found in small amounts in many vegetables, grains and seed oils, and is abundant in oatmeal, spirulina, oil of borage seed, evening primrose, and blackcurrent seed. GLA is used by the body as a kind of hormone that has important beneficial effects on the brain.

3. **Oleic acid** is an Omega-9 mono-unsaturated fatty acid. It is the most abundant of all fatty acids, and is found in most plant-based foods (nuts, seeds, grains, vegetables and their oils, fruit, pulses). Olive oil is rich in oleic acid. There is no oleic acid in dairy milk. However, the long chain fatty acid 18:1 in milk breaks down to oleic acid once consumed. In this way, dairy milk provides *less than one teaspoon* of oleic acid in ½ quart (1 pint) of dairy milk – *you get more oleic acid in one teaspoon of olive oil than in a pint of milk!* The body uses oleic acid for many important life-enhancing tasks, but it does not play any major role in brain development.

4. **AA (arachidonic acid)** is an Omega-6 mono-unsaturated fatty acid. A new-born baby gets AA from mother's milk. After the age of one, the human body makes its own AA, so we do not need it from the diet. AA is a major fatty acid in the brain and it fulfills many important brain functions. The body uses LA (linoleic acid) to make AA whenever needed and it does not like to receive AA in the diet. AA can be harmful to health when consumed and supplementation of AA should only be done under medical supervision. Here is an extract from the book *Brain Building Nutrition* by Dr. Michael Schmidt:

'The typical American diet, rich in Omega-6 fatty acids and low in Omega-3 fatty acids, is precisely the formula one would use to promote inflammation of the brain and alter brain chemistry in a negative way. We should consume foods that are low in AA (arachidonic acid) and low in linolenic acid while balancing our Omega-3 fatty acid intake. PGE2 is a highly inflammatory substance. [AA in the diet converts to PGE2 in the body]. *It can cause swelling, increased pain sensitivity, blood platelet clumping, spasm of blood vessels, and an overactive immune system. Elevated PGE2 has been found in a number of problems affecting mood, behaviour, and nervous system function.'* [25]

AA is found mainly in dairy milk, meat, and eggs, but virtually none is found in plant based foods (small amounts of AA are found in peanuts and black walnuts).

Most diets in developed nations are much too high in Omega-6 fats and much too low in Omega-3 fats. The human brain has evolved on a diet that had approximately equal amounts of Omega-6 and 3 (between ratios 2:1 and 1:1). A ratio of 1:1 is thought to be ideal for optimum health. With dairy milk you get harmful Omega-6 fat (because of AA) and no Omega-3 fat. This poor fat ratio can be a major contributor to bad health.

In a study presented to the *American Association for Cancer Research* in April 2005, Dr. Elaine Hardman warned about the dangers of eating a diet high in Omega-6 and low in Omega-3. The study showed that giving infant girls Omega-6-rich food can greatly increase their chances of getting breast cancer later in life. She said: *Mothers may inadvertently be setting up their daughters to develop breast cancer 50 years from now.* [88]

In another study commissioned by the *Daily Mail* newspaper in the UK schoolchildren were given fish oil capsules rich in DHA and the results were dramatic. All the children in the study showed marked improvements in their studies and behaviour, and some benefited dramatically by becoming calmer and doing much better at school. Commenting on the study, Dr. Madeleine Portwood said: *'This study demonstrates that essential fatty acids can make a huge difference to children's performance regardless of current ability. I now strongly recommend all parents try to include more essential fatty acids in their children's diet.'* [101]

The point here is that dairy milk provides no significant amount of essential fatty acids, but many kinds of non-dairy milks are rich in health-promoting fatty acids.

But what kind of fat is best for the brain? All the research shows that the brain thrives on DHA fat. This is the only fat the brain needs from the diet to develop and stay healthy. The brain does also need other fats, but the body makes such fats, as needed. The brain is made entirely of body cells. Some of these cells are saturated and some unsaturated. But all the cells in the brain (whether saturated or unsaturated) are made from *unsaturated* fats.

The argument that we need saturated fat in the diet because the brain is mostly made of saturated fat is an erroneous argument. Worse still is to suggest that we need *animal saturated fat* in the diet (as provided, for example, by dairy milk) for good health or for brain development – this is simply not so.

DHA (docosahexaenoic acid) is a critical fatty acid found in abundance in the brain. Our bodies can make DHA from ALA (alpha-linolenic acid) but this process is often very inefficient, and as we get older we become less capable of making DHA. Thus, we ideally need to get DHA from the diet. Note: do not confuse DHA with DHEA (a hormone). DHA is a healthy fatty acid that should be part of everyone's diet.

> *'Children who receive adequate DHA have been shown to have better visual acuity and IQ than children who receive inadequate amounts. These are periods* [of childhood] *when pre-formed DHA must be provided since the body during these periods is unable to make enough. As we age we make less DHA and it may be needed from the diet throughout life. …as a staple milk provides neither the right kind nor the right balance of fats. For children, in whom the brain is still forming, regular consumption of dairy products fill them with protein and fat, but the fat is not conducive to peak brain formation.'* [25]

For non-vegetarians, cold water fish such as salmon, mackerel, herring, and sardines provide sources of DHA. (Fish get their DHA from consuming algae). Also, fish oil supplements usually contain good amounts of DHA.

For vegetarians and vegans, some forms of seaweed (such as hijiki, nori, and kombu) and algae-rich foods contain DHA, and spirulina has small amounts. Also, plant-based DHA supplements are increasingly becoming available. Omega-3 flaxseed oil is excellent for good health, but it contains no DHA. Therefore, vegetarians and vegans should ensure they consume DHA-rich foods, or take a suitable DHA supplement (whether or not consuming flax seeds or taking Omega-3 oil supplements). Research shows that for good health you cannot rely on the body making enough DHA from the consumption of alpha-Linlenic acid.[25]

DHA's presence in breast milk may explain why breast-fed babies have a demonstrably higher IQ over babies fed formula without DHA. An emerging body of research led an expert committee of the World Health Organization to recommend that DHA be included in infant formulas at levels comparable to those of mothers' milk. Yet DHA levels in the breast milk of American women rank among the lowest in the world, and the FDA has only recently allowed DHA to be added to U.S. infant formulas. The DHA level of breast milk in Japanese women is estimated to be about three times that of American women.

The benefits of DHA are not limited to infant development. Supplementation may be helpful to anyone with a low DHA intake, especially for supporting a healthy nervous system. DHA has been associated with optimal memory function, visual acuity, and maintaining a positive mental state.

So is dairy milk good for brain development? This can now be answered quite simply by stating the fact that dairy milk contains no DHA and no fats (saturated or unsaturated) that serve the brain. If, as a parent, you are concerned about brain development in your child, *depriving the child of dairy milk will enhance brain development* for the following reasons:

1. It will help to redress the ratio of Omega-6 and Omega-3 fats in the diet by reducing Omega-6, which is high in dairy milk.

2. It will help to encourage the child to consume more healthy alternatives to dairy milk, since hunger will not be sated with dairy milk. Many non-dairy milk recipes in this book are rich in Omega-3 oils.

3. It will help to improve the general health of the child, as dairy milk causes nothing but harm and ill-health.

These three factors, combined with food or supplements rich in DHA, will give your child the best chance of developing a healthy brain at a critical stage in brain development.

In his world-famous book, *Baby and Child Care*, Dr. Benjamin Spock wrote, '*I no longer recommend dairy products. ... The essential fats that are needed for brain development are found in vegetable oils. Milk is very low in these essential fats and high in the saturated fats that encourage artery blockage and weight problems as children grow.*'

Is dairy milk good for growing bones and teeth?

The bones and teeth are being formed during childhood and teenage years, setting the stage for the years ahead. During this period it is critical to develop strong *healthy* bones and teeth through good nutrition, exercise, and the avoidance of dairy milk. A full examination of this subject is given in the chapter **Dairy Milk Effect on Osteoporosis.**

Researchers from the *University of Sydney and Westmead Hospital* discovered that consumption of dairy foods, **especially early in life**, increases the risk of hip fractures in old age:

'Consumption of dairy products, **particularly at age 20 years**, were associated with an increased risk of hip fractures... metabolism of dietary protein causes increased urinary excretion of calcium.' Source: American Journal of Epidemiology 1994;139

For an excellent free guide on this subject go to:

http://www.pcrm.org/health/prevmed/building_bones.html where you can get a *'Parent's Guide to Building Better Bones'* issued by the *Physicians Committee for Responsible Medicine*, USA.

Bone mass and bone density reach their peak by about age 25 and plateaus for about 10 years, after which bone density is gradually lost. The rate of bone density loss for women can increase **as much as tenfold** during the first six years after menopause. The imperative here (particularly for children) is to switch to non-dairy milk before it is too late, i.e. before the body stops growing. If milk is bad for adults, it is much worse for growing children.

A word of caution for parents

Virtually any kind of food you care to mention has a good side to it and a dark side. As this book is about milk, the dark side to soybeans should be mentioned: soybeans contain substances that can inhibit digestion such as phytic acid, polyurones, arabinoxylanes (special pentosanes), toxic lectins and mutagenic phyto-estrogens. Phyto-estrogens can also impair sex-hormone metabolism. Don't let this put you off soy as it has many attributes. The same kind of story could be told about oranges, bananas, beef, lettuce, anything. The point is that *any kind of food should be consumed in moderation.*

As soy milk is readily available in supermarkets do not fall into the trap of substituting dairy milk for soy milk and then just giving soy milk to your children every day. An excess consumption of soy milk (as with any other food product) is unhealthy, particularly where children are concerned. When giving non-dairy milk to children do it in *moderation*, and give them *variety* by rotating through a different type of non-dairy milk every week or so, or by blending different types of non-dairy milks.

Regarding infant milk-feeding, the *Canadian Pediatric Society* (www.cps.ca/english/CPSP/Studies/Rickets.htm) advises that *all infants* who are being breastfed should also be given a vitamin D3 supplement of appropriate dosage - not only those who may receive insufficient sunlight. Breastfed babies should not be given other supplements unless advised by a health professional because all the nutrients required for good health are contained in mother's milk. Babies under two who are not being breastfed at all should be given specially formulated baby milk, and any *additional* supplementation (including vitamin D) should only be given under the supervision of a healthcare professional.

The American Academy of Pediatrics goes further and says: *'It is recommended that all infants, including those who are exclusively breastfed, have a minimum intake of 200 IU (5 mcg) of vitamin D3 per day during the first 2 months of life. In addition, it is recommended that an intake of 200 IU of vitamin D3 per day be continued throughout childhood and adolescence, because adequate sunlight exposure is not easily determined for a given individual. These vitamin D3 intake guidelines for healthy infants and children are based on the recommendations of the National Academy of Sciences.'*

For children aged over two years old, it is better to avoid vitamin D and calcium supplements altogether for the reasons explained in the chapter **Dairy Milk Effect on Osteoporosis.**

Giving milk to infants

Weaning is a gradual process that begins when you start to replace milk with solid foods. Infants should not be given solid foods before the age of four months except on the advice of a health professional. A mixed diet should be offered by the age of six months, at which stage babies need a source of iron in their diet as breast or formula milk can no longer provide enough. Especially if there is a family history of allergies, when you begin weaning your baby, introduce one food at a time and leave a few days between each new food. This way, you will be able to tell if your baby is allergic or sensitive to any particular food.

For infants under one there are only two good sources of milk: the left breast and the right breast, period. *Dairy* milk is bad for infants of any age. Infants don't need any kind of milk (apart from human milk) while still breastfeeding. Infants need many nutrients that they get in mother's milk, including calcium, vitamin D and fat. Dairy milk is a bad source for these nutrients. If human milk is not available, use infant formula milk that does not contain dairy milk.

There is no shortage of research showing that breast milk is always best when compared to formula milk or dairy milk. Here are some extracts:

Formula-fed babies, at the age of three months, were secreting low levels of serum antibodies [in response] *to cow milk antigens contained in their formula.*[2]

Those who consumed cow's milk were fourteen times more likely to die from diarrhea-related complications and four times more likely to die of pneumonia than were breast-fed babies. Intolerance and allergy to cow's milk products is a factor in sudden infant death syndrome.[41]

After the first year of life the child requires no [dairy] *milk of any type. The child, like us adults, can thrive without cow milk ever crossing his/her lips.*[23]

Infants given baby formula containing cow's milk developed symptoms of allergic rejection to cow milk protein before one month of age. The recommended therapy is to avoid cow's milk.[42]

When scientists analyzed data from diabetic children they discovered an absolute cause and effect relationship between dairy milk consumption and childhood diabetes.[126]

Infant formulas based on dairy milk are loaded with harmful protein hormones. When consumed, this creates antibodies (histamines) which cause diarrhea, coughing, congestion, cramps, stomach ache, mucosal congestion, and other symptoms. *Many scientists and doctors have hypothesized that Sudden Infant Death Syndrome (SIDS) is actually an allergic reaction to milk hormones. Babies who drink* [dairy milk] *formula are actually drinking milk which contains milk proteins.*[60]

Wet-nursing better than infant formula

If breastfeeding or expressing your own milk is impossible consider letting your child drink the milk from another lactating woman. She can use a breast pump so that you may buy her human milk. However, it is appreciated that this is not easily arranged as the use of a breast pump is not so straightforward.

Alternatively, let your baby be wet-nursed. Most women can produce enough breast milk for two babies at the same time. This too, may not be so easy to arrange as you would need to trust the wet-nurse and be confident she is free of disease.

A wet-nursing arrangement may sound outlandish but is infinitely better than using infant formula, which should be an ***absolute last resort***. Infant formula is better than dairy or non-dairy milk; nevertheless, infant formula is very much inferior to human milk as it lacks vital messenger substances which the baby needs for good health. Also, infant formulas of all types tend to be high in phosphorus which is bad for babies. Another problem is that boiling tap water for mixing with infant formula powder does not remove nitrates, sodium, and other harmful substances found in all tap water (better to use sterilized/distilled water). If you feel you must use infant formula, check out the latest news on internet by doing a search for 'infant formula.'

Of all humans, babies need the most calcium because their bones are still weak and need to be strengthened much more. And mother's milk does, of course, contain all the calcium (and other nutrients) babies need in their first two years. Babies fed on mother's milk are perfectly able to increase bone-mineral density.

Breast feeding should continue until the baby is at least two years old. If you absolutely must use infant formula, it is best to avoid an infant formula based on dairy milk or soy. In the case of soy formula the problem is that some commercial brands contain high concentrations of soy genistein, which has been shown to inhibit intestinal growth.[63] Also, soy formula contains phyto-estrogens which in a baby can be harmful. Either use a soy formula low in genistein, or use an 'elemental formula' that is soy and dairy free.

According to the **American Academy of Pediatrics** babies shouldn't have dairy milk (if at all) until they are at least one year old. Babies do need milk, but not the pasteurized milk from cows produced by the dairy industry. They need *human* breast milk. And, if for some reason this is unavailable, they need the next best thing, and that is *non-dairy* iron-fortified milk *specially formulated* for babies, and prepared with pure distilled water.

Dairy milk should not be given to children of any age, particularly if under two. Worse still, never give a baby or a child low-fat cow's milk because of it being 'less fattening.' Low-fat and non-fat milk is even worse for health than whole milk, as explained in the chapter ***Dairy Milk Effect on Weight Loss***. Babies need to consume fat in their diet, as provided in breast milk or infant formula milk, for several important reasons. For example it enables fat-soluble vitamins to be assimilated into the body.

In general nutritional supplements for a breastfeeding baby under one are not necessary. For children aged over one, supplementation of certain nutrients may be advisable – but always do this with the guidance of a health professional and be sure to use the dosage appropriate for the age of the child.

For babies under two, when breastfeeding is no longer possible (or being phased out) infant formula milk should be given instead if a wet-nursing arrangement is not possible. Do not replace breast milk with dairy milk or non-dairy milk. However, small amounts of non-dairy milk may be given *in*

addition to formula milk. *Cow's milk allergy is common in infancy and childhood. An appropriate cow's milk substitute is necessary for feeding babies.* [26] Fig. 4 gives a summary of the milk options for infants.

Fig. 4
Milk options for infants

Type of milk:
A = Dairy milk.
B = Other animal milks, e.g. goat's milk.
C = Non-dairy milks made from nuts, as given in this book, e.g. almond milk, peanut milk, etc.
D = Non-dairy milks made without nuts, as given in this book, e.g. rice milk, soya milk, etc.

Type of milk	Contains nuts?	Age: up to 1 year	Age: 1 – 2 years	Age: 2 – 4 years	Age: over 4 years
A	no	Avoid	Avoid	Avoid	Avoid
B	no	Avoid	Avoid	Avoid	Avoid
C	yes	Avoid	Avoid	See note **1** below	See note **2** below
D	no	Avoid	See note **3** below	Okay in moderation	Okay

Notes relating to Fig. 4

1. In this age group non-dairy milk made from nuts may be introduced gradually if no family history of nut allergies. (Note: non-allergic children should avoid peanuts and peanut milk until aged 4 so as to minimize risk of creating an allergy). ***If there is a history of nut allergy in the family avoid giving nut-based milks to any child in this age group.*** When giving a nut-based milk to a child for the first time watch carefully for any allergic reactions. A small amount of non-saturated oil may be added, such as olive oil or Omega-3 oil. Do not exceed the supplementation dosage applicable to the child's age. Consult a health professional if unsure.

2. In this age group non-dairy milk made from nuts may be introduced gradually if no family history of nut allergies. If there is a history of nut allergy in the family, have child tested for allergies before giving nut-based milk. When giving nut-based milk to a child for the first time

watch carefully for any allergic reactions. A small amount of non-saturated oil may be added, such as olive oil or Omega-3 oil. Do not exceed the supplementation dosage applicable to the child's age. Consult a health professional if unsure.

3. In this age group non-dairy milk made without nuts may be introduced gradually, but *not as a substitute for human milk or infant formula milk*. Pumpkin seed milk for example, may be given to children aged 1 - 2 to *supplement* breast milk or formula milk (*not as a substitute or replacement*).

4. Any kind of non-human *animal* milk, including dairy milk, is bad for humans, particularly babies and young children.

5. Infants under 6 months old should only be given mother's breast milk. If this is not possible consult a medical doctor or a child health professional.

6. Nut allergies in children can be a major concern. Therefore, avoid nut-based milks for anybody allergic to nuts, regardless of age.

7. Mothers who are breast feeding in first six months of baby's life should avoid (or moderate) their consumption of dairy milk, egg, citrus fruit, wheat, peanuts, tree nuts, sesame, fish and shellfish, as 'traces' of these foods may be passed onto the baby and cause allergies in later life.

The increase in food allergies is likely to be caused by a small number of foods. These include dairy milk, egg, citrus fruit, wheat, peanuts, tree nuts, sesame, fish and shellfish. The introduction of such foods should be avoided in first 6 months. There is little agreement about when peanuts and nuts can safely be introduced, but in atopic families, their introduction should be delayed until after three years of age. All babies should initially be weaned on to foods that have a low risk of inducing allergy, such as rice, fruits, and vegetables. Source: The Anaphylaxis Campaign, UK. www.anaphylaxis.org.uk

Dairy milk and breastfeeding do not mix

A pregnant woman should avoid dairy milk because antibiotics, cow hormones, and harmful substances in milk get passed into the unborn child.

Just as important, a mother should not consume dairy milk after birth. Many of the harmful substance in dairy milk can pass into the infant through breast milk. Worse still, the hormones in dairy milk inhibit the production of human milk. This happens because the hormones in dairy milk are similar to the hormones produced by a breastfeeding woman. This upsets the woman's body chemistry, making the body reduce or shut down the production of human milk.

Also, it is well known that the act of breastfeeding helps a woman become slimmer and regain her figure by releasing oxytocin, leptin and prolactin. These natural hormones work in concert inside the mother's body to suppresses appetite and get rid of surplus body fat.[150] The sooner the mother can regain her figure and fitness, the sooner she can be active to protect her baby, or flee with the baby in the face of danger (this is how the human species has evolved).

A woman's body chemistry is finely tuned during breastfeeding months so that she is able to produce milk, breastfeed and look after the infant. If the mother consumes dairy milk at this time, the cow hormones will interfere with the human hormones oxytocin, leptin and prolactin. This happens because cow hormones are more similar to human hormones than any other animal, and are able to mimic human hormones. This confuses the delicate body chemistry of a breastfeeding woman, causing havoc.[150]

So by consuming dairy milk, a breastfeeding mother may suffer three major consequences, with possible life-long effects for both mother and baby:

1. Harmful substances in dairy milk can pass into the baby through breast milk, impairing the health of the baby.

2. The mother will be less able to breastfeed as a result of a dwindling supply of breast milk. This has disastrous consequences: (i) By switching to infant formula the baby's health can be affected. (ii) Research shows that mothers who do not breastfeed are more likely to get breast cancer. (iii) Lack of breastfeeding can affect the bonding between mother and child.

3. **The mother will be more likely to remain overweight, perhaps never again regaining a slim healthy figure.**

The imperative here is for pregnant women and new mothers to completely avoid dairy milk. All pre-natal classes and hospital maternity wards should be telling new mothers that dairy milk is strictly off bounds!

Dairy Milk Effect on Weight Loss

The dairy industry, with a multi-million dollar advertising budget, does its best to portray whole milk as a non-fattening product. The inescapable truth is that **dairy milk is very fattening.**

'The vast majority of scientific studies show that dairy milk either causes weight gain or else has no effect at all on weight or body fat. Non-fat milk is 55 percent sugar, while whole milk is nearly 50 percent fat, as a percentage of calories. Neither one is a formula for weight loss.' Source: Dr. Amy Joy Lanou, Ph.D., senior nutrition scientist of Physicians Committee for Responsible Medicine, Washington DC, USA.

The above statement is backed up by a major study by the *Harvard Medical School,* published in the June 2005 issue of *Archives of Pediatrics and Adolescent Medicine.* This analyzed milk intake data from more than 12,000 children from 1996-1999 and concluded that the more milk children drank, the more weight they gained.

Also, as explained in the previous chapter, breastfeeding mothers who consume dairy milk will find it much harder to regain their previous figure or become slim. This is so because dairy milk interferes with a woman's production of oxytocin and leptin, hormones which get rid of surplus body fat, and which suppress food cravings and overeating. [150]

Many people are overweight or do not want to gain surplus body fat. Also, many people are concerned about not consuming too much saturated fat. As a consequence, there is a huge market for low fat varieties of milk that is as big as the market for whole milk.

Clearly, people believe that low fat milk must be better for you because it contains less saturated fat. It would seem a logical conclusion to draw; however, it would be a false conclusion.

Why low fat milk is more fattening

Consider this: *low fat milk is actually more fattening than regular whole milk!* Here's why low fat milk is both more fattening and unhealthier:

1. Higher consumption. By consuming low fat milk as an alternative to whole milk, people usually end up consuming *more milk* than otherwise. This happens from a false sense that low fat milk is 'better'. As a result, you end up consuming more calories than just sticking to whole milk.

2. More calories. Low fat milk contains almost the same amount of calories as regular whole milk. See the comparison table on the next page:

Fig. 5
Calories & fat in dairy milk

(All figures approximate)

8 Fluid ounces (1 cup or 272mL)	Country	Calories	Grams fat	Fat Calories	Grams Sat. Fat
3% whole	USA	150	8	48%	5
2% low-fat	USA	120	5	38%	4
1% low-fat	USA	100	3	27%	2
Skim	USA	80	trace	5%	trace
1% buttermilk	USA	100	2	18%	1
dry(no fat, reconstituted)	USA	80	trace	5%	trace
Canned Evaporated undiluted whole	USA	340	20	53%	17
Lactaid,1% lactose treated	USA	100	2	18%	2
Whole Goat's	USA	168	10	54%	6
Whole milk	UK/EU	145	8.2	55.1%	5.2
Semi-skimmed	UK/EU	105	3.9	27.6%	2.3
Skimmed	UK/EU	77	0.2	2.3%	0.1

Some Variations in dairy milk terminology		
(Each row below refers to the same kind of milk)		
UK/EU	USA	Canada
Full cream (up to 4%)	Whole (up to 4%)	Full cream (up to 4%)
Whole (3%)	Regular (3%)	Homo or Regular (3%)
Unhomogenized	Unhomogenized	Whole
Semi-skimmed	1% low fat	1% low fat
(Not widely sold)	2% low fat	2% low fat
Skimmed	Skim	Skim

In the Fig. 5 above we see that in the USA *'2% milk'* only has about a fifth less calories than whole milk. This small difference in calorie consumption is soon eroded from a false sense of security that results in a higher consumption of low-fat milk. If you are more likely to consume such milk by virtue of it being low fat, you are better off consuming a smaller amount of whole dairy milk.

> **You only need to consume a little more low fat milk (about a quarter of a cup more per day) to get more calories compared to consuming whole milk!**

This is aptly illustrated in a major study published in June 2005 *(Longitudinal Study of Adolescents)* which looked at 12,829 children and concluded that skim and 1% milk were more fattening than whole milk. The study found that those consuming more than three daily servings were about 35 percent more likely to become overweight than those who drank one or two. The study concluded: *'Children who drank the most milk gained more weight, but the added calories appeared responsible. Contrary to our hypotheses, dietary calcium and skim and 1% milk were associated with weight gain, but dairy fat was not. Drinking large amounts of milk may provide excess* [fattening] *energy to some children.* [127]

This does not mean that dairy fat in whole milk is non-fattening, but it does mean that low-fat milks can be more fattening.

4. Excess calcium. As explained in the chapter *Dairy Milk Effect on Osteoporosis* all forms for dairy milk are bad for bones because of high acidity and calcium. Low fat and non-fat dairy milk contain about 10% *more* calcium than whole milk and much more indigestible protein. This harmful cocktail makes low fat milks highly acidic and significantly more harmful to health by increasing the risk of osteoporosis.

3. Little nutritional difference. Apart from the difference in fat content, the nutritional comparison between whole milk and low fat varieties of milk is about the same (apart from calcium, see previous point). The milk industry itself readily admits that all varieties of whole and low-fat milk contain about the same amount of nutrients (including protein and calcium). Given this, you would think they contain similar amounts of pesticides, herbicides, antibiotics, hormones, and other pollutants, since the only difference is the amount of fat removed. But this is not so, read on.

4. More harmful substances. Low fat milk actually contains *more* lactose, casein and other harmful substances compared to whole milk. Here is what the *Physicians Committee For Responsible Medicine*, USA, has to say:

> *'When people switch to low fat milk varieties (to reduce their fat intake), this delivers lactose in much larger amounts: skim milk and low fat milk products are usually supplemented with additional milk solids, sugars and other derivatives to give them substance and make them more appealing.*
>
> *Especially among elderly people, switching to low-fat milk (with its higher levels of lactose) brings on severe diarrhea and other gastro-*

intestinal symptoms. Many people in western developed countries eat all types of foods indiscriminately and may have come to accept chronic flatulence, constipation and bloating as 'normal'. However these are not normal and should be investigated.' [64]

In another study it was found that each daily glass of low fat milk or skim milk [non-fat milk] was associated with a 20 percent increase in serious ovarian cancers. Researchers hypothesize that galactose, a component of the milk sugar lactose, may damage ovarian cells, making them more susceptible to cancer. [54]

5. More fattening. Low fat milk is *more* fattening (not less fattening) than whole milk, even though it contains less fat. How can this be? Here is a scientific explanation: when we consume fat the enzymes in the food we eat serve to break down the fat so that it can be digested and used by the body. Thus, when *whole* milk is consumed, the enzymes in the milk help to break down and metabolize (burn up) the fat. With low fat milk the skimming process takes away the enzymes. As a consequence, the little fat that does remain behind does not get digested properly and it gets stored as surplus body fat.

6. More hunger. The pasteurizing process in milk turns the lactose into beta-lactose that is far more soluble and therefore more rapidly absorbed into the blood stream. The sudden rise in blood sugar is followed by a fall leading to low blood sugar, hypoglycemia, which induces hunger. If more pasteurized milk is drunk to satisfy the hunger, then the cycle is repeated: hyperglycemia, hypoglycemia, hunger, more milk, etc. The end result is obesity. Obesity has become one of the most common diseases of childhood. **Pasteurized milk causes obesity even if it is skimmed.** Pigs are regularly fattened with skimmed milk for this reason.

7. Extra bad for heart. As mentioned in the chapter *Dairy Milk Effect on Health,* homogenized milk can cause illness in several ways. It does this by helping fat soluble toxins in the digestive system get through to the bloodstream – some of these toxins end up in arterial plaque. Also, some of the saturated fat in dairy milk gets stored in the plaque. These two factors are part of the jigsaw that contributes to arterial furring and heart disease. As low-fat varieties of milk are also homogenized, *the harm caused by homogenized milk also applies to low fat milk.* You would think that homogenization in low fat milk is less severe because there is less homogenized fat in the milk. But this would be a false conclusion for the following reasons:

- When whole milk is changed to 2% milk it does not mean that 98% of the fat has been removed. In Fig. 5 above we see that whole milk contains 5g of saturated fat, and 2% milk contains 4g of saturated fat. So this means that only about a fifth of the saturated fat has been removed (not 98 %!). Put another way, 80% of the saturated fat in whole milk goes into 2% milk. So when removing some of the fat from whole milk to create 2% milk, the total fat content is reduced by about 35% (from 8g to 5g) in the skimming process. This means the harmful homogenization factor has only been reduced by about 35%.

Non-fat dried milk is added to all kinds of low fat milk. Unlike the cholesterol in fresh pasteurized milk, which is not so oxidized, the cholesterol in non-fat dried milk is mostly oxidized and it is this rancid cholesterol that promotes heart disease by providing a sticking agent for the build up of plaque (oxidized cholesterol is used in research to cause atherosclerosis).

- Like all spray dried products, non-fat dried milk has a high nitrite content. When they make low fat powdered milk (for adding to low fat liquid milk), first of all it is forced through a tiny hole at high pressure, and then blown out into the air. This causes a lot of nitrates to form and the cholesterol in the milk is oxidized. Nitrates are toxic and are linked to stomach cancer and cancer of the esophagus among others. This means low fat varieties of milk contain more cancer-causing nitrates than whole milk.

8. More galactose. Low-fat and skim milk have much more harmful galactose than whole milk. In the following table we see that low-fat has about a third more lactose (and hence galactose) than whole milk:

	Whole	Low-fat	Skim
Fat	49%	31%	2%
Protein	21%	28%	41%
Lactose	30%	41%	57%

Many studies show a strong association between milk-rich galactose and diseases such as cataracts and heart disease. Please see the section on 'galactose' in the chapter *'Dairy Milk Effect on Health.'*

The conclusion we come to then, is that low fat dairy milk of any variety is not a healthier option compared to whole milk, even if you want to lose surplus body fat. When you take into account the *combined* effect of the above factors, low fat milk is actually more fattening (and more harmful to health) than whole milk!

Skim milk

When it comes to skim milk (non-fat milk) the situation is even worse! As shown in the above table, skim milk has about twice the lactose/galactose compared to whole milk, greatly increasing the harm caused by galactose.

Furthermore, the amount of indigestible protein in skim milk is about double the amount in whole milk – this greatly increases the amount of minerals that do not get absorbed into the body. Additionally, the extra high acidity in skim (non-fat) milk puts you at greater risk of osteoporosis compared to whole milk because of the harmful calcium yo-yo effect (see appendix four). The net result is that the nutritional value of skim milk is significantly less than whole milk.

Skim milk then is even worse for your health than whole milk or low-fat milk. But that's not all: even skim milk contains 0.5 grams of fat and 90 calories in a cupful (8 fl oz). The point is this: skim milk has been pasteurized and homogenized, and it contains just about all the same junk as whole milk. Consuming skim milk is as harmful or worse to health as consuming any kind of dairy milk, except that you don't get as much saturated fat per cupful.

Harmful cholesterol

In March 2004 researchers in Brazil studied the effects of skim dairy milk consumption compared to soy milk consumption using a double-blind randomized crossover study. After 3 months each participant had spent 6 weeks on soy and six on skim in random order. When the double-blind codes were deciphered and analyzed it became clear that soy milk had won hands down.

When the subjects were drinking soy milk, their bad cholesterol went down and their good cholesterol went up (exactly the reverse of what happened when they were drinking dairy milk). The amount of rancid fat circulating in their blood stream (a further risk factor for heart disease) was also reduced by drinking soy milk.[65]

> **A glass of skim milk (non-fat dairy milk) has 6% *more* calories than an equal portion of regular soymilk**

The imperative here is to give up skim and low fat milk because they are worse for health compared to whole milk. They have higher amounts of non-digestible protein and lactose, and lower amounts of folic acid and vitamin B, a particularly harmful combination of factors.

According to Dr. William Grant, a Nasa Research Scientist, this combination promotes a build-up of homocysteine, a promoter of heart disease, stroke, and dementia. This view is reinforced by many studies, including a study published in the *Lancet Medical Journal* (January 2005) which says that a quarter of all heart attacks could be caused by high levels of homocysteine. This can explain why even some people who are apparently healthy, slim, and non-smoking, get heart attacks – they have high homocysteine levels.

The NDM Plan

The *NDM (Non-Dairy Milk) Plan* is based on consuming flax seeds or chia seeds combined with non-dairy milk. This provides a highly effective way to lose surplus body fat. The *NDM Plan* is based on three key points:

- It is filling and satisfying without being fattening.
- It is delicious and nutritious because of the flavour and nutrients in non-dairy milk combined with the super-healthy seeds.
- It compliments any dietary regime, which means that it can fit in with any life-style or weight-loss program you may be following.

Before looking at *The NDM Plan* in more detail the following is a brief comparison of dairy and non-dairy milk in terms of achieving optimum body weight.

Dairy Milk

- **Saturated fat.** Whole milk is high in saturated fat which gets stored as body fat.

- **Other dairy milk varieties.** Low-fat dairy milk is more fattening than whole milk, and non-fat (skim) milk may be less fattening than whole milk but is worse for your health. For a fuller explanation see the chapter *Dairy Milk and Related Products.*

- **Energy.** Dairy milk offers virtually no energy for the reasons given in the chapter *Dairy Milk Effect on Physical Fitness.* A lack of energy discourages physical activity which means you burn less calories and put on more weight. Also, a lack of energy usually makes you hungrier, leading to overeating.

- **Health.** Dairy milk promotes poor health in a variety of ways as explained in *Part One* of this book. This in turn affects the way that *all the food you eat* is metabolized. Food generally will be used less efficiently, making more of it end up as body fat. Poor health also makes a person lethargic, more inclined to over-eat, and less inclined to become fit and slim. Poor health can trap you into a vicious circle of weight-gain (or weight-loss combined with flabby muscles, poor complexion, and illness).

Non-dairy Milk

- **Saturated fat**. Non-dairy milk is mostly low in saturated fat which, in any event, does not get stored as body fat.

- **Other non-dairy milk varieties**. All varieties of non-dairy milk are low in calories compared to whole milk. But more importantly, a greater proportion of the calories in non-dairy milk end up being burnt as energy (or used as nutrition) instead of being stored as body fat. Here is a calorie comparison table:

Fig. 6
Calorie Comparison table

(All figures approximate)

8 Fluid ounces (1 cup or 272mL)	Calories	8 Fluid ounces (1 cup or 272mL)	Calories
3% whole, USA	150	Macadamia Milk	120
2% low-fat, USA	120	Millet Milk	63
1% low-fat, USA	100	Oat Milk	65
Skim, USA	80	Pea Milk	7
Whole milk, EU	145	Peanut Milk	95
Semi-skimmed, EU	105	Pecan Nut Milk	115
Skimmed, EU	77	Pine Nut Milk	105
Whole milk, EU	145	Pumpkin Seed Milk	90
Semi-skimmed, EU	105	Quinoa Milk	62
Almond Milk	96	Rice Milk	62
Brazil Nut Milk	109	Sesame Seed Milk	99
Cashew Nut Milk	92	Soybean Milk	29
Chestnut Milk	32	Spelt Milk	64
Coconut Milk	59	Sunflower Seed Milk	95
Hazelnut Milk	105	Tiger Nut Milk	44
Hemp Seed Milk	94	Walnut Milk	109

Note: The calorie content of non-dairy milks in the above table is a rough calculation, based on dividing the calories of the main ingredient by six to allow for 5 parts of water and 1 part of left over residue. The calorie content of any condiments or sweetening agent has not been taken into account.

- **Energy.** Non-dairy milk offers plenty of energy because a large part of the fat and carbohydrate content gets converted to energy rather than ending up as surplus body fat.

- **Health.** Non-dairy milk provides a wide variety of nutrients that promote good health, with little or none of the harmful pollutants, pesticides, dioxins, and other harmful factors found in dairy milk. The molecular structure of saturated fat in dairy milk is different to the molecular structure of saturated fat in non-dairy milk, as explained in the chapter *Non-Dairy Milk*. Consequently, the saturated fat in non-dairy milk gets converted into healthy *unsaturated* fat which the body can then use for essential nutritional purposes. This in turn affects the way that *all the food you eat* is metabolized. Food generally will be used more efficiently, making less of it end up as body fat. Good health also makes a person more energetic, less inclined to over-eat, and more inclined to become fit and slim. Good health puts you into a virtuous circle for attaining optimum body weight and a good figure, whether masculine or feminine.

The NDM Plan in five simple steps
(Suitable for women and men)

Step 1: Drink water. Half an hour before a meal drink a glass of purest drinking water to satisfy any feelings of thirst.

Step 2: Prepare NDM drink.

- Pulverize the seeds using a grain-mill or coffee-grinder. Make enough to last 3-7 days and always keep the pulverized seeds in an airtight bag or container in the refrigerator. Do not grind a large amount as the seeds deteriorate quickly once ground.

- Mix one heaped teaspoon of ground flax seeds or chia seeds into a cup of warm (not boiling hot) **non-dairy milk**. As an *occasional* alternative to the NDM drink, you can add the ground flax/chia seeds to a smoothie or a shake, or just about anything else you may be consuming.

Step 3: Consume before meal. Stir the pulverized seeds into the warm non-dairy milk and consume straight away, about half and hour before any main meal (do this *after* step 1, not before). You may repeat this before every main meal, but not more than three times a day so as not to overdo the amount of flax or chia seeds consumed. If you wish, you may add some flavouring to the drink such as coffee, carob powder, or whatever you like. The ground seeds combined with the liquid milk will swell inside your stomach, giving you a satisfying feeling of fullness. This in turn will help prevent over-eating, reduce your consumption of fattening foods, help you avoid unhealthy snacks, and provide good nutrition.

Step 4: Understand how it works. Realize that flax seeds and chia seeds undergo a dramatic swelling effect once ground and mixed with a fluid, increasing in volume by almost double into a gel-like substance that is digested slowly. This is exactly what you want as it is non-fattening, nutritious, and prevents the harmful ups and downs of blood-sugar levels.

Best of all, this is the easiest and most effective way of controlling your impulse to eat. The swelling of the pulverized seeds inside your stomach is *perfectly natural and safe* and will do nothing but good. Use the *NDM Plan* with any other dietary regime you may wish to follow as there will be no conflict.

Step 5: Eat nutritious food. The *NDM Plan* is intended to compliment, not replace, a healthy varied diet. The best way to lose surplus body fat is to eat a well-balanced and nutritious diet rather than fasting or eating insufficient food.

This means eating a mix of fruit, vegetables, salads, nuts, seeds, and pulses every day, and not less than five days a week. This offers a low Glycemic Index diet that is alkaline and perfectly compliments **The NDM Plan**. Generally you should try to eat as little cooked food as possible – the cooking process, particularly in the case of meat, creates mutagens. These are substances that make body cells mutate and develop into cancer.

Fresh food such as fruit, salads, nuts and seeds should form the bulk of your diet. This provides the body with enough fatty acids and carbohydrates for good health. If you make your body go without a steady flow of fatty acids and carbohydrates you will soon feel deprived, depressed and depleted (and no doubt depraved!). Your body is objecting strongly to being starved of essential nutrients, and you are telling your body there is a food shortage.

Any kind of restricted diet or fasting stimulates your body into saving fat and increasing cravings to eat. The body does this as a survival mechanism because it 'thinks' you face conditions of famine. The body saves fat as a way of storing emergency energy.

But if sufficient fat and carbohydrate is eaten regularly (in the form of a varied and nutritious diet) your body will not object to losing surplus body fat. On the contrary, if sufficient fatty acids and carbohydrates are consumed regularly, the body will find no need to conserve body fat.

You should make it a golden rule to eat a big mixed salad everyday. Include in the salad as much sprouted seeds as you can, such as alfafa, mung, raddish, adzuki, quinoa, millet, and others. Sprouted seeds are packed with all the nutrients you need for good health. By also adding a generous helping of a salad-dressing made with a good quality oil, you will always look forward to eating salad.

Regarding pulses, give favour to peas, lentils and chickpeas, and eat beans and grains sparingly. This does not mean beans and grains are 'bad', just that they should be eaten in moderation because they contain phytic acid which inhibits absorption of protein, minerals and trace elements. Also, beans and grains get poorly digested and consequently can cause a pot belly over time. Look at disadvantaged people in under-developed countries who *mainly* eat a diet based on grains or beans and you will notice they mostly have pot bellies (this, in spite of the amount of energy expended in daily life). If you must eat grains give preference to whole grain foods, and go for variety rather than always eating the same kind of grain.

By eating a nutritious varied diet that avoids dairy milk you will not go hungry, develop food cravings, or over-eat, and consequently you will not store surplus body fat. Over time, your body will lose its surplus body fat until you reach your optimum weight. Consuming the non-dairy milks given in this book are ideal as part of a nutritious varied diet because they are satisfying, filling, and full of vitamins, minerals, enzymes, healthy fatty-acids and non-fattening carbohydrates.

***

Flax and chia seeds are both delicious and nutritious, each in their own unique way. Once the seeds **are ground up**, mixed with a liquid and consumed, they swell up inside you and solidify, a little like gelatin. Don't let this put you off – if you wish to lose surplus body fat in a safe and effective manner these seeds are a godsend.

Flax and chia seeds are bursting with healthy nutrients and when combined with non-dairy milk as a drink, you get a big range of nutrients that virtually amounts to a 'meal' in itself. Here is some background information on both flax and chia seeds.

Flax Seeds

Flaxseed cultivation reaches back to the remotest periods of history. It has been found in all temperate and tropical regions for so many centuries that its geographical origin cannot be identified, for it readily escapes from cultivation and is found in a semi-wild condition in all the countries where it is grown.

The plant fibre of this wonderful product of nature has been found *woven into cloth* in ancient Egyptian tombs. The picture here shows the beautiful blue/white flowers that grow from flaxseeds.

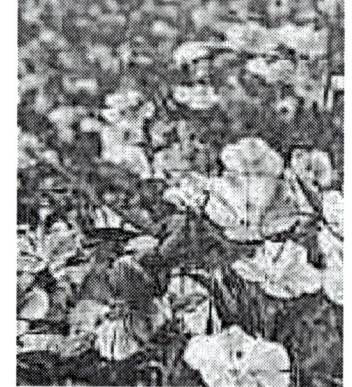

Flax seeds are by far the richest source of alpha-linolenic acid (ALA), the parent compound of the Omega-3 fatty acids. In comparison, fish contain only trace amounts of ALA. Omega-3 is an essential fatty acid because it cannot be synthesized by the body. Research indicates that ALA improves immunity, and may lower the risk of stroke and other cardiovascular diseases. Both the *Food and Agriculture Organization* and the *World Health Organization* recommend an increased daily intake of Omega-3 fatty acids, as most people tend to get too much Omega-6 in their diet but not enough Omega-3.

Flaxseeds are also rich in L-glutamic acid (an excellent nutrition for the brain, and used to treat mental deficiencies in adults) and Linoleic Acid, a valuable Omega-6 oil. About 90% of flaxseed oil is unsaturated, making it ideal for just about any dietary or weight-loss regime.

Lignans in flaxseeds are 200 to 800 times more concentrated than any other lignan source. Lignans (phytochemicals that protect against certain cancers) are shown to play an ever increasing role in numerous aspects of human health. Also, the soluble fibre in flaxseeds acts to clean out the digestive tract and protect the body against cancer.

Flaxseeds contain good amounts of calcium, magnesium, manganese, potassium, and phosphorus, thus providing a good mix of minerals for protecting bone density and healthy teeth.

Chia seeds

The chia plant is a summer annual that belonging to the mint family (Lamiaceae). It has been cultivated for centuries by the Aztecs of Mexico and the Indians of Southwest America: the tiny chia seeds formed part of their staple diet. In fact they were so highly prized that for a time they were used as currency.

Aztec warriors would eat chia during hunting trips, and the Indians of the Southwest USA would eat only chia seed mixed with water as they ran from the Colorado River to the Pacific Ocean to trade products. Chia was one of the main components of not only the Aztec diet, but also of another great Pre-Columbian civilization that developed in Mesoamerica, the Mayas.

The chia seed offers a natural source of Omega-3 fatty acids, antioxidants, dietary fibre, and a complete source of dietary protein, providing all the essential amino acids. Compared to other seeds and grains, the chia seed provides the highest source of protein, giving between 19 to 23 percent protein by weight. One of the unique qualities of the chia seed is its ability to absorb more than **nine times** its volume in water or other liquid. This ability can prolong hydration and retain electrolytes in body fluids, especially during exertion or exercise. Normal fluid retention ensures electrolyte dispersion across cell membranes, maintaining fluid balances, and aiding normal cellular function.

The gel-forming property of the chia seed tends to slow digestion and sustain balanced blood sugar levels, which can be helpful in preventing or controlling diabetes. (Even whole, water-soaked chia seeds can be easily digested and absorbed). **The NDM Plan** provides a rapid transport of chia nutrients to the tissues for use by the cells. Chia also facilitates the growth and regeneration of tissue during pregnancy and lactation, and aids the formation of muscles for athletes and bodybuilders. For the dieter, this means feeling full with no more peaks and valleys in blood sugar levels.

Using the **NDM Plan**, the chia or flax seeds will cause a slow release of carbohydrates and an equally slow converting of carbohydrates into glucose (blood sugar) for energy. The outer layer of chia seed is rich in mucilloid-soluble fibre. When chia or flax seeds are pulverized and mixed with fluid and digested, the gel that forms creates a physical barrier between the carbohydrates and the digestive enzymes that break them down. The carbohydrates are digested eventually, but at a slow and uniform rate. No insulin surge occurs to lower the blood sugar level after consumption.

Other benefits of chia seeds include:

- Promising signs from research that chia may prevent and/or overcome Type 2 (non-insulin dependent) diabetes.

- Chia seeds contain high levels of both Omega-3 and Omega-6 oils, both needed for good health.

- Chia seeds contain greater alpha-linolenic acid concentrations than any other seed or grain. This substance lowers the risk of heart disease, blurred vision and numbness among many other health benefits.

- Native people have used chia gel on wounds, for colds and sore throats, for upset stomachs, body odors, prostate problems, and even constipation.

- Chia seeds contain large amounts of B vitamins and calcium. By volume, one ounce of chia contains two percent B-2 (riboflavin), 13 percent niacin, and 29 percent thiamin, plus trace amounts of all B vitamins. Chia seeds have five times more calcium than dairy milk but without the fat and other harmful substances you get in dairy milk.

- Chia is an excellent source of fibre and contains strong antioxidants for good health. The most important antioxidants in chia are chlorogenic acid, caffeic acid and flavanol glycosides. Since oxidation is significantly delayed, chia shows a great potential within the food industry as an additive for the prevention of food deterioration.

***

Dairy Milk and Related Products

In giving consideration to dairy milk, it is valid to ask whether all dairy products are harmful to health. Clearly, different dairy products will have different proportions of nutrients, casein, lactose, etc. Therefore, the harmful effects of dairy products will vary from product to product.

Some dairy products, such as plain live yogurt, whey, kefir, cultured curds, and some kinds of cheese are relatively low in acidity and less harmful to human health than the milk they were derived from. This is so because the lactose sugar is partly neutralized by the bacteria and enzymes. Also, some kinds of non-processed cheese have smaller amounts of harmful casein than others. These products can have a place in the diets of some people provided they are consumed in moderation.

When it comes to the staple dairy products such as milk, butter, cream, and most types of cheese, they all produce undesirable acidic effects in the stomach, in varying degrees, and they all contain some degree of harmful compounds derived from dairy milk, e.g. antibiotics, pesticides, toxins, hormones, PCB's, and so on.

Let's remember that the more acidic a food is, the worse it is for health. This is so without exception. Acidity in food causes the body to age and deteriorate, and is at the root of just about all ill-health.

Some may argue that butter, cream, cheese, ice-cream, and yogurt have a place in the human diet if consumed in moderation. This argument has some merit because some products are less acidic, others have virtually no lactose (less lactose intolerance), and they are generally consumed less (in volume and frequency). But consider this:

Each bite of hard cheese has TEN TIMES whatever was in that sip of milk because it takes ten pounds of milk to make one pound of cheese. The same goes for ice cream (12 times!). The same goes for butter (21 times!). All the pollution, harmful chemicals, hormones, etc. in dairy milk get highly concentrated in other milk-based products, and although not consumed in the same volume they are nevertheless very unhealthy.

Are other kinds of animal milk as bad as dairy milk?

The short answer is ***yes, but not quite as bad*** because they contain no IGF-1 (the harmful bovine growth hormone). Goat's milk and other types of animal milk are not good for human consumption because they are not designed for the human species. Goat's milk is unhealthy because it has about 10% more lactic acid (and hence 10% more galactose) compared to dairy milk. Also, several studies show that goat's milk is more difficult to digest than dairy milk. Since goat's milk is similar to dairy milk nutritionally (but more expensive) it is difficult to understand why anybody would buy it.

Casein is another factor (see chapter **Dairy Milk Effect on Health**). Casein is mucus-causing and acid-causing, and is the main component of protein in dairy milk. Casein is truly bad news – it coats the organs and respiratory system causing congestion and chronic illness. But casein is not limited to cow's milk – it's also found in other animal milks in *higher amounts*! Compared to *human* milk, cow's milk contains 7 times as much casein, sheep milk 12 times, horse milk 3 times and goat's milk 8 times as much.[151] For this reason alone, all types of animal milk should be avoided.

In the first year of life, a new-born human will thrive on human milk, but would die if only fed dairy milk. Equally, a baby calf will thrive on dairy milk, but would die if only fed human milk. This was aptly illustrated when, in May 2005, some tiger cubs were fed *human* milk because the mother of the cubs would not feed them. In spite of intensive efforts that involved giving the cubs plenty of human milk plus nutritional supplements, the cubs died because their livers could not accept human milk.[102]

All kinds of animal milks are bad for humans

Quite simply, all kinds of animal milk are bad for human adults, including human milk! Offer a cow or bull some dairy milk to drink and it will be rejected. Similar tests with other animals give the same results. Some domesticated cats will drink dairy milk because they have been conditioned to do so or because they are too hungry to desist. Wild cats will not.

On the whole, adult animals of any species will not drink milk (unless starving), whether it be from their own species or another species. Why is this so? Because the nutritional content of milk is only suitable for the baby of the species. It is known that if a baby orphan elephant is given cow's milk it will die in a matter of days. If an adult human is fed *human* milk (and nothing else), he/she would die more quickly than being given water only. Note for example that human milk is super-rich in galactose (even more than dairy milk) – this is perfectly healthy (and essential) for a human baby, but for a human adult galactose in this concentration is toxic. Human adults are the only creatures on earth known to regularly drink animal milk.

A detailed analysis of the merits and de-merits of the various kinds of dairy products is beyond the scope of this book. Suffice to say that dairy milk (among dairy products) is by far the worst culprit in terms of human health.

Are all kinds of dairy milk harmful to human health?

To do this question justice, an important distinction should be made between the three main kinds of dairy milk. See Fig. 7.

Fig. 7
Main Kinds of dairy milk

- **Raw unpasteurized organic:** Difficult to find as sales of unpasteurized milk are outlawed in many places. Such milk would have to be obtained from cows fed on non-polluted, organic pastures. Both the cows and the milk would have to be thoroughly tested for disease and contamination, making the milk less viable and more expensive on a commercial level.
- **Pasteurized organic:** Pasteurized milk from cows fed on non-polluted, organic pastures and organic grains. Antibiotics not given as a matter of course (only if ill). No hormones given.
- **Pasteurized non-organic:** Regular pasteurized milk from cows fed on commercial feed and mass produced with antibiotics and other chemicals for maximum milk production.

Unpasteurized milk

There is a world of difference between *raw unpasteurized organic milk* and regular commercial *pasteurized milk*. The latter is at best junk food, devoid of any redeeming features. Whereas unpasteurized milk obtained from un-stressed, *disease-free* cows (fed on good quality, unpolluted pastures) can be a source of nutrition for some people if consumed in moderation.

Clearly, unpasteurized dairy milk is better than pasteurized because the pasteurization process has a dramatic effect on the digestibility and nutritional content of milk. As we have seen, pasteurization involves boiling the milk several times to very high temperatures. Then when the milk is consumed it no longer contains enzymes to aid protein digestion, or beneficial bacteria that stop the milk from putrefying inside the human gut.

But the choice of *raw unpasteurized milk* is somewhat hypothetical because the selling (or even giving away) of unpasteurized milk is outlawed in most countries. In any event, because of stringent hygiene requirements (to make sure unpasteurized milk is free from disease) it would be uneconomical to produce on a commercial scale.

In the book "*The Untold Story of Milk*" the author Ron Schmidt makes a strong case for raw milk. He counters the argument that pasteurization is necessary because raw milk has harmful pathogens by saying that harmful pathogens only arise from the poor way cows are fed and milked. Here is an extract from the book *The Untold Story Of Milk* (newtrendspublishing.com):

"Domesticated animals were first used for milk 8,000 to 10,000 years ago, as a genetic change affecting mostly people in Europe, the Middle East, and parts of Africa enabled them to digest milk as adults. Milk from domesticated animals then began to become important as a human food. With domesticationt, fewer wild animals were available; as groups of

people roamed less, they hunted less, eating more grains and vegetables. In some cultures, milk replaced animal bones as the chief source of calcium and some other minerals. In indigenous cultures milk was often used as cultured or clabbered milk. This is similar to homemade raw yogurt, and it is partially predigested — much of the lactose (milk sugar) has been broken down by bacterial action. When drinking fresh milk [pasteurized or raw], this process must be accomplished over a period of several hours in the stomach; yogurt or clabbered milk is much more easily digested. Adaptations in evolution are always the effects of particular causes. Humans developing the ability to digest milk into adulthood possessed a survival advantage; such change is the basis of evolution. Human beings evolved the ability to easily digest raw milk because raw milk from healthy, grass-fed animals gave them an adaptive advantage; it made them stronger and more able to reproduce."

Clearly, in past centuries when dairy milk was consumed raw, from cows that grazed unpolluted pastures, it fulfilled a sought after role in human nutrition (particularly if you face a daily risk of starvation). But today's pasteurized milk is a different product that does not contribute towards human nutrition, and worse still, is actually harmful to our health.

Does that mean it's good to consume *raw* dairy milk? The answer is a firm NO because of the mucus forming properties of dairy milk, the saturated fat, the effects of lactose intolerance and milk allergy. Note that **all kinds of milk** (whether raw or pasteurized) increase the risk of osteoporosis. However, as mentioned, provided the raw milk has come from disease-free contented cows, fed on green unpolluted pastures, and provided it is consumed in moderation, having been carefully tested for harmful pathogens, such milk may occasionally be a source of nutrition for some people (if you can get it).

Organic milk

What about *pasteurized organic milk*? This is a big and growing industry in the developed world, and is part of a world-wide trend to 'buy organic' in the belief that it is somehow better for your health.

Is *pasteurized organic milk* less harmful than non-organic pasteurized milk? The answer is *yes,* but only just. Some studies are showing that organic milk is higher in vitamin E, antioxidants, and Omega-3 fatty acids (the saying 'you are what you eat' applies to cows as much as to humans).

The killer blow for organic milk

Food regulations require that organic milk be produced without the addition of hormones, herbicides, pesticides, and antibiotics. In the USA organic milk must additionally be certified free of rBGH. This powerful drug was discussed in the chapter *Dairy Milk effect on Health.* It is well known that rBGH increases the amount of IGF-1 in pasteurized milk. But what is not generally realized is that all cows (whether or not organic) produce IGF-1 in their milk in abundance.

IGF-1 is a growth hormone and a main component of mother's milk in any mammalian species. The purpose of IGF-1 is to help the baby grow as quickly as possible. Hence, organic dairy milk is loaded with IGF-1, even though it may contain less IGF-1 than milk containing rBGH.

This means organic dairy milk in any country of the world contains bovine IGF-1, and when consumed by humans it plays havoc with the body, promoting many kinds of illness including cancer (for more information on IGF-1 see the chapter *Dairy Milk effect on Health).*

IGF-1 leads to insulin resistance, diabetes, fluid retention, carpal tunnel syndrome, gynecomastia (enlarged breasts), lowered output of the body's own growth hormone, abnormal bone growth in the wrists, hands and feet, and tumor growth.[66]

Additionally, organic dairy milk contains traces of herbicides and pesticides as these cannot be completely eradicated from pastures, even though such chemicals may not be used on the pastures used by *organic* cows.

It should also be realized that although antibiotics are not given to organic cows as a matter of course, *they are given* whenever needed through illness, which can be quite often.

Furthermore, does 'organic' mean the milk comes from smaller farms where cows are led to pasture on a daily basis? Or does it only mean the cows are fed organic food that is pesticide-free? The controversy over these questions is raging within the dairy industry (and within many countries), and no doubt the controversy will continue.

What does all this mean? It means that organic pasteurized milk is going to be lower in (but not bereft of) some hormones, antibiotics, herbicides, pesticides, and other drugs. And it means that organic milk does not necessarily come from cows free of stress.

In reality here is little difference between organic and non-organic dairy milk. Both provide harmful IGF-1, get poorly digested, are mucus forming, produce lactose intolerance, have little nutritional benefit (because of poor absorption), promote osteoporosis and obesity, and do not provide good energy. Additionally, organic milk is highly acidic as it contains just as much indigestible protein as non-organic milk – this high acidity prevents valuable nutrients in the diet from being assimilated and used by the body.

Specialty milks

There is a growing trend to produce 'specialty milks' that address niche markets and specific groups of people. I have even seen 'GM Free' milk advertised on the basis that such milk comes from cows not given genetically modified feed. Quite apart from the politics and arguments about the environment, GM Free milk is just as unhealthy as regular milk.

Specialty dairy milks are typically packaged differently and may be fortified with nutrients. For example, in several countries 'Omega-3 enhanced milk' was launched in 2005 so as to appeal to mothers with young children concerned about getting enough Omega-3 oil in the diet. In fact, the amount of omega-3 contained in such milks is very small, and to some extent, the very high temperatures of the pasteurization process serve to oxidize and hydrogenate any oils contained in the milk, making them less than healthy.

Omega-3 dairy milk is created by adding fish oil to cow feed, and some dieticians and scientists are questioning the wisdom of feeding fish to cows, who are by nature herbivorous (echoes of mad cow disease come to mind!). For this reason omega-3 milk will not appeal to vegetarians, vegans, and other groups of people.

To get round the objection of feeding fish to cows, some dairy producers are instead feeding flax seeds to cows. Flax seeds are rich in omega-3 oil, but here we hit another snag: flax seeds contain no DHA, an essential fatty acid required for brain and nerve development. Hence, in this scenario the whole raison-detre for offering omega-3 milk is nullified.

Note that omega-3 *with* DHA is readily obtained from many varieties of fish, algae and sea foods. Omega-3 *without* DHA is easily obtained from a variety of nuts, seeds, and plant oils (walnut, canola, olive, wheat germ, flax, soy, hemp and others). Less than a teaspoon of olive oil or fish oil provides more omega-3 than a pint of omega-3 dairy milk.

The trend to disguise dairy milk as flavoured, sugared, and even carbonated drinks is destined to grow as large soft drink and confectionary companies form alliances with dairy milk producers. Companies such as Coca-Cola, Mars, Pepsi, Quaker, and Bravo are all involved with dairy milk products. According to Bravo chief executive Roy G. Warren, the flavored-milk industry has grown from about $750 million in 1995 to $2 billion in 2004. Bravo had $3.3 million in revenue in 2004, with 2005 sales expected to be at least $13 million.

On 30 July 2005 the Washington Post reported that 'the newcomers in the [supermarket] dairy aisle include Cookies & Cream, Milky Way, 3 Musketeer, Bubble Blast, Starburst, Orange Sparkle and MooBerry – and Nesquik is selling "milkshakes" in vanilla, caramel and other flavours.'

The tragedy here is that children are being seduced into consuming dairy milk products at a vulnerable time in their lives when dairy milk does the most harm.

Another new trend is the so called 'medicinal' or 'therapeutic' milks that are being used as a way of selling more milk. For example New Zealand scientists have developed 'anti-thrush milk' by injecting chemicals into cows to make them produce anti-bodies in their milk that fight thrush. Neil Brown of *Dairy Farmers of New Zealand* said: *'If we add value to the milk and make it even healthier and let people benefit from it, it's got to be good and if it puts money in farmers pockets it's better still.'* Source: OneNews, 12 June 2005.

This is a travesty because so called medicinal milks impose the consumption of medication on people that may not need it, and the long-term effects of consuming unnecessary medication may be harmful in unforeseen ways. Worse still is the likelihood that this will encourage an even greater consumption of dairy milk with all the associated ill-health this causes (a feint whiff of irony?).

A picture of seduction

- When you enter a supermarket you enter a carefully choreographed world where *every last detail* is planned to entice shoppers to spend money. As you approach the refrigerated section that contains dairy milk you see a big selection of dairy milk cartons, all professionally packaged and arranged for maximum appeal. The long rows of colourful milk cartons project an air of fresh coolness and reassurance which plays on the unconscious mind.

- As you gaze for a few moments at the rows of milk cartons carefully displayed to attract maximum custom, you occasionally see people taking a milk carton from the good-looking display. The people buying milk are a mix of nice ordinary people: a family, a housewife, a vicar, a teenager, and a business man. You think: *Can so many people not know the truth about milk?* You look closely at a few cartons and you see a cornucopia of health-promoting messages: *lactose free, low fat, natural, organic, healthy, fruit flavoured, good for bones, etc.*

- You unconsciously make an association between these health-promoting messages, the cool enticing display of milk cartons, and the people buying milk (*'they cannot all be wrong about milk'*). Deep down in your mind you think to yourself: *If dairy milk were truly bad for health the supermarket wouldn't be allowed to sell it! Anyhow, I use so little it won't make any difference.'* This picture of seduction is reinforced by television, magazine, bill-board and other advertising seen in recent days promoting dairy milk. You buy the milk.

Different versions of this *picture of seduction* are played out daily, millions of times all over the world. Many people have vaguely heard that milk may be fattening or that it causes lactose intolerance, but it does not stop them being seduced into buying yet more milk. The message to take on board is simple: don't be seduced! If you have dairy milk delivered to your house, just cancel it – don't get beaten by inertia.

If at present you cannot make non-dairy milk at home, you may simply buy non-dairy milk instead of dairy milk. Supermarkets and health food stores are increasingly selling a wide variety of non-dairy milks such as rice milk, soy milk, tiger nut milk, oat milk and almond milk.

The point to remember is that however the milk may be packaged, carbonated, or disguised with flavouring, it does not change the basic nature of dairy milk: **all kinds of pasteurized dairy milk** promote poor health and illness by virtue of containing acidic protein, harmful hormones, mucus forming casein, and many other unhealthy substances as mentioned throughout Part One of this book. And never forget that dairy milk in all its forms promotes osteoporosis, prostate cancer, and other serious diseases.

Non-dairy milks offer a simple and healthy alternative, making it easy to avoid dairy milk altogether. The imperative here is to avoid the trap of being seduced into consuming a 'better' kind of dairy milk. ***All kinds*** of dairy milk are bad for health.

Dairy Milk Effect on Physical Fitness

Is dairy milk bad for physical fitness?

Dairy milk is bad for physical fitness because it causes poor health generally. When you are overweight, not well, feeling lethargic, or coughing and wheezing from mucosal congestion (or just feeling under par) there is much less motivation to be physically active.

More specifically, dairy milk has a direct impact on physical fitness in four ways:

1. It reduces the body's energy.
2. It prevents efficient breathing.
3. It weakens bones.
4. It makes exercise harmful to health.

How does dairy milk reduce the body's energy?

Energy (i.e. calories) can be derived from fat, protein, and sugar, and dairy milk has all three ingredients. However, dairy milk is an extremely poor source of energy for humans, for the following reasons:

Fat. Dairy milk provides saturated fat (unless low fat milk is used) which the body can break down into energy should it need to. However, as we know to our cost, the fat from dairy milk usually gets stored as surplus body fat, causing obesity, clogged arteries, and many other health problems. A glass of whole milk contains about 160 calories. A glass of skim milk, having much of the fat removed, has about 90 calories. So you can see that about half the calorie content of dairy milk is contained in the fat. As fat gets stored rather than burnt, it has little effect on energy requirements for everyday activities. That is why athletes avoid fatty foods when they want lots of energy for a forthcoming event.

Protein. The body is able to break protein down into energy as a last resort, when little carbohydrate or fat is available in the human body. The body does this by stripping protein from your organs and other body parts (it cannot directly convert the protein from food into energy). So for all practical purposes, the protein content of dairy milk cannot be regarded as a source of energy.

Sugar:

- **Lactose intolerance.** Dairy milk contains sugar (i.e. carbohydrate) in the form of lactose. This lactose is broken down by the digestive system and turned into blood sugar. The blood sugar (i.e. glucose) is then taken by the blood stream to the cells in your body where it is burnt to produce energy. Unfortunately, as already mentioned, many people are lactose intolerant. Furthermore, large amounts of dairy milk would have to be consumed to get enough energy from lactose for everyday activities.

- **Poor oxygenation.** The human body gets its energy from body cells that burn oxygen. When you move your hand you are making the cells in your hand muscles burn oxygen. When body cells do not get enough oxygen you will feel tired and lacking in energy. Dairy milk interferes with the efficient oxygenation of body cells. It does this by coating the digestive organs of the body with unwelcome casein mucus (including the kidneys). As a result, the kidneys do a poor job in keeping the red blood cells well oxygenated. This in turn makes it more difficult for red blood cells to carry oxygen to all the cells in your body. As a result, the cells in your muscles do not get enough oxygen to produce the energy that you need for daily life. The end result is lethargy, insufficient energy, and poor health.

- **Associated health problems.** Lactose from dairy milk is not a good source of energy for human beings because of all the other health problems associated with dairy milk. Energy for daily activities, sport, and exercise, is best obtained form low-glycaemic carbohydrate foods such as fresh fruit, nuts, seeds and vegetables. Dairy milk does have a low-glycaemic rating, but this does not mean it is healthy to consume, it simply means that the lactose in the milk gets absorbed slowly by the body. All the home-made milks described in this book have a low-glycaemic rating as they are based on nuts, seeds, plants and pulses, and are therefore excellent sources of energy without the associated health problems that you get with dairy milk.

As dairy milk gives a feeling of fullness when consumed it reduces the desire to consume energy-producing foods such as fruit, vegetables, nuts, seeds and pulses, and whole grain foods. Because of this and the fact that dairy milk does not provide muscle energy, you are made to feel less energetic as a result of consuming dairy milk.

How does dairy milk prevent efficient breathing?

As mentioned in the chapter **Dairy Milk Effect on Health** the casein in milk causes a thick dense mucus that clogs and irritates the body's entire respiratory system. Dairy milk is unique in being able to cause significant and chronic mucosal congestion in humans.

This in turn makes you more vulnerable to many illnesses associated with the airways such as bronchitis, chest infections, coughs, colds, aggravated asthma, and so on.

To become physically fit you have to be physically active either in your daily activities or as part of an exercise program. But you cannot do this effectively if your breathing is impaired. Dairy milk consumers become breathless or wheezy more quickly than people who avoid dairy milk. The point here is that to become physically fit you have to do regular exercise that is sufficient to make you breathe more quickly. If you cannot do this comfortably, you will be held back from becoming physically fit.

To test yourself try running for a short period of time, or take the stairs instead of the elevator. People who are physically fit can breathe easily even when breathless from physical exertion.

How does dairy milk weaken bones?

This question is fully answered in the chapter *Dairy Milk Effect on Osteoporosis*. Here is a brief summary to this question:

Dairy milk is high in calcium and indigestible protein. For these reasons, dairy milk more than any other food causes a harmful *calcium yo-yo effect*. The yo-yo effect refers to calcium that goes in and out of the bones causing erosion of bone-making cells. As bone cells are eroded their numbers dwindle. When this happens your bones become weaker because bone-making cells can no longer make enough new bone to keep up with the rate of decomposition of old bone. Gradually, this causes bones to become more porous and susceptible to fracture.

To develop and maintain good physical fitness you need healthy muscles and bones. If your muscles/bones are weak you will be much less inclined to be physically active, making you less physically fit. By consuming dairy milk your bones may have higher bone mineral density in the short-term, but this increases the risk of weaker bones in the long-term, making you less physically fit. Having high bone mineral density *does not* make you fitter or healthier than having normal bone mineral density. Dairy milk consumers with high bone mineral density may be as strong as or stronger than non-dairy consumers with lower bone mineral density, but they will be at higher risk of getting osteoporosis later on in life.

How does dairy milk make exercise harmful to health?

When you exercise it triggers a series of events that become more pronounced the more exercise you do:

Exercise causes microfractures in the bones. This in turn stimulates the manufacture of new bone to fill up the microfractures. And this in turn triggers hormones that extract more calcium from the diet than usual (normally only about a third of calcium is extracted, the other two thirds do not get absorbed into the blood). The body tries to squeeze more calcium from the diet because it is needed for making the new bone material to fill the microfractures.

In a healthy, varied diet that avoids dairy products, getting this extra calcium is no problem. There is plenty of calcium in fruit, vegetables, salads, nuts, seeds, and pulses, and the body will take exactly as much as it needs and no more. But when a physically active person consumes dairy milk, the hormones released by exercise act to flood the bloodstream with too much calcium. This in turn exacerbates the harmful calcium yo-yo effect (see appendix four). The net result is that the consumption of dairy milk has made exercise cause the bones to age more than otherwise.

Why is too much exercise harmful?

Note: At the end of this chapter *The Low G.I. Workout*[tm] plan summarizes the best way to exercise.

There is increasing evidence that too much exercise can be bad for bones (and bad for health) for two reasons:

1. Over-exercising creates free-radicals

According to Dr. Peter Axt (Fulda University) and Dr Michaela Axt-Gadermann (a medical doctor), both from Germany, the one key difference between the 'lazy' and those who exercise was that the more active body produces more *free radicals* - unstable oxygen molecules that are believed to speed the ageing process. Dr Michaela Axt-Gadermann said *'Laziness* [in the sense of avoiding too much exercise] *is important for a healthy immune system because special immune-cells are stronger in times of relaxation than stress. During relaxation or 'down time', your metabolism is less active, which means the body produces fewer free radicals. If you do a lot of sport or are permanently stressed, then your body will produce more free radicals and that is one reason why your life could be shortened.*[117]

2. Over-exercising increases risk of osteoporosis

Doing less exercise does not increase the risk of osteoporosis because osteoporosis is caused by a *lack* of bone-making cells. *Bone-loss with age cannot be explained by declining physical activity levels.*[118]

If osteoporosis was about a lack of exercise all healthy, but physically inactive, people would have osteoporosis, which is not the case. A lack of exercise does indeed make bones lose calcium **but not osteoblasts** (bone-making cells). Of course, extreme starvation, complete inactivity, and no sunlight/vitamin D can result in a loss of bone-making cells, but just about any kind of activity carried out to extreme can be harmful.

Exercise stops bones from losing calcium and increases their capacity to absorb more calcium. This in turn makes bones stronger, but not necessarily healthier. To be clear, weight-bearing exercise makes bones stronger by maintaining calcium – if bones do not get exercised (as for example in space) they rapidly lose calcium.

If we are normally active (i.e. if we do not over-exercise) our bones will be healthy. This means the bones will be sufficiently strong for normal everyday living, and will be long-lasting without any risk of osteoporosis.

If we are over-active (i.e. if we over-exercise) our bones will be dense but unhealthy. This means the bones will be unnecessarily dense for normal everyday living, and be at greater risk of osteoporosis (at a future date) from erosion of bone-making cells.

Once you are grown up, a lack of exercise does not accelerate the erosion of bone-making cells because less calcium is processed by the bones – this in turn reduces the risk of osteoporosis. If one lacks exercise, one can easily increase bone mineral density by doing more exercise.

Over-exercise accelerates the erosion of bone-making cells and therefore increases the risk of osteoporosis. Once your bone-making cells are depleted you get osteoporosis, you lose bone mineral density, and the condition is irreversible. (For more information on osteoporosis see the chapter *Dairy Milk Effect on Osteoporosis)*.

Any degree of exercise causes microfractures in the bone which stimulate osteoblasts to increase their bone-making activity. This in turn increases the death-rate of osteoblasts and the risk of osteoporosis. [119] Good physical fitness is therefore best achieved by finding a balance between under and over-activity. Too little activity results in calcium loss, muscle atrophy, and other health-related problems, but it does not increase the risk of osteoporosis. Too much activity results in (i) calcium gain, (ii) muscle and bone density gain, (iii) health related problems associated with over-aging of the body generally, and (iv) increased risk of osteoporosis in particular.

Over-exercising makes bones stronger in the short term, but *permanently* weaker in the long-term.[120] This is why professional athletes are more prone to osteoporosis in old age. What happens is that the more you exercise, the more microfractures you create in the bones. These microfractures cause damage to bone cells, forcing osteoblasts to go into action to fill the microfractures with new bone material. This in turn erodes osteoblasts, thus aging the bones more quickly.

So when you see 'super-fit' professional sports people with strong bodies and bulging muscles you are looking at bodies that are beyond their age – these are people who are at *greater* risk of getting osteoporosis.

Postmenopausal women are often advised to embark on strenuous exercise programs and take calcium supplements as a way of keeping osteoporosis at bay. Such advice is not only incorrect, strenuous exercise and calcium supplements actually hasten the onset of osteoporosis! [121]

How does dairy milk affect physical activity?

As stated, physical activity creates microfractures in the bone. This in turn stimulates hormones to make the bones absorb more calcium (because it is needed for repairing the microfractures). As part of this process, the hormones make the bloodstream absorb as much calcium as possible from the diet, and this calcium is then sent into the bones.

If you are consuming a healthy and varied diet of fruit, vegetables, salads, nuts, seeds, and pulses, the body will get exactly the right amount of calcium, whatever the exercise. But if you consume dairy milk, the hormones produced as a result of exercise will force the bloodstream to absorb more calcium from the milk than otherwise.

This in turn will result in too much calcium going into the bloodstream, accelerating the harmful calcium yo-yo effect (see appendix four). This is why athletes and people who are over- training or doing vigorous exercise must be extra careful to avoid dairy milk at this time.

In fact, anybody who is doing intense physical training or involved in any kind of rigorous physical activity should avoid dairy milk, high calcium foods, calcium and vitamin D supplements. This is essential to prevent any unnecessary processing of calcium and erosion of osteoblasts. The imperative here is to **not** absorb any more calcium than is needed to maintain adequate bone density for normal day-to-day activities. This is easily achieved by avoiding dairy milk, consuming little or no dairy products, and eating a healthy varied diet.

Female athletes have an additional reason for avoiding dairy milk: estrogen levels are decreased in women because intense physical exercise makes the body produce less estrogen. The same applies to men, but to a smaller degree. So over-exercise has two effects on the body which act together to increase the risk of osteoporosis by increasing the harmful calcium yo-yo effect:: (i) It increases microfractures and hence the level of calcium processed into bones, and (ii) It reduces estrogen and hence the calcium yo-yo effect is accentuated, as explained in appendix three.

The consumption of dairy milk in the life of an over-exerciser acts to feed calcium to the harmful calcium yo-yo effect, like adding petrol to a fire.

If a woman stops having a monthly period (because of over-exercise or the menopause) it means estrogen levels are depleted. At this time the calcium yo-yo effect will be more pronounced and it is therefore particularly important to avoid dairy milk.

How much exercise is best for avoiding osteoporosis?

It is often said that *exercise is very important for slowing the progression of osteoporosis*. Others go even further and say that *mild exercise does not protect bones, and that moderate exercise reduces the risk for osteoporosis*. Both these statements are incorrect.

Exercise does not prevent osteoporosis, it makes osteoporosis more likely for the reasons explained above. However, *moderate exercise* is essential for good health for the reasons that follow.

We define *moderate exercise* as being exercise that is not too little to cause muscle atrophy, and not too much to cause osteoporosis. We are talking about a sensible middle-ground that is enough to keep the body fit enough for normal day-to-day activities. Fitness experts typically describe moderate exercise as *'physical activity that is taken for at least three days a week and for at least 90 minutes a week.'* Clearly, a degree of common sense is required here, as the amount and type of exercise you do will depend on many factors (the kind of work you do, your lifestyle, your sporting interests, etc). The point to always remember is that any exercise (however little) makes bone cells age, and life-style osteoporosis is *entirely* caused by the aging of bone cells – nothing else.

Moderate exercise is essential for good health and here are just some of the reasons:

- It prevents muscles and other parts of the body from atrophying. The saying '**use it or lose it**' is apt.

- It reduces the risk and incidence of many diseases (but not osteoporosis).

- It increases the body's immunity and ability to fight off disease.

- It makes you feel better physically and mentally by oxygenating the body and improving self-esteem.

- It makes the body more supple, more attractive to look at, and more healthy generally.

- It is good for mental agility by increasing the amount of oxygen supplied to the brain. Exercise may also slow down the loss of dopamine in the brain (a neurotransmitter that helps to prevent the shaking and stiffness that can come with old age).

- It increases muscle strength, balance and coordination. With greater muscle strength, one can often avoid falls and situations that cause fractures.

- It helps to prevent obesity, not because you burn calories during exercise, but because surplus body fat in converted to muscle. As a result, you look and feel slimmer, but more importantly, your muscles are able to store more energy. By storing more energy, you become more active generally, and hence burn more calories generally.

What kind of exercise is best?

We have established that any kind of physical activity makes the bone matrix *age more quickly* by eroding osteoblasts. But then, just being alive makes the body age. The purpose of exercise is to keep the body fit enough for normal everyday living – no more, no less. This is the best way to fight osteoporosis and keep the body healthy into old age. It's about moderation in all things – in what we eat, how we live, and how we exercise.

When it comes to the bones, traditional advice says that *'exercise plays an important role in the retention of bone density in the aging person.'* Clearly, you need to exercise all parts of the body so as to maintain sufficient bone density for everyday living. Increasing bone density too much is anti-productive as it erodes osteoblasts, bringing forward the day you get osteoporosis.

Some health professionals advise that you should do below-waist exercise so as to keep the hip and thigh bones strong. In this way you build a bigger 'calcium store' for servicing the whole body. While it is true that the hip and thigh bones serve as a kind of calcium warehouse, it is not correct to say that below-waist high impact exercise is specifically beneficial for bones. This is so because any kind of exercise is bad for bones unless it is moderate, i.e. enough to keep the body fit enough for everyday living, but no more than this.

Hence, traditional advice to do high impact exercise (e.g. strenuous running, prolonged stepping aerobics, intense activity sports) for the sake of your bones is ***incorrect***. It is based on two misunderstandings:

1. It is known that calcium cannot be assimilated properly into bones without the body being physically active, **but it does not follow** that greater calcium assimilation keeps osteoporosis at bay. On the contrary, every time calcium is assimilated, it erodes osteoblasts and brings nearer the day you may get osteoporosis.

2. Research shows that high impact exercise increases BMD (bone mineral density) more than low impact exercise:

We examined data from over 5,000 EPIC participants aged 45-74 who had attended for a second health check. We found that reported time spent on high impact physical activity was strongly and positively associated with higher ultrasound levels [higher BMD]. *Our results suggest that participation in high impact activities may help preserve bone density and reduce the risk of fracture for people in mid-life. However, this would not be appropriate for older people, who have thinner bones, as these activities could increase the likelihood of falls and fractures.* Source: British Medical Journal, January 2001, 322(7279): 140-146.

This kind of research aptly illustrates the misunderstanding: high impact exercise increases BMD **but it does not follow** that a higher BMD combats osteoporosis. On the contrary, the higher BMD caused by high impact exercise has eroded more osteoblasts than necessary and hastened the onset of osteoporosis.

Weight bearing, below-waist exercises, **done in moderation**, are worthy and beneficial for general good health and for keeping the bones sufficiently strong for everyday activities. Over-doing these kinds of exercises will indeed increase bone density but at a terrible price: erosion of osteoblasts and, in the long run, permanently weaker bones.

> **Before starting a program of exercises you are not used to, consult a physician. Any exercise program should start slowly and build up gradually. Women who already have osteoporosis of the spine should be careful about exercise that jolts or puts weight on the back, as it could cause a fracture. All exercise should be moderate.**
> **Over-exercising or exercise addiction is harmful and as serious as any other compulsive form of behavior.**

Exercise should be regular, life-long, and always done in moderation. Both children and adults should lead active lives from as young an age as possible. Intense high impact exercise is okay in short bursts or once in a while but **not as a regular routine** because it ages the bones.

All kinds of exercise are beneficial providing it is not a sustained intense exercise repeated for long periods of time. For example, for some people playing an *occasional* game of football or squash can be good for health. There is a world of difference between playing tennis, say, two or three times a month (okay for bones), and training/playing vigorous tennis several hours daily for six days a week (bad for bones).

Children of all ages should be inspired and encouraged to do sport by using the principles of the ***Low G.I. Workout*** rather than using peer pressure, bullying and coercion (often the case in school curriculums). There is no sport that cannot be adapted to the principles of the ***Low G.I. workout***.

Professional athletes and sportspeople are at greater risk of osteoporosis than the population at large because their reservoir of bone-making cells will be depleted. For these people, it is critical to avoid dairy milk, calcium and vitamin D supplements, and to not train more than absolutely necessary.

No part of the body should be neglected when it comes to doing exercise. But generally it should be gentle to moderate – not enough to make you exhausted or make the body ache, but enough to work up a sweat and make you a little breathless. This provides important cardio-vascular exercise, and body sweating releases toxins through the skin that would otherwise stay inside you. The key is to lead a physically active life generally.

Sweating through exercise helps keep bones healthy because you *lose* excess calcium in sweat. This in turn reduces the harmful calcium yo-yo effect that weakens bones (appendix four). This is proven by the fact that osteoporosis is worse in cold climate countries.

'This calls attention to another component of milk: calcium. Sweat glands are an important calcium excretor. In cold climates the amount of calcium excreted by sweating is small, in the tropics it can be several times the quantity excreted by the kidneys.' [145]

This raises an interesting question. On the one hand we are saying that vigorous high-impact exercise is bad for bones because it increases the harmful calcium yo-yo effect. And on the other hand we are saying that the sweating caused by the vigorous exercise reduces the harmful calcium yo-yo effect. Does one cancel out the other?

Unfortunately, no. Over-exercising increases the amount of calcium processed *in the bones*, thus eroding bone-making cells. Sweating helps reduce the amount of excess calcium *in the bloodstream*, thus reducing the amount of calcium that causes harmful calcification around the body. Clearly, the loss of calcium through sweat will to some extent ameliorate the harmful calcium yo-yo effect but not enough to 'cancel out' the erosion of bone-making cells caused by over-exercise.

> **Always stop doing exercise if you feel nausea, have blurred vision, faintness, pain in chest, severe shortness of breath, muscle pains, or heart palpitations. Never exercise through a pain.**

A good physical activity is **normal-to-quick walking or gentle jogging** as this exercises many parts of the body, including the cardio-vascular system. If your daily routine is physically sedentary, make sure you walk every day for 30 – 60 minutes (more if possible). Generally, *walking* is about the best kind of exercise for humans as this is what we are designed for.

Strength training exercise is also important: push-ups, pull-ups, weight-lifting, and walking with weighted vests. These kinds of exercises help to keep muscles and joints in good shape and prevent loss of bone density. If you lose too much bone density through lack of exercise you will become weak and be less energetic from smaller muscles (but you will not be increasing your risk of osteoporosis). You therefore want to keep just sufficiently active to maintain good bone density and muscles for normal every day living (but no more than this, so as to minimize erosion of osteoblasts and maximize the life-span of your bones).

Activities such as yoga, swimming, horse-riding, cycling, archery, and isometrics are sometimes criticized as they are said to be low-impact and do not involve weight bearing exercise below the waist. However, this does not matter as they help to preserve your bones and keep osteoporosis at bay. Also, they can be good for cardiovascular fitness, so if you wish, include any such activities in a regular and varied regimen. Cycling and rowing in particular are good examples of activities that provide excellent all round exercise, a good cardio-vascular workout, and low-impact on the bones. We need to change our concept of sport and associate low-impact with *good for bones*, and high-impact with *bad for bones*.

When bone density is lost through insufficient exercise, the potential population of bone-making cells is not lost. This has been proven from many research studies showing that bone density lost from lack of use can be rebuilt with weight-bearing activity. Further proof of this can be found in any physiotherapy hospital where patients, immobilized for long periods, are made to recover their bone mineral density through appropriate exercise. If it were true that lack of exercise brings about osteoporosis, such recoveries would not be possible.

The Low G.I. Workout[tm]

To be clear, we are not advocating a charter for doing less physical activity. This is about doing physical activity **the right way** for optimum bone health. It's more about *how* you do exercise rather than the *amount*. Instead of doing strenuous repetitive exercise to the point of exhaustion, you should be doing a wider repertoire of gentle exercises so that all parts of the body are serviced. Exertion should be enough to work up a mild sweat or make you a little breathless, and it should be done on a regular basis. This kind of low-impact, gentle, intelligent exercise will age the bones the least and keep you physically fit for normal everyday activities.

We have all heard about *The Low G.I. Diet* (based on the low Glycemic Index ratings of foods). Now we have **The Low G.I. Workout**[tm] (based on principles that combat bone aging). The table that follows gives an explanation. *The Low G.I. Workout*[tm] stands for *The **L**ow **G**entle **I**ntelligent **W**orkout* and is for ***everybody***: people of all ages and however fit or unfit you may be. See Fig. 8 on the next page.

Fig. 8: The Low G.I. Workout™

Low	**Low** impact exercise is best as it minimizes microfractures that hasten bone ageing and osteoporosis. 'Low impact' means not high enough to cause pain, aching, exhaustion, or trauma. Low impact can be mixed with short bursts of high impact activity, but the less the better.
G	**Gentle** exercise is best as it prevents injury and trauma. Gentle does not mean soft, superficial or inconsequential. It means exercising within your comfort zone combined with minimizing ***but not avoiding*** microfractures caused by weight-bearing impacts.
I	**Intelligent** exercise is smart exercise. It means using your intelligence and common sense to find a middle ground between over-exercising and under-exercising. ***Be intelligent*** by always exercising in *moderation*. The exercise should be enough to work up a sweat or become a little breathless. This ensures general good health while minimizing erosion of bone-making cells.
Workout	**Workout** every part of your body for general good health. Alternatively, exercise different parts of the body on different days in rotation. Good workouts can include any mix and match of the following: walking, gentle jogging, dancing, skating, floor exercises, strength exercises using weights, push-ups & pull-ups, swimming, and any sport or aerobic exercise, provided it is low impact and within your comfort zone.

Dairy Milk and So Called Myths

The dairy industry, and in particular the milk industry, is a *very large* business. As a result, the production, marketing and selling of dairy milk is well established all over the world. Most countries have national bodies and associations that represent dairy farmers and milk producers – they act vigorously to defend and promote milk, and to lobby politicians, nutritionists, and other bodies at every opportunity.

What follows is a list of so called 'myths' that the milk industry refer to when defending and promoting the consumption of dairy milk. These so called myths can be found in the propaganda issued by milk marketing associations, and in their websites. Here are some of these so called myths, followed by my comments:

▶**Dairy industry comment:**

MYTH: Allergy to cows' milk is common in young children.

Only two to three per cent of the population are truly allergic to milk. Cows' milk allergy is mainly a condition of infancy and around nine out of ten of those affected grow out of it by the age of three. If anyone has a concern, they should consult a medical doctor and not rely on High Street or mail order allergy tests. It is unwise to exclude dairy products from the diet without specialized advice from a State Registered Dietician.

Author's comment:

Milk allergies are extremely common and are caused by the inability of the immune system to accept certain milk proteins, including casein and whey. You never 'grow out of them' – in fact, as you get older your body's enzymes make less lactase and rennin, making you more allergic or sensitive to dairy milk as you age.

Typical symptoms include itchy red rash; hives; eczema; swelling of lips, mouth, tongue, face or throat; allergic "shiners" (black eyes); abdominal pain and bloating; diarrhea; vomiting; gas/wind; cramps; runny nose; sneezing; watery and/or itchy eyes; coughing; wheezing; shortness of breath. People get these symptoms in varying degrees, often not associating the symptoms with dairy milk. Indeed, milk allergies are so common that they can be deemed to affect almost everybody who consumes dairy milk. If an allergic reaction is described as an acute reaction requiring emergency treatment or hospitalization then it can be argued that milk allergies are not common. If an allergic reaction is described as a symptom that makes you feel uncomfortable, below par, or unwell in some way, then milk allergies are extremely common.

▶ **Dairy industry comment:**

MYTH: Drinking milk causes calcium to be leached from the body.

It has been suggested that the consumption of milk and dairy products increases the rate of calcium loss from the body and therefore increases the risk of osteoporosis. Several studies have confirmed that calcium is well absorbed from milk and that much more calcium is absorbed from one glass of milk than from a portion of most vegetable foods.

Supporters of the 'calcium leaching' idea bolster their case with statistics to show that osteoporosis is more prevalent in countries where a dairy culture exists, e.g. northern Europe. However, this can be explained by the fact that countries in the northern hemisphere have a limited number of months each year during which sunlight exposure is sufficiently strong to generate vitamin D synthesis in the skin - vitamin D is necessary for the absorption of calcium. Also, in industrial countries, the general lifestyle tends to be less active and thus osteoporosis tends to be more prevalent.

Author's comment:

Dairy milk does not help to prevent osteoporosis because the calcium in dairy milk combined with the high acidity of milk protein causes the blood to be overloaded with calcium. This in turn causes calcium to go in and out of the bones, eroding bone cells, and leading to osteoporosis. (For a full explanation please see appendix four).

To argue that osteoporosis is high in countries with little sunlight is a false argument. Osteoporosis is high in all countries with high dairy milk consumption, including countries that are not in the Northern Hemisphere. For example, Eastern Europe has the highest rate of dairy milk consumption and osteoporosis in the world, yet there is no shortage of sunshine in this region. Furthermore, dairy milk in countries in the Northern Hemisphere is fortified with vitamin D, and therefore it cannot be said that the high incidence of osteoporosis is due to lack of vitamin D from sunlight.

Osteoporosis is indeed high in industrial countries where a sedentary lifestyle is more common, but it does not follow that dairy milk is good for bones. Osteoporosis is high in dairy milk consumers wherever they live.

Osteoporosis is not due to a deficiency of calcium in the diet, or even to a loss of calcium from the body. Osteoporosis happens when there is a lack of bone-making cells, and dairy milk is the principal dietary cause because it acts to erode bone-making cells every time milk is consumed.

▶ **Dairy industry comment:**

MYTH: Drinking milk causes excess mucus production.

It has been suggested that milk and dairy products increase mucus production, and that avoiding milk will therefore alleviate the respiratory symptoms associated with colds. However, there is no good scientific evidence to support this. In one test, people given flavoured milk and soy drink found no real difference between the two. Milk does tend to leave a slightly filmy coating in the mouth or throat, but this is the result of milk's texture and perhaps a little saliva production but not mucus.

Author's comment:

Just about everybody who consumes dairy milk suffers from mucus congestion, even though some people may not make the link between the two. This can easily be tested. Simply give up consuming dairy milk for 3 or 4 days and you will begin to feel less mucus congestion.

Mucus congestion is caused by casein, a protein component of dairy milk broken down and digested by the enzyme rennin. Unfortunately, by the age of three, rennin is virtually non-existent in the human digestive tract. As a result, the casein does not get broken down and digested – instead this thick coarse substance decomposes and sticks to mucous membranes and clogs the airways and other parts of the body. Countless studies have shown this to be a fact, and it is nonsense for the milk industry to suggest otherwise. For a full explanation please see the chapter ***Dairy Milk Effect on Osteoporosis***.

▶ **Dairy industry comment:**

MYTH: Drinking milk is directly linked to cardiovascular disease.

Foods such as milk, that provide some fat and for which lower fat alternatives exist, are often singled out when dietary advice is given. This may lead to the assumption that a direct link has been shown between milk intake and heart disease, but this is not the case. Milk contains several components that may actually help protect against heart disease. For example, the DASH (Dietary Approaches to Stop Hypertension) eating plan including low fat dairy products may help to reduce the risk of heart disease by its beneficial effect on blood pressure, blood lipids, and blood homocysteine levels. Findings from epidemiological studies such as the Caerphilly Cohort Study (May 2005) demonstrate that intake of dairy foods or dairy food nutrients (e.g. calcium, potassium, magnesium) is inversely associated with stroke.

Author's comment:

The DASH eating plan referred to above (issued by the US Dept. of Health) is simply a list of menus designed to reduce blood pressure. Dozens of food items are listed, and one of these food items is *'low fat or fat free milk as a source of calcium'*. There is nothing in the DASH eating plan that says or implies that *'dairy products may help to reduce the risk of heart disease by its beneficial effect on blood pressure, blood lipids, and blood homocysteine levels.'*

Regarding the Caerphilly Cohort Study (J Epidemiol Community Health 2005;59:502-505) it examined the effects of dairy milk consumption on a random sample of 764 men and concluded that *'high milk consumption may not increase the risk of heart disease and stroke.'* But the study method did not include a control group of non-dairy milk consumers for comparison, and consequently the findings are suspect. A study comparing, say, 700 (random) milk consumers with 700 (random) non-milk consumers would have been a more valid approach. There are no independent epidemiological studies that demonstrate that intake of dairy milk does not increase the risk of heart disease or stroke. But there are several independent epidemiological studies that show how the consumption of dairy milk *does contribute* to heart disease and stroke. The reader is invited to search Google on Internet by entering **milk "heart disease"** and checking the results.

Many studies show that saturated fat, as found in dairy milk and dairy products, contribute towards heart disease and stroke. Furthermore, the homogenized fat in dairy milk is particularly harmful because of the way it contributes to the build up of plaque in arteries, making a stroke or a heart attack more likely.

▶ **Dairy industry comment:**

MYTH: Drinking soybean 'milk' is healthier than cows' milk.

Strictly speaking soybean 'milk' is not even milk; it is a drink of plant origin. It is naturally low in calcium, which is why some brands are fortified, and it contains phytate, a strong inhibitor of the absorption of several minerals including iron. Although it is often claimed that soy helps to reduce the rise of cancer, recent studies have indicated that soy could have the opposite effect - and be cancer promoting. The long-term effects of soy consumption by Western populations are at present completely unknown.

Author's comment:

There are various dictionary definitions of 'milk' such as: *'any of several nutritive milk-like liquids'* (Princeton). It is perfectly valid to refer to *'soybean milk'* or *'oat milk'* in such terms since the source of the milk is being made clear in the name of the product. Soybean milk has a rich mix of valuable nutrients as explained in the recipe section of this book.

Many foods contain some degree of phytates, including soybeans, and phytates do indeed inhibit absorption of some minerals, but it does not follow that dairy milk is good for you!

For the scientifically minded here is the position: research into soy protein shows that although mineral absorption may be less efficient compared with animal protein sources, overall mineral balance has not been found to be adversely compromised. Ingestion of soy protein may result in metabolic effects which could actually improve retention of some minerals such as calcium. With lower daily losses, requirements for these minerals are lower. The positive effects of soy protein ingestion on reducing mineral losses should be taken into account when the impact of soy protein on mineral status is evaluated. For example, soy protein is less hypercalciuric than animal protein and does not inhibit vitamin D activation as does phosphate-rich animal protein (Breslau et al, 1988; Portale et al, 1986). Consequently, despite a lower bioavailability of calcium from soy protein, less calcium is lost in the urine and thus mineral balance may not be adversely impacted.

▶ **Dairy industry comment:**

MYTH: Lactose intolerance is widespread.

Lactose intolerance (an inability to digest the milk sugar, lactose, properly) does not mean that you should avoid all dairy products. On the contrary most lactose maldigesters can tolerate a certain amount of lactose and so can enjoy hard cheese (which is virtually lactose-free), yogurts and small quantities of milk. The gradual reintroduction of dairy products in progressively greater quantities tends to improve your ability to tolerate lactose.

Author's comment:

Everybody is lactose intolerant, some more than others. For some young and fit people, the degree of lactose intolerance may be so mild that it is hardly noticeable, e.g. a slight feeling of lethargy, or indigestion, or feeling bloated. For others, lactose intolerance causes severe illness. Dairy milk contains more lactose than other dairy products and is therefore the worst offender. When dairy milk is consumed by a human, it is broken down in the stomach by an enzyme called 'lactase'. As we get older, we gradually (or completely) lose this lactase. The less lactase we have, the more lactose intolerant we become. That is why older people instinctively tend to shun dairy milk. It therefore does not make to suggest that the *'gradual reintroduction of dairy products in progressively greater quantities tends to improve your ability to tolerate lactose.'* There is absolutely no evidence that consuming *more* dairy milk will somehow make you more able to tolerate lactose; this will only exacerbate the problem.

Poor absorption of lactose may more than double the risk of ovarian cancer in women.[45]

▶ **Dairy industry comment:**

MYTH: Milk is a major contributor to fat intake.

FACT: Foods such as milk, that provide some fat and for which lower fat alternatives exist, are often singled out when dietary advice is given. This may lead to the assumption that a direct link has been shown between milk intake and heart disease, but this is not the case. Milk contains several components that may actually help protect against heart disease FACT: Lactose intolerance (an inability to digest the milk sugar, lactose, properly) does not mean that you should avoid all dairy products. On the contrary most lactose maldigesters can tolerate a certain amount of lactose and so can enjoy hard cheese (which is virtually lactose-free), yogurts and small quantities of milk. The gradual reintroduction of dairy products in progressively greater quantities tends to improve your ability to tolerate lactose.

On average, whole milk contains 4 per cent fat, semi-skimmed 1.7 per cent and skimmed only 0.1 per cent. The Guideline Daily Amount for fat intake for women is 70g per day and 95g for men. Milk only supplies around eight percent of the fat in the diet. Therefore milk is not a major contributor to fat intake.

*The Guideline Daily Amounts are official government figures for the predicted daily consumption by an average adult of normal weight eating a diet conforming to UK Department of Health recommendations.

Author's comment:

It is a gross distortion of the truth to say that *'Milk only supplies around eight percent of fat in the diet.'* The Dietary Guidelines clearly recommend that no more 10% of calories should come from fat. In the case of Whole Milk, 48% of calories come from fat which is way above the recommended 10%. In the case of '2% milk' it amounts to deception to imply that you somehow only get '2% fat' when in fact 80% of the fat is saturated fat, giving you a whopping 38% calories from fat!

Even *1% Milk* (the equivalent of semi-skimmed milk in the UK/EU) provides 27% calories from fat, which is nearly three times the maximum amount recommended by Dietary Guidelines. Furthermore, in Whole milk for example, 63% of the fat in milk is saturated fat, which is way above any dietary guidelines!

On average, [UK] adults consume a third of a pint of milk a day. As semi-skimmed milk [1% milk], this provides just over 90 kilocalories and has 3.4 grams of fat, 60 per cent of which is saturated. Source: Which? Magazine, UK, www.which.co.uk.

There are about 35 grams of fat in a quart of milk. If you drink one quart (two pints) of whole milk per day, this alone will give you over one-third of your daily quota of fat as recommended by the American Heart Association.

But although whole milk is a major contributor of *bad fat* intake, low-fat varieties of dairy milk are even worse for your health (see chapter ***Dairy Milk Effect on Weight Loss***).

▶ **Dairy industry comment:**

MYTH: The protein in milk (animal protein) is not good for you.

FACT: On average, whole milk contains 4 per cent fat, semi-skimmed 1.7 per cent and skimmed only 0.1 per cent. The Guideline Daily Amount* for fat intake for women is 70g per day and 95g for men. Milk only supplies around eight percent of the fat in the British diet. Therefore milk is not a major contributor to fat intake. The Guideline Daily Amounts are official government figures for the predicted daily consumption by an average adult of normal weight eating a diet conforming to Department of Health recommendations.

For scientific references please contact The Dairy Council's nutrition team.

FACT: Calcium is contained in the non-cream portion of milk and so when milk is skimmed all the calcium remains. In fact, pint for pint, skimmed and semi-skimmed contain slightly more than whole. Milk provides almost 40 per cent of the calcium in the British diet.

The protein in milk is very good for you, as it is a high quality animal protein. The protein from animal sources, e.g. milk, eggs and meat, provides all the indispensable amino acids that we cannot make by ourselves. Some studies have also shown that it may help protect against cancer.

Author's comment:

The protein in dairy milk is bad for you because it causes a multitude of diseases and ill health arising from poor digestion of the protein. For a full discussion on protein see the chapter '***Dairy Milk Effect on Protein***'

Milk protein cannot be digested properly and is harmful to health for the following reasons:

- It is badly digested because humans lack rennin, an enzyme required for digesting the casein protein in milk. As a result, casein putrefies into mucus which coats the digestive system, impeding proper digestion generally.

- The RDA (Recommended Daily Allowance) for protein is about 20 grams (less than 1 ounce) for children, and about 40 grams (about 1 ½ ounces) for adults. This tiny amount is easily obtained from plant foods. Virtually all vegetables and many fruits contain protein, such as green vegetables, beans, pulses, potatoes, bananas, grains (rice, wheat, quinoa, etc), seeds, soy foods, and many other products. Animal protein provides *'ready-made protein'* whereas plant protein provides *'amino acids for making protein.'* The human body prefers to receive plant protein because then it can make exactly the right amount of protein that it needs. *Excess protein is bad for you.* With animal protein, the body has to break the protein down to amino acids – it then uses some of the amino acids to make the amount of protein it needs *and it discards the excess amino acids.* As the excess amino acids are discarded they stick to valuable minerals before being excreted through urine and sweat. So this excess protein is not digested and it causes harm to the body by acting as a mineral robber.

- When dairy promoters argue that getting so called 'complete protein' from plant foods needs careful planning, this is a false argument. The amino acids from plant protein remain in your body for days at a time. Therefore, by consuming a variety of plant based foods, you will get all the essential amino acids required for the body to make the protein that it needs, *with no harmful excess.*

- When milk is pasteurized it is boiled to very high temperatures. This kills a variety of enzymes that would otherwise help you digest the protein in milk. As a result, when pasteurized milk is consumed, it is badly digested, it putrefies inside the body, and it causes illness and disease as a consequence.

- Eating a low protein diet is key to developing and preserving strong bones, and combating osteoporosis. The high content of badly digested animal protein in dairy milk is a major contributor to osteoporosis in the world today.

> *Hospitals in the USA and other developed countries are filled with people who have eaten too much dietary animal protein. It is nearly impossible to live in America and not over-burden your body with protein if you consume dairy products.*

- In many people, the antigenic proteins in dairy milk can 'leak' out into the bloodstream through the intestinal lining, and incite allergic reactions in lungs and joints – exacerbating asthma and rheumatoid arthritis. This can also cause intestinal bleeding leading to anemia in children.

- The dairy industry says that protein from dairy sources provides all the indispensable amino acids that we cannot make by ourselves. So what? The protein from plant sources *also* provides all the indispensable amino acids that we cannot make by ourselves.

▶ **Dairy industry comment:**

MYTH: There is a link between milk consumption and diabetes.

It is sometimes suggested that there is a link between the development of Type 1 (or juvenile onset) diabetes and the consumption of cows' milk. It is important to recognize that this is just one of several theories about the cause of diabetes. At present there is no conclusive proof one way or the other. Milk is not the only food that has been linked to diabetes - trials in animals suggest that wheat and soy protein have a greater potential to induce Type 1 diabetes. The Dairy Council recommends breast-feeding for the first few months of an infant's life, cows' milk should not be introduced as a main drink until the child is one year old.

Author's comment:

All the latest research into this subject is pointing to the fact that dairy milk *does* contribute to diabetes in children, and hence adults. There are many studies that corroborate this, and here are just a few:

1. *A study from Arizona State University found that the early ingestion of dairy milk-based formula increases the risk of diabetes.*[67]

2. *Many studies have linked dairy milk consumed by babies to subsequent diabetes. Now, Finnish researchers have added to the case against cows' milk by studying children from birth.*[68]

3. *Exposure to bovine proteins [in dairy milk] is a trigger for insulin-dependent diabetes mellitus.*[69]

4. Dr. Hans-Michael Dosch is a senior scientist in immunology at Toronto's Hospital for Sick Children. He has spent years investigating the effect of dairy milk on infants at risk of diabetes. He says: *'Early exposure to a lot of cow milk in formula seemed to be associated with a higher risk of developing auto-immune or juvenile diabetes.'*[70]

5. In a study of 40 countries it was found that dairy products were predictors of elevated incidence in rates of diabetes, whereas among dietary

items of plant origin there were inverse predictors. There was a direct correlation between animal sources and positive associations of type 1 diabetes.[71]

6. *Introduction of dairy products and high milk consumption during childhood may increase the child's risk of developing juvenile diabetes.*[72]

7. *More than 20 well-documented previous studies, have prompted one researcher to say the link between milk and juvenile diabetes is very solid.*[73]

There are no studies to indicate that soy induces diabetes, as suggested by milk industry lobbyists. On the contrary, all the research suggests the opposite.

Diabetes occurs when the blood stream gets overloaded with glucose. But when it comes to soy, research into its effect on diabetes has found *less* glucose in the urine of diabetics who consumed soybeans. This could indicate that their cells were able to absorb more glucose. Also, soluble fibre found in soy may help to regulate glucose levels. Here are some examples of research into this subject:

1. *Several types of gel fibre or so-called "soluble" fibre, such as that contained within soybeans, apples, and legumes, exert a beneficial effect on controlling blood glucose in diabetic patients.*[74]

2. *Soy products play a beneficial role in obesity and diabetes.*[75]

3. *Soy cuts insulin and cholesterol risks in diabetic women.*[76]

4. *Soy may be extremely useful in managing blood sugar levels for diabetes. The complex carbohydrates found in soy are slowly digested and produce low blood sugar and insulin responses. This means that the glucose from a soy-based meal is released gradually into the bloodstream, assisting in keeping the blood sugar level within the normal range.*[77]

5. Dr. Mark Messina and his associates in their book ***The Simple Soybean and Your Health*** (Avery Publishing, New York, 1994) look at the many amazing nutritional advantages provided by soy foods, highlighting the latest studies that have found soy foods helpful in preventing many forms of cancer, heart disease and osteoporosis, and in controlling diabetes.

6. *Soy protein is slowly becoming a staple in America's pantries because of its potential health benefits. Now there is surprising evidence of soy's therapeutic power in preventing two of the biggest complications facing people with type 2 diabetes: kidney disease and heart disease.*[78]

Soy Caution

Any food consumed to excess is bad for you. Even drinking too much water can kill you! The same goes for soy or anything else. Consumed in moderation, soybeans (or soybean milk) is perfectly safe, nutritious and healthy. But soy is rich in *isoflavones*, a weak form of the estrogen hormone. When soy is consumed to excess, some studies have shown that the concentration of *isoflavones* can be bad for health.

Therefore it is best to consume soy *wholefoods* such as tofu, soybean milk made from soybeans, soy yoghurt, edamame, tempeh, miso, cooked soybeans, and any soy foods that do not contain the protein isolate derived from the soybean through chemical extraction. It is best to avoid soy foods that contain **soy protein isolate** as it contains concentrated *isoflavones*. Examples of soy foods to avoid are soy protein powder supplements, soy energy bars; or hot dogs, ice cream, chips, and cookies made from soy protein isolate.

Criticisms leveled against soy by the milk industry are centered around studies of soy foods with concentrated *isoflavones*, or foods made with **soy protein isolate**.

▶ **Dairy industry comment:**

MYTH: Consumption of milk and other dairy products causes cancer.

There is no persuasive evidence to support the myth that consumption of milk and other dairy products causes cancer. On the contrary, intake of dairy foods may reduce the risk of some cancers, notably colon cancer. Moreover, several dairy food components such as vitamin D, calcium, conjugated linoleic acid (CLA), and sphingolipids may potentially protect against cancer.

Author's comment:

Naturally, vitamin D, calcium, conjugated linoleic acid (CLA) and sphingolipids may potentially protect against cancer, **but it does not follow** that dairy milk protects against cancer. More specifically, dairy milk does not protect against or reduce the risk of colon cancer. The milk industry likes to quote a study carried out by doctors from *Brigham and Women's Hospital and Harvard Medical School*, USA (*Journal of the National Cancer Institute, July 2004*). This study concluded that the consumption of dairy milk reduced the risks of colon cancer. But the study **only compared dairy milk to other calcium-laden foods such as yogurt or cheese.** This study compared the effects of different *dairy* products; it did not compare cancer patients who consumed dairy milk with cancer patients who consumed non- animal calcium-rich foods.

Furthermore, the researchers readily admitted that as the study was *only based on ten people*, it was not conclusive and more research was necessary. The point here is that calcium from whatever source, once absorbed into the body, helps to prevent colon cancer. There is no evidence that dairy milk as such helps prevent colon cancer.

The *Brigham study* is the only known study that puts dairy milk in what could be called a 'favourable light' and naturally the milk industry is milking it for all it's worth. Numerous other studies show that dairy milk *causes* cancer. Here are some of the more recent studies:

- *Consumption of dairy products leads to an increased risk of lymphatic cancer (non-Hodgkin's lymphoma or NHL).*[79]

- *IGF-I has been identified as a key factor in the growth of cancer. IGF-I is identical in humans and cows. Drinking dairy milk increases IGF-I levels, leading to cancers such as breast cancer, gynecological cancers, and other types of cancer.*[80]

- *Women who consume two or more glasses of* [cow's] *milk a day have twice the risk of a certain form of ovarian cancer than those who rarely or never consume milk. Intakes of lactose and dairy products, particularly milk, were significantly associated with the risk of serious ovarian cancer.*[81] This was a study headed by Susanna Larsson at the *Karolinska Institute* in Sweden, in which researchers studied more than 60,000 women.

- *We studied more than 13 000 women participants and found that those who ate the most saturated fat were almost twice as likely to develop breast cancer as those who ate the least. Saturated fats are found mainly in full-fat milk, meat and products such as biscuits and cakes.* Source: *The Lancet*, July 2003, 362(9379):212-214.

According to Dr. Michael Lam (USA) MD, MPH, ABAAM, CNCT, several studies have confirmed that milk fat is a recognized source of *carcinogenesis* because of the saturated fat content of milk, and because milk is an ideal carrier for chemical carcinogens. Dr. Lam sites ovarian cancer as an example: *'Its incidence parallels dairy eating patterns around the world. The culprit seems to be galactose, the simple sugar broken down from the milk sugar lactose. Animals fed galactose develop ovarian cancer at a much higher rate than control groups. About 10% of the U.S. population lacks the enzymes to metabolize galactose.'* Source: www.LamMD.com.

PART TWO: ALL ABOUT NON-DAIRY MILK

***

Why Choose Non-Dairy Milk?

As far back as the 1930's soybean and nut milks were being recognized for their excellence: *'Cow's milk is not suited for human consumption. Milk causes constipation, biliousness, coated tongue, headache, and these are the symptoms of intestinal auto-intoxication. Soybean milk, and nut milks are excellent substitutes, and have practically the same analyses, and the danger of disease is removed.'* Source: Jewthro Kloss, 'Back to Eden' 1939.

In the above extract it is interesting to note that in the 1930's dairy milk was practically a different product: no harmful homogenization, less pesticides and pollutants, little or no pasteurization (less acidic), and much less intensive dairy farming (less mastitis, less antibiotics). But even then, when dairy milk was *less* harmful to health, some enlightened people were already aware that it had no redeeming features.

Here are ten good reasons for choosing non-dairy milk:

1. Avoidance of dairy milk. The avoidance of all kinds of animal milk, and in particular dairy milk, has to be the best reason for choosing non-dairy milk. The moment you give up or greatly reduce the consumption of dairy milk, you will be on a path to better health. Not only will your health improve generally, you will feel more energetic and full of life, your thinking will be clearer as a result of feeling better, and you will breathe more easily as your airways get freed up.

2. More nutritious. Non-dairy milks are bursting with a host of vitamins, minerals, health-promoting oils, life-giving enzymes, and much more.

Enzymes are fundamental to all living processes in the body, necessary for every chemical reaction and the normal activity of our organs, tissues, fluids, and cells. All the vitamins, minerals, and hormones we rely on need enzymes to work.

Pasteurized dairy milk contains no enzymes. Only plant enzymes initiate digestion in the stomach, which is why the protein in dairy milk is always poorly digested. The plant enzymes in non-dairy milk enhance nourishment, and spare the pancreas from doing all of your digestion. Please see *Part three* of this book for more details of the nutritional benefits of non-dairy milk.

3. More variety. *'Variety is the spice of life'* and the same goes for what you eat and drink. ***A healthy diet is a varied diet*** because this gives the body a wide spectrum of nutrients to exploit. In this book you can choose from over twenty different kinds of milks and enjoy a variety of delicious flavours and super-healthy nutritional cocktails all the year round.

4. More convenient. Making milk at home is quick and easy, and you will soon know how to make your favourite milks in minutes, without reference to the book. This saves time and money as you will no longer have to go out and buy milk. And should you run out of milk, you can make more anytime. Virtually all the ingredients for making non-dairy milk are readily available in supermarkets, and they can be stored at home for weeks or months at a time. If travelling away from home you could even take the ingredients with you, ready mixed. Then when you get to your destination, all you need is water!

5. Better Protein. Humans have evolved to thrive on a low protein diet. We only need a tiny amount of protein to stay healthy (about 1 ½ ounces per day). Excess protein from dairy milk and animal-based foods causes bad health because the excess protein acts to rob the body of valuable minerals. Furthermore, animal protein is never digested efficiently, causing carcinogens as it passes through the intestines. Eating a varied diet of plant-based foods provides plenty of protein with no excess amounts that can cause ill health. Most of the non-dairy milk recipes in this book provide good sources of protein that is easily digested. For more information on protein please see the chapter '***Dairy Milk Effect on Protein***'

6. Less fattening. Compared to whole dairy milk, most non-dairy milks are less fattening. This is why:

- Saturated fat in dairy milk mostly gets stored as *body fat*. Whereas saturated fat in non-dairy milk mostly gets stored and used up as *energy*. This is so because the saturated fat in animal milk is mainly made up of long chain fatty acids (14:0, 16:0, and 18:0 carbon atoms). This kind of fat gets stored as body fat. But the saturated fat in non-dairy milks is mainly made up of medium-chain fatty acids (8:0, 10:0, and 12:0 carbon atoms). This kind of fat gets converted into unsaturated fats, assimilated into the body, or burnt as energy in day to day activities. As a result, saturated fat in animal milk (compared to the same amount of *saturated fat* in plant milk) is much more likely to lead to obesity.

- The carbohydrate content in plant milks tends to have a low Glycemic Index which means that the calories are more likely to get used up as energy instead of being stored as fat. However, in dairy milk the carbohydrate content (i.e. lactose) also has a low Glycemic Index, but it gets poorly digested and this results in many calories getting stored as body fat instead of being burnt off as energy. The poor digestion of lactose arises from a combination of lactose intolerance, however mild, and the poorly digested protein present in all pasteurized milk.

- The total calorie count in non-dairy milks is usually lower than the total calorie count in dairy milk, given an equal amount of liquid volume. Furthermore, the calories in non-dairy milk can be easily reduced anytime just by adding water without much change in the taste. If you do this with dairy milk, it can taste 'watery'. Note that if comparing the calorie count of nuts with the calorie count of dairy milk, consideration must be given to the water dilution in nut milk, and the amount of calories that get left behind in the okara. When these factors are taken into account, nut milk usually has less calories than whole dairy milk.

> *'Reducing dietary fat to levels necessary for the control of cholesterol cannot be achieved if a child drinks whole milk.'* Charles Attwood, M.D., Dr. Attwood's Low-Fat Prescription for Kids.
>
> *'Milk fat has been identified as a cholesterol-elevating fat because it contains cholesterol and is primarily saturated.'* Journal of Dairy Science, 1991: 74(II).
>
> *'Milk and high fat dairy products contribute considerably to dietary fat intake.'* Journal of the American College of Nutrition, 2000 April, 19:2 Supplement.

But what about low fat and non-fat dairy milk? How do they compare when it comes to fat? If comparing such milks with non-dairy milks, there is no simple answer. Some non-dairy milks will have more fat and some less fat, compared to low fat dairy milk. But consider this: most non-dairy milks have *very little saturated* fat anyway, and the little they do have tends to get used by the body instead of being stored as fat. Hence, even if the total calorie count in non-dairy milk is higher than, say 1% milk, it does not mean you will lose more weight consuming the 1% milk. In any event, you can add water to any home-made milk to make it thinner and reduce the calorie count.

Furthermore, do you really want to consume low fat or non-fat dairy milk just to avoid a few calories, given the harm it does to your health? If you are not convinced that low fat and non-fat dairy milk is truly harmful to health, you may wish to review the chapters **Dairy Effect on Weight Loss** and **Dairy Milk and related products.**

To summarize, the saturated fats in cow's milk are different to the saturated fats in non-dairy milks. They are different in the following respects:

Saturated fat in dairy milk	Saturated fat in non-dairy milk
Contains some of the herbicides, pesticides, antibiotics, hormones, and other pollutants that reside in the animal.	Does not contain any harmful chemicals or pollutants, unless they have been put into the soil or sprayed onto the plants. Even then, the saturated fats inside the plant are unlikely to be affected by such pollutants because of the metabolic process of the plant.
Goes solid at room temperature. Such fats are more likely to clog your arteries than non-saturated fats.	Does not go solid at room temperature unless hydrogenated (mixed with hydrogen in the air). Typically, vegetable lard and some margarines contain hydrogenated vegetable oil. The saturated fats in plant-based milks are not hydrogenated.
Likely to contain harmful cholesterol, thus contributing to raised serum cholesterol and heart disease. The latest research shows there is no relationship between the level of cholesterol in the blood and the incidence of atherosclerosis. But the same research shows this not to be the case when oxidized or rancid cholesterol is consumed, as in the case of pasteurized cow's milk.	Does not contain any cholesterol, and therefore does not raise serum cholesterol or contribute to heart disease.

Most dairy milk is high in saturated fat, unless specifically removed. These saturated fats mostly get stored as surplus body fat (because of their molecular structure) rather than being used for nutrition or energy.	Most plants and non-dairy milks contain little or no saturated fats. Any saturated fats they do contain have a different molecular structure (**short and medium chain triglycerides**) making them less likely to get stored as body fat and more likely to be broken down to unsaturated fats and used for nutrition or energy.
The saturated fats in pasteurized cow's milk are not anti-viral, antibacterial or anti-fungal, and therefore promote disease and obesity. They also promote harmful cholesterol in the body.	The relatively small amount of saturated fats in plant-based milks can have an anti-viral, antibacterial and anti-fungal role when consumed in the natural state, thus contributing to good health. *'Trials have confirmed that coconut oil does have an anti-viral effect and can beneficially reduce the viral load of HIV patients.'* Source: Dr. Conrato S. Dayrit, Emeritus professor of pharmacology, University of the Philippines.

7. Okara. The left over Okara that you get from most of the milk recipes is just as nutritious as the milk itself. Additionally, the okara provides valuable fibre and other nutrients not passed into the milk. This is a major benefit of making your own milk, as the okara can be used in just about any recipe you can think of. It mixes equally well into savoury dishes as it does in desserts, ice cream and smoothies. This adds bulk, texture, and nutrition to whatever you are making. Okara tends to soak up the flavour and juices of whatever it is added to, so you can think of is as a super-nutritious 'bulking agent'. Whenever you are cooking, always think 'okara'.

8. More humane. The consumption of non-dairy milk provides an ideal alternative to dairy milk. In developed countries up to 40% of dairy cows suffer from mastitis causing *constant* pain in the udder to 20% of the cows. In less developed countries the figures are worse. Many dairy cows are never allowed to graze – instead they are forced to live in small enclosures all their lives. Here is an extract from *'Advocates For Animals'* (www.advocatesforanimals.org.uk):

'The image of dairy cows living an idyllic life, happily munching away on grass in open green fields is, sadly, far from being a reality. Most dairy cows suffer terribly during their unnaturally short intense lives.

Most dairy cows graze on pasture during spring and summer months and are housed indoors in cowsheds during the winter. The practice of keeping dairy cows indoors for most of the year is increasing. In some cases, cows are kept indoors all year - this is known as zero-grazing.

Dairy cows are the most over-worked of all farm animals, forced to produce higher and higher milk yields. To produce milk, the cow must become pregnant and give birth. The modern dairy cow must remain lactating, which means being in a constant cycle of pregnancy. She is first impregnated, usually artificially, at 15-18 months, giving birth nine months later when she is just over two years old. After about 12 hours her calf is taken away from her forever, so that her milk can be extracted and sold for human consumption. Separation of mother and infant causes acute anxiety and suffering to both animals - calves can be heard calling for their mothers long after they have been separated. Impregnated again, just two to three months after each calving, cows are simultaneously lactating and pregnant for at least seven months of the year. They will produce up to 10,000 litres of milk during each lactation.

The demand for the massive over-production of milk has had severe welfare implications for dairy cows and has resulted in a number of so-called production diseases.

Mastitis is a painful bacterial infection of the udder that causes inflammation and swelling. The udder becomes hard and hot with an abnormal discharge. Studies show that over one-third of the UK dairy herd suffers from mastitis. [Similar or worse figures apply in other countries]. The cow is often lame in one or both hind legs with swollen joints. Body temperature can be high and in some cases pregnant cows will abort or produce a stunted calf. Mastitis can lead to depressed appetite, dehydration and severe diarrhea. It can be fatal.

Poor hygiene in cubicle houses and poorly designed and maintained milking machines are major contributors. Milking occurs two to three times per day and is fully mechanized. Automated milking machines extract milk by a method known as vacuum pulsation. This can weaken tissue and make the teats more prone to infections like mastitis.

The financial cost of mastitis to farmers is often high, with millions of doses of antibiotics (often penicillin) being used to treat it every year. The cost to cows in terms of pain and suffering is much harder to quantify.

A cow's udders can be so huge and swollen that they force her hind legs apart, causing a distortion of the hind limbs. Her foot becomes predisposed to damage and inflammation causing considerable suffering and pain.

She is also often forced to stand with her hind feet in the passageway behind the cubicle where manure and urine collect. This can soften the cow's hooves and encourages infection.

Yield-boosting starchy high-protein feeds that increase milk output can lead to ruminal acidosis, too much acid in the cow's rumen. This in turn leads to inflammatory substances being released into the blood, which supplies the sensitive laminae of the cow's feet. The feet become hot, swollen and inflamed, causing and exacerbating lameness.

Scientific surveys have shown a mean annual incidence of lameness of over 50%, with practically all cows showing signs of foot damage by the time they are slaughtered.

Dairy cows typically suffer from a range of diseases: BSE, ketosis, milk fever, grass staggers, viral pneumonia, salmonellosis, bovine virus diarrhea, brucellosis and endometritis. Most of these diseases result in terrible suffering. They are caused and exacerbated by the cows being pushed too hard to produce huge milk yields.

Most dairy cows are impregnated by artificial insemination (AI). An increasing number are being bred using a procedure known as embryo transfer. This is so painful that, when being undertaken, the law requires that an epidural anesthetic be administered. Embryo transfer is used to multiply quickly the 'highest quality' cows. These cows are given drugs to cause 'superovulation', so that their egg cells can be retrieved and used for embryo transfer to lower quality surrogate mothers.

Cows that do not produce enough milk are often killed after only one lactation. Other cows may be killed if they are not easy to handle, become ill or have calving problems.

By the time she is just five years old, a cow is worn out by the strain of constant production and is slaughtered as a 'spent' or 'cast' dairy cow. She may be so run-down and emaciated that her back and hip bones protrude. A cow's natural lifespan should normally be as much as 25 years.

BST or Bovine Somatotropin is a genetically-engineered version of a cow's own growth hormone and is injected into the cow to increase milk yield. It usually causes long-lasting swellings at the injection site, doubles the length of the period of catabolic stress experienced by lactating cows after calving and increases the chances of a cow contracting mastitis. These health and welfare issues led to an EU ban. However, BST is still being used in several countries, including the USA, whose dairy products are still being imported into the EU.

Organic dairy farming can cause less suffering to dairy cows. However, conditions for the cows are far from ideal, with many animals often suffering from diseases such as mastitis and lameness. In order to lactate, the cows still need to be made pregnant. Male calves are still a by-product and are usually taken away from their mothers within 24 hours, and many are shot. There is no such thing as 'humane milk' - the only truly welfare-friendly type of milk is non-dairy and obtained from plants.'

9. No harmful cholesterol.

Cholesterol is vital to life. We need cholesterol because it plays a major role in forming cell membrane structures, i.e. keeping our cells healthy. We can get cholesterol in two ways: the body makes it, and we can get it from animal products such as meat and dairy milk. *No plant foods contain cholesterol* – this includes all fruit, vegetables, cereals, grains, pulses, seeds, nuts, etc. Problems arise when we eat bad cholesterol (i.e. cholesterol that has been oxidized by heating, such as pasteurization) as this can clog arteries and increase the risk of a heart attack or stroke.

'It takes only a small amount of cholesterol in the blood to meet our needs. If you have too much cholesterol in your bloodstream, the excess is deposited in arteries, including the coronary arteries, where it contributes to the narrowing and blockages that cause the signs and symptoms of heart disease.' Source: **National Heart, Lung, & Blood Institute, USA (http://www.nhlbi.nih.gov/chd).**

In fact, an ideal diet would be a diet with no cholesterol at all. Our bodies make all the cholesterol we need. (The amount of cholesterol that our liver makes *daily* is equivalent to the amount of cholesterol in about five chicken eggs). In fact, our body always makes a mix of HDL and LDL (good and bad) cholesterol, and it keeps both types of cholesterol in balance so as to avoid harm from LDL cholesterol. Put simply, LDL is necessary for carrying cholesterol into the bloodstream, and HDL carries cholesterol out of the bloodstream, so we need both LDL and HDL.

But when we consume the kind of saturated fat provided by dairy milk, this encourages the body **to make more LDL (bad) cholesterol than it needs** or can get rid of, and as a consequence the surplus cholesterol gets stuck to artery walls, causing heart disease and stroke. (Note: the bloodstream is obliged to dump the excess cholesterol wherever it can because it is not water soluble and hence won't dissolve, and because the blood stream is always compelled to keep HDL and LDL in balance).

This is why even vegetarians who eat a low or nil cholesterol diet can suffer from harmful cholesterol – the culprit is the *animal saturated fat* in cow's milk (and other animal foodstuffs). After all, vegans who consume no cholesterol or animal fat are known to be healthier than the population at large.

Incidentally, it is known that low HDL cholesterol levels are related to osteoporosis in both men and women. [167] This does not mean that low HDL causes osteoporosis – it means that people with osteoporosis are likely to have consumed a diet high in animal fat (e.g. dairy milk) thus causing low HDL cholesterol levels. Most regular dairy milk consumers have low HDL cholesterol levels, and equally, most regular dairy milk consumers have a high incidence of osteoporosis. Given that dairy milk is the biggest dietary cause of osteoporosis (see appendix two) it is the common link between low HDL cholesterol levels and osteoporosis.

In a much acclaimed book 'The Okinawa Way', the authors state: *The type of saturated fat in dairy products is also the worst offender for making cholesterol in the body. Perhaps it's no surprise that the Scandinavians have an epidemic of heart disease with their high dairy products consumption.*[91]

Some people have argued that *animal* food products are not the cause of excess cholesterol in the population at large. That in fact, the cause is related to the consumption of hydrogenated and industrially processed vegetable fats rather than the consumption of animal fat.

This is not so for the following reasons:

• *Saturated fat and cholesterol in the food you eat make your blood cholesterol level go up. Saturated fat is the main culprit, but cholesterol in food also matters. Reducing the amount of saturated fat and cholesterol in your diet helps lower your blood cholesterol level.* Source: American Heart Association (www.americanheart.org).

• Both *animal saturated fat* and *trans fatty acids (created through hydrogenation)* cause elevated levels of harmful cholesterol in the blood. But the main cause of excess harmful cholesterol is the former rather than the latter. This is so because only a tiny amount of trans fatty acids are consumed compared to the amount of *animal saturated fat* consumed by most people. Furthermore, 'fatty foods' generally contain much more saturated fat than trans fatty acids. However, trans fatty acids, even though consumed in smaller amounts compared to saturated fat, are very harmful – they act to prevent the body from making DHA, a critically important fatty acid required by the brain.

• Clearly, not all fats in animal-based foods are bad for health. Equally, not all fats in plant-based foods are good for health. As mentioned, trans fatty acids are very harmful. These are vegetable fats that have been mixed with hydrogen in the air (through whipping or heating processes) to make them thicker. Like most animal saturated fats, trans fatty acids encourage bad LDL cholesterol to clog up arteries, but they also reduce the level good HDL cholesterol in the blood. ***But if vegetable trans fatty acids are bad for you it does not follow that animal fats are good for you.*** This kind of non-sequitor is often used by the dairy and meat industry to justify the content of saturated fat in animal-based foods.

The only fats we need for optimum health are the unsaturated and saturated fats found naturally in plant-based and sea-based foods. This is how the human species has evolved. To suggest that animal saturated fats do not cause furring in arteries or do not promote bad cholesterol is simply erroneous.

The sterol marvel

We have said that human cells need cholesterol for life. Equally, plant cells could not exist without their equivalent to cholesterol, called 'sterol'. Whenever we consume plant-based foods we consume a small amount of sterols.

Plant sterols have been used since the 1950's to help lower harmful cholesterol levels in humans – this is why doctors and nutritionists recommend a diet high in fruit and vegetables. The reason sterols can lower bad cholesterol is that they have a similar molecular structure to dietary cholesterol, and by being similar they get absorbed into the intestine *in place of bad cholesterol.* In other words, sterols stop bad cholesterol from getting into the blood steam to cause health problems.

In a study reported in *The American Journal of Medicine* it reviewed 16 published trials that administered plant sterols to almost 600 people, and it was found that bad (LDL) cholesterol was lowered by up to 23%! The point is this: dairy milk (particularly whole milk) promotes bad cholesterol in the body because it contains both animal saturated fat and cholesterol. Plant milks, however, contain no cholesterol and no animal saturated fats. Additionally, plant milks contain sterols which help reduce any harmful cholesterol you may have.

Another important point is that if no boiling temperatures are used when making non-dairy milk, the nutritional integrity is kept intact. This means the integrity of the natural plant fats get preserved instead of being converted into hydrogenated fat or trans-fatty acids. This also means the sterols get preserved.

When you analyze the nutritional content of the nuts, seeds, pulses and plants used in the non-dairy milk recipes, just about every recipe will contain a mix of vitamins, minerals, enzymes, and fats. But these fats are all good fats because they get stored as energy rather than as surplus body fat, and because they get used by the body to make the healthy kind of fats we need for good health.

10. More healthy. Last but not least, a good reason for choosing non-dairy milk is your own good health. On the one side, by giving up dairy milk you will become less prone to illness and you will feel better generally. And on the other side, by consuming non-dairy milk, you will benefit from the super-nutrition contained in the milk. The wide spectrum of vitamins, minerals, enzymes, soluble fibre, and health-promoting fatty acids, all combine to provide an ideal and natural way to get these nutrients.

In July 2003, the US FDA said: **'*Scientific evidence suggests but does not prove that eating 1.5 ounces per day of most nuts, as part of a diet low in saturated fat and cholesterol, may reduce the risk of heart disease.*'**

This book is even more relevant for you if you're allergic to nuts. Less than half the milk recipes in this book involve using nuts. A person allergic to nuts should never try to 'compensate' by consuming more dairy products or dairy milk. *Everybody* benefits by giving up dairy milk regardless of other factors – this is the imperative!

Also, by switching to a different non-dairy milk every so often, you benefit from a greater variety of nutrition. For example, pumpkin seed milk is high in zinc and is excellent for keeping the prostate healthy in men. The best way to start is to browse through the milk-making possibilities in *Part three*, and become familiar with making just one or two recipes to begin with. Then, over time, experiment with other varieties by buying and storing the appropriate ingredients. As flavour and texture varies tremendously from milk to milk, keep an open mind about your preferences until you have tried them all.

***

Almond Milk

(For milk recipe please see *Part Three*)

Reaching a height of 3-7 m (9-22 ft) the almond tree has beautiful pink or white flowers that bloom in early spring. The dry, leathery almond fruit surrounds the almond nut which is harvested when the fruit dries and splits open.

The almond tree probably originated in the Near East but now grows all over the world. The familiar sweet almond nut has the largest share of the nut trade world-wide. It is sold in many guises, such as almond flour, almond flakes, roasted almonds and blanched almonds.

Almonds are grown commercially mostly in Southern Europe, Western Asia, California, South Australia and South Africa.

Milk made from almonds has a delicious light nutty flavour, and it makes a refreshing drink straight from the fridge. It can be used just like regular milk, or as a 'non-dairy milk' in just about any recipe.

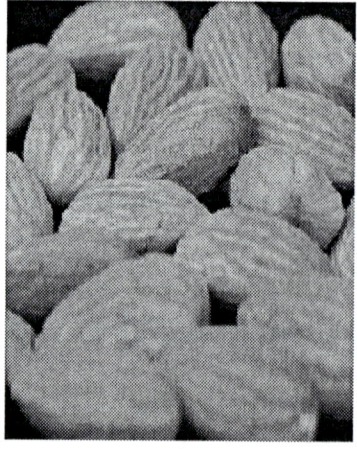

Storage

Almonds without their shells can be stored for up to 1 month if kept airtight in a cool dark dry place, or up to a maximum of 12 months in the refrigerator if kept air tight. Almonds can be frozen for 2-3 years depending on temperature.

Nutritional benefits

Almonds are particularly nutritious in **protein, iron,** vitamin **E, zinc,** and **vitamin B2**. They also have valuable amounts of **magnesium, potassium,** and **folate**.

For weight-conscious people, almond milk is low-fat and low-carbohydrate, and is therefore ideal as part of any weight loss proramme. Among the nut family, almonds privide the richest source of calcium. Also, almonds are the best whole-food source of vitamin E, in the form of alpha-tocopherol, which may hclp prevent cancer. Vitamin E is important for keeping joint and muscle tissue healthy and free from 'wear and tear'. Think of vitamin *E* as going with *E*xercise.

A study carried out by Dr. Gary Fraser (City of Hope Medical Center and Loma Linda University in California) found that eating a modest quantity of almonds daily (approximately 2 ounces or 40 almonds) resulted in increased unsaturated fats intake with *no significant changes in body weight*. Long-term daily consumption of almonds also improved micronutrient profiles and eating patterns of free-living healthy individuals. The lack of weight gain was especially evident in more obese subjects, and some actually *lost small amounts of weight*.

Almonds contain more magnesium than oatmeal or even spinach, making a valuable contribution to good health: magnesium is needed for healthy bones, and for more than 300 biochemical reactions in the body. It helps maintain normal muscle and nerve function, keeps heart rhythm steady, and is involved in energy metabolism and protein synthesis. One ounce (about 23 almonds) provides more than a quarter of your daily needs for magnesium.

Here is a list of the main nutrients in almonds:

Note: 'Value' column shows value per 100 grams of edible portion. Divide by six to work out approximate value per 100 grams of milk.

Almond nuts, not roasted	Units	Value	Almond nuts, not roasted	Units	Value
Calories	kcal	578	Manganese	mg	2.535
Protein	g	21.26	Selenium	mcg	2.8
Fat Sat. 3.881 Mono. 32.15 Poly. 12.214	g	58.24	Thiamin	mg	0.241
Calcium	mg	248	Riboflavin	mg	0.811
Iron	mg	4.30	Niacin	mg	3.925
Magnesium	mg	275	Pantothenic acid	mg	0.349
Phosphorus	mg	474	Vitamin B-6	mg	0.131
Potassium	mg	728	Folate	mcg	29
Zinc	mg	3.36	Vitamin A, IU	IU	5
Copper	mg	1.110	Vitamin E	mg	25.87

Extract from USDA National Nutrient Database for Standard Reference, Release 17 (2004)

***

Brazil Nut Milk

(For milk recipe please see *Part Three*)

Brazil nuts are the largest of the commonly consumed nuts. They resemble, but are only distantly related to, the American chestnut. Everything about these nuts is big: from the tree on which it grows in the world's largest rainforest, to the huge fruit (see picture) in which this large nut appears. The massive tree that produces this nut can reach a height of 150 feet, towering over the dense foliage of the Amazon River basin. Peru, Bolivia, Colombia, Venezuela and the Guyanas, as well as Brazil, are home to this tree, which is propagated entirely by the chance sowing of the seeds, usually by animals.

A mature Brazil nut tree can produce between 250 and 500 pounds of nuts per year. Brazil nut trees do not begin to produce nuts in significant quantities until after about 12 to 15 years. The majestic Brazil nut tree grows wild in the tropical rain forests, and most attempts to cultivate it elsewhere have been unsuccessful.

Brazil nuts can be eaten raw, roasted, salted or unsalted. They are popular in ice cream, chocolate, bakery dishes and confectionery items.

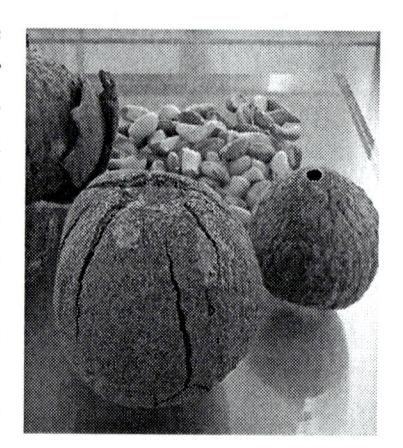

Storage

Once out of their shells, Brazil nuts should be kept refrigerated as they tend to spoil quickly. Nuts without shells will stay fresh for several months in the fridge if sealed tight. Nuts in their shells will stay fresh outside the fridge for several months if kept in a cool dark place.

Nutritional benefits

Brazil nuts are nutrient-dense, which means that in relation to their size, they contain a wide variety of nutrients. Brazil nuts are, in fact, stuffed full of significant nutrients, including protein, fibre, selenium, magnesium, phosphorus, and thiamin. They also have good amounts of vitamin E, vitamin B6, calcium, iron, potassium, zinc, and copper.

Brazil nuts are high in arginine (an amino acid that plays a role in blood clot formation) and flavonoids – important antioxidant compounds believed to be protective against both heart disease and cancer.

Just one ounce – about eight Brazil nuts – provides 20% of the RDA (Recommended Daily Allowance) for magnesium and for phosphorus. And just one Brazil nut provides more than the RDA for selenium. You would have to take more than 15 times the RDA for selenium to exceed the recommended upper daily limit.

Note that as you are getting selenium from a natural *food source* rather than as a supplement, you're unlikely to overdose on selenium in Brazil nuts unless you consume dozens daily over a long period. And since Brazil nut milk is diluted to 5 parts of water, you won't be overdosing on selenium unless you were to drink more than two or three pints a day over a long period! Furthermore, extreme overdosing on selenium will cause nausea and diarrhea, so you will soon know it. Nevertheless, selenium supplements should not be taken if consuming Brazil nuts or Brazil nut milk on a regular basis.

Selenium has significant protective effects on our heart and immune system. According to several studies of cancer patients, selenium may reduce incidence of cancers of the lung, prostate, colon and rectum. In addition, epidemiological studies indicate that people who live in areas of low-selenium soils have more cancer and heart complaints than those located in high-selenium soil areas.

When researchers at Cornell University and the University of Arizona, USA, pooled results from 5-year studies (designed to assess the effects of selenium supplements at 200 mcg daily) they came up with some startling findings: compared with the rest of the population, participants had 63% fewer prostate cancers, 58% fewer colorectal tumors, and 46% fewer lung cancers. Overall, their death rate from cancer was 39% lower than the average.

While it is true that Brazil nuts are high in fat, the fat is mostly unsaturated. They contain alpha-linolenic acid which converts to Omega-3 fatty acids in the body; it is the Omega-3 fatty acids which scientists feel may reduce the risk of heart disease by controlling cholesterol and keeping arteries clear.

Here is a summary list of nutrients in Brazil nuts:

Note: 'Value' column shows value per 100 grams of edible portion. Divide by six to work out approximate value per 100 grams of milk.

Brazil nuts	Units	Value	Brazil nuts	Units	Value
Calories	kcal	656	Manganese	mg	1.223
Protein	g	14.32	Selenium	mcg	1917.0
Fat Sat. 15.137 Mono. 24.548 Poly. 20.577	g	60.262	Vitamin C	mg	0.7
Calcium	mg	160	Thiamin	mg	0.617
Iron	mg	2.43	Riboflavin	mg	0.035

Magnesium	mg	376	Niacin	mg	0.295
Phosphorus	mg	725	Pantothenic acid	mg	0.184
Potassium	mg	659	Vitamin B-6	mg	0.101
Zinc	mg	4.06	Folate	mcg	22
Copper	mg	1.743	Vitamin E	mg	5.73

Extract from USDA National Nutrient Database for Standard Reference, Release 17 (2004)

***

Cashew Nut Milk

(For milk recipe please see *Part Three*)

The cashew-nut tree is a fast grower and an evergreen tropical tree, and is related to the mango and pistachio trees. It can grow to a height of at least 12 m (40 ft). It is a hearty tree, with an umbrella-like canopy, and it has a rather messy look with its gnarled stem and crooked branches. Lower branches rest near the ground and may root, further augmenting its spreading form. The leaves of the cashew tree are four to eight inches long and two to three inches wide. Its aromatic flower-clusters are a yellowish pink.

The cashew nut is attached to the lower portion of the cashew apple which is *pear* shaped. The cashew nut (seed) hangs at the bottom of the apple in a hard shell, and is c-shaped.

Harvested nuts in their shells are usually dried in the sun for a few days. Properly dried nuts can be stored for 2 years before being shelled in the factory. As the shells of cashew nuts contain a toxic substance that can cause blisters, they have to be heated and washed before the cashews inside can be removed. As a consequence, so-called 'raw' cashews are not truly raw - they have been heat processed in order to remove the delicious nut from the toxic shell. Most of the vitamins and minerals survive this process because the nut is heated while still protected by a hard shell.

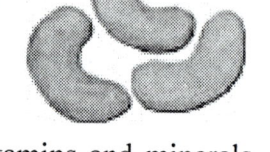

However, modern mechanical techniques have enabled some producers to open the shell cleanly every time without ever exposing the cashew nut to the toxic resin in the shell (and without using any heat at all). Such cashews, although hard to find and more expensive to buy, taste sweeter and are more nutritious than their cooked counterparts.

The cashew tree is native to South America where it flourishes in Brazil and Peru. In the sixteenth century, Portuguese traders introduced the tree to

India where it is now an important export crop equal to that of Brazil. Other countries that grow and export cashews include Sri Lanka, China, Malaysia, the Philippines, Thailand, Colombia, Guatemala, Venezuela, the West Indies, Nigeria, Mozambique, Tanzania, and Kenya. The United States is the largest importer of cashew nuts.

Storage

As with all nuts, once out of their shells they should be stored in airtight containers and be refrigerated or frozen.

Nutritional benefits

Cashew nuts are packed with proteins, fats, vitamins and minerals. The protein content is about 15.3g per 100g of cashews, due to its high concentration valuable amino acids.

The healthy fatty acids in cashews are mostly unsaturated. In 100g of cashews the total fat content is about 40 g of which about a fifth is saturated, a fifth is polyunsaturated, and the rest is monounsaturated (some Omega-3, but mostly Omega-6 oil).

In terms of vitamins and minerals, cashews are rich in vitamin E, magnesium, phosphorus, potassium, and small amounts of calcium, vitamin B, iron, zinc and selenium. Cashews are also a good source of folate (folic acid) which helps prevent cancer and anemia, and helps in the formation of red blood cells for good health. Here is a list of the main nutrients in cashew nuts:

Note: The table refers to cashew nuts heat treated to safely remove from shell but not further roasted. The 'Value' column shows value per 100 grams of edible portion. Divide by six to work out approximate value per 100 grams of milk.

Raw cashew nuts	Units	Value	Raw cashew nuts	Units	Value
Calories	kcal	553	Manganese	mg	1.655
Protein	g	18.22	Selenium	mcg	19.9
Fat Sat. 7.783 Mono. 23.797 Poly. 7.845	g	39.425	Vitamin C	mg	0.5
Calcium	mg	37	Thiamin	mg	0.423
Iron	mg	6.68	Riboflavin	mg	0.058
Magnesium	mg	292	Niacin	mg	1.062
Phosphorus	mg	593	Pantothenic acid	mg	0.864
Potassium	mg	660	Vitamin B-6	mg	0.417

Sodium	mg	12	Folate	mcg	25
Zinc	mg	5.78	Vitamin E	mg	0.90
Copper	mg	2.195	Vitamin K	mcg	34.1

Extract from USDA National Nutrient Database for Standard Reference, Release 17 (2004)

***

Chestnut Milk

(For milk recipe please see *Part Three*)

Chestnuts (also called '*sweet chestnuts*') have a long history of cultivation in Europe. During Roman times, the chestnut was the basis of a vital economy in the Mediterranean Basin, as well as rural and mountainous areas of Southern Europe.

The systematic cultivation of chestnuts probably started after the Roman Empire, in medieval times. Cultivated forms of chestnuts included hundreds of varieties, selected for specific uses such as candying, roasting, boiling, drying, flour and butter. The native habitat of the chestnut extended throughout the Northern Hemisphere and is found in China, Korea, Japan, Southern Europe and North America. The entire Eastern half of the US was once covered with wild chestnut trees and served as a year-round source of food for humans and animals.

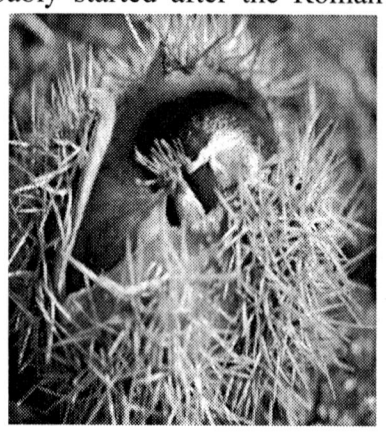

In the first half of the 20th century (by 1950) blight destroyed 3.5 billion American chestnuts. What had been the most important tree in the American Eastern forest was reduced to insignificance. No comparable devastation of a species exists in recorded history. It is thought that the blight was caused by the introduction of Oriental varieties of chestnuts. Today, efforts are being made to re-introduce a disease resistant variety of American Chestnut.

Storage

The chestnut milk recipe is made with *raw* chestnuts (either fresh or taken from frozen stock). Chestnuts are delicious eaten raw and they do not need to be cooked in any way except as a way of removing the skins. Frozen raw peeled chestnuts can be bought in supermarkets and from specialist suppliers. Simply store the frozen chestnuts in the freezer, and use up gradually, as and when you want to make chestnut milk. If storing *unpeeled* fresh chestnuts, always keep refrigerated.

When using frozen peeled chestnuts, some may still have traces of chestnut skins that failed to be completely removed. Therefore, always wash thoroughly and inspect each chestnut before use – remove any traces of remaining skins. If any chestnuts have marks that look like mould, either discard or cut off. Any slight 'burn' marks on frozen chestnuts can be ignored, as this arises from the mechanized peeling process. A mould mark goes *into* the chestnut, whereas a burn mark is jut on the surface.

Nutritional benefits

Chestnuts have a remarkable nutritional composition that sets them apart from other nuts and makes them an outstanding food source, which can be a dietary staple. The nuts are about 50% water when fresh, which makes them highly perishable. They contain complex carbohydrates, are very low in fat at about 1%, and have reasonable quantities of vitamin C, potassium, calcium, iron, vitamins B1 and B2.

The protein in chestnuts is high quality, and is easily assimilated by the human body. Also, they provide a good source of energy without being 'fattening', and chestnut milk makes an ideal and delicious non-dairy milk for the whole family. Here is a list of the nutrients in chestnuts:

Note: The 'Value' column shows value per 100 grams of edible portion. Divide by six to work out approximate value per 100 grams of milk.

Raw, peeled 'European' chestnuts	Units	Value	Raw, peeled 'European' chestnuts	Units	Value
Calories	kcal	196	Manganese	mg	0.336
Protein	g	1.63	Vitamin C	mg	40.2
Fat Sat. 0.235 Mono. 0.430 Poly. 0.493	g	1.158	Thiamin	mg	0.144
Calcium	mg	19	Riboflavin	mg	0.016
Iron	mg	0.94	Niacin	mg	1.102
Magnesium	mg	30	Pantothenic acid	mg	0.476
Phosphorus	mg	38	Vitamin B-6	mg	0.352
Potassium	mg	484	Folate	mcg	58
Zinc	mg	0.49	Vitamin A	IU	26
Copper	mg	0.418			

Extract from USDA National Nutrient Database for Standard Reference, Release 17 (2004)

***

Coconut Milk

(For milk recipe please see *Part Three*)

Coconut trees (also called *coconut palm trees* or *coco palms* to distinguish them from the many other varieties of palm trees) grow in the tropics all over the world. They are widely cultivated in Malaysia, Sri Lanka, India, and parts of Florida and the Caribbean.

Coconut trees typically grow to a height of 20 – 30m (60 – 100 ft), and each tree can produce between 100 and 200 coconuts a year. The coconuts grow in clusters of pods, and each coconut is surrounded by a thick layer of fibrous plant material which acts to protect the coconut when it eventually falls to the ground. A coconut has three 'eyes' the biggest of which can be punctured to pour out the juice. By also puncturing one of the smaller eyes, the juice will pour out more easily as air pressure will be released.

The coconut tree has a long history of providing people with useful materials: palm leaves for shelter and clothing, and palm-tree trunks for construction. Also, the white flesh of the coconut has provided a staple food for generations of people living in the tropics. Today, the oil of the coconut is used in many foods, medicines, cosmetics and toiletries. Even the sap of the coconut tree has been used as a fermented alcoholic beverage.

Modern research has found a common link between coconuts and human milk – both are rich in ***medium chain fatty acids*** (known as MCFA's) which have important antimicrobial properties. MCFA's have antibacterial, antimicrobial, and antiprotozoal properties that make up the building blocks of a healthy immune system.

Coconut oil that has been kept at room temperature for a year has been tested for rancidity, and showed no evidence of it because of its antimicrobial properties.

Storage

Fresh coconuts in the shell retain good quality up to a month in the refrigerator. Unshelled coconut flesh is best kept immersed in water and used within 4-5 days (or freeze and use within a year).

Nutritional Benefits

It used to be thought that because coconut oil is saturated it is therefore bad for your health – but this is not so. Past research was often based on hydrogenated coconut oil, rather than virgin coconut oil, thus giving a false impression that it was fattening and bad for health. Also, it was not realized that some saturated fats end up as surplus body fat and others get burnt as energy or broken down to unsaturated fats, depending on their atomic structure.

Modern research shows coconuts to be a valuable source of healthy nutrition. About a third of the white coconut flesh is fat, and most of this fat (92%) is technically classed as *saturated*. However, this saturated fat is mostly made up of MCFA's (fatty chains that get burnt up as energy rather than being stored as body fat). Because of this, coconut oil/fat is increasingly used in weight-loss regimes.

Furthermore around 50% of these MCFA's are made up of lauric acid, the most important essential fatty acid in building and maintaining the body's immune system. Apart from coconut oil, the only other source of lauric acid found in such high concentrations is human milk.

Coconut milk recipe provides an excellent source of nutrition in any weight loss regime because the saturated fat is made up of short-and medium-chain fatty acids that are easily and quickly assimilated by the body – they are not stored as fat in the body like the long chain fatty acids in dairy products.

'Coconut oil is likely to be a beneficial oil for the prevention and treatment of some heart disease. Additionally, coconut oil provides a source of antimicrobial lipid for individuals with compromised immune systems and is a nonpromoting fat with respect to chemical carcinogenesis. Replacing the fats you now eat with coconut oil may be the wisest decision you can make to lose excess body fat. We often think that the less fat we eat, the better. However, you don't necessarily need to reduce your fat intake, you simply need to choose a fat that is better for you, one that doesn't contribute to weight gain. You can lose unwanted body fat by eating more saturated fat (in the form of coconut oil) and less polyunsaturated fat (processed vegetable oils). One of the remarkable things about coconut oil is that it can help you lose weight. Yes, there is a dietary fat that can actually help you take off unwanted pounds. Coconut oil can quite literally be called a low-fat fat.' Mary G. Enig, Ph.D., USA.

'In tests, animals which ate just a little pure unsaturated oil were fat, and animals which ate a lot of coconut oil were lean. The anti-obesity effect of coconut oil is clear in all of the animal studies, and in my friends who eat it regularly. I personally found that eating more coconut oil lowered my weight, and eating less caused it to increase.' Raymond Peat (scientist and biochemist), Ph.D. P.O. Box 5764, Eugene, OR 97405, USA.

The coconut milk recipe contains a mix of the juice from the coconut and the white flesh, and is rich in a variety of vitamins and minerals.

To summarize, although high in saturated fat, coconut milk is a good source of nutrition in any weight loss regime because the fat mostly gets burnt as energy instead of being stored as fat. It is highly nutritious, good for your bones, and it helps build up a strong immune system to fight off disease and illness. Much research is currently being done on the high nutritional value of pure coconut oil (i.e. the 'saturated' coconut fat), and you can benefit from this now by making and consuming coconut milk on a regular basis. Here is a list of the main nutrients in coconuts:

Note: The 'Value' column shows value per 100 grams of edible portion. Divide by six to work out approximate value per 100 grams of milk.

Raw coconut flesh	Units	Value	Raw coconut flesh	Units	Value
Calories	kcal	354	Manganese	mg	1.500
Protein	g	3.33	Selenium	mcg	10.1
Fat Sat. 29.698 Mono. 1.425 Poly. 0.366	g	31.489	Vitamin C	mg	3.3
Calcium	mg	14	Thiamin	mg	0.066
Iron	mg	2.43	Riboflavin	mg	0.020
Magnesium	mg	32	Niacin	mg	0.540
Phosphorus	mg	113	Pantothenic acid	mg	0.300
Potassium	mg	356	Vitamin B-6	mg	0.054
Sodium	mg	20	Folate	mcg	26
Zinc	mg	1.10	Vitamin E	mg	0.24
Copper	mg	0.435	Vitamin K	mcg	0.2

Extract from USDA National Nutrient Database for Standard Reference, Release 17 (2004)

***

Corn Milk

(For milk recipe please see *Part Three*)

An important food plant that is native to America, corn is thought to have originated in either Mexico or Central America about 7,000 years ago. It played a major role in native American cultures for its sustenance as food, as material for shelter, as fuel, decoration and more. Corn also played a central role in the Maya, Aztec and Inca civilizations.

When Christopher Columbus and other explorers came to the New World, they found corn growing throughout the Americas, from Chile to Canada, and it was brought back to Europe by Spanish and Portuguese explorers who later introduced it throughout the world.

Corn that is cultivated today falls into two main categories: ***sweet corn*** and ***field corn***. Sweet corn, which was not widely cultivated until the mid-1800s, is harvested at an immature stage, so that its kernels are tender and juicy. Field corn, on the other hand, is picked at a mature, predominantly starchy stage, dried to a more hardened state, and used in a multitude of ways: as livestock feed, whiskey making, fuel, paper and plastics, to name a few.

Corn milk requires ***sweet corn*** that is picked and used fresh so that the corn is soft, juicy, and sweet – tinned or frozen sweet corn cannot be used for milk. The new varieties of 'supersweet corn' are also ideal for making milk. Note that although the **Master Recipe** calls for a sweetener to be added, you may find this unnecessary as the natural sweetness of the corn may suffice.

When buying, the leaves on the cob should be green and tight fitting. If you press a fingernail into a kernel of corn milk should come out. Corn deteriorates very quickly after picking. Do not store – keep refrigerated if not making milk immediately. Note that you can get *white* sweet corn or *yellow* sweet corn. Always give preference to *white* sweet corn as this is much better for making milk. Sweet corn that is more than four or five days old from the date it was picked should not be used. Ideally, make the milk as soon as the corn is picked.

Blanching

The corn must be blanched before making milk. Remove the leaves, and put the whole corn-on-the-cob into a large pot of boiling water for just one minute (cut cob in two if too big). Then remove and immediately immerse in cold water for 30 seconds. Then dry, scrape the kernels off the cob and put into blender. Blanching the sweet corn will not reduce its nutritional value, but is essential as it removes any bacteria, insects, or agricultural chemicals that may be present, making the milk safe to consume. Also, blanching will make it easier to remove the kernels.

Nutritional benefits

Freshly picked sweet corn is packed full of healthy nutrients. It provides a good source of thiamin (vitamin B1), pantothenic acid (vitamin B5), folate, dietary fiber, vitamin C, phosphorous and manganese.

The natural sweetness of the corn will be digested slowly because of the fibre which helps stabilize blood sugar levels, and this provides a good source of energy. Corn is also good for the heart because it contains significant amounts of folate which helps to lower levels of harmful homocysteine.

Fresh sweet corn is high in beta-cryptoxanthin which is thought to lower the risk of developing lung cancer. A study published in the September 2003 issue of *Cancer Epidemiology, Biomarkers and Prevention* found that those eating the most crytpoxanthin-rich foods showed a 27% reduction in lung cancer risk.

Corn is a good source of thiamin, providing about one-quarter (24.0%) of the daily value in a single cup. Thiamin is critical for brain cell/cognitive function and therefore fights Alzheimer's disease. Other research shows that corn is high in anti-oxidants which help prevent cancer.

Here is a list of the main nutrients:

Note: The 'Value' column shows value per 100 grams of edible portion. Divide by six to work out approximate value per 100 grams of milk.

Fresh white sweet corn	Units	Value	Fresh white sweet corn	Units	Value
Calories	kcal	86	Vitamin C	mg	6.8
Protein	g	3.22	Thiamin	mg	0.200
Total fat	g	1.18	Riboflavin	mg	0.060
Calcium	mg	2	Niacin	mg	1.700
Iron	mg	0.52	Pantothenic acid	mg	0.760
Magnesium	mg	37	Vitamin B-6	mg	0.055
Phosphorus	mg	89	Folate, total	mcg	46
Potassium	mg	270	Folate	mcg	46
Zinc	mg	0.45	Vitamin A, IU	IU	1
Copper	mg	0.054	Vitamin E	mg	0.07
Manganese	mg	0.161	Vitamin K	mcg	0.3
Selenium	mcg	0.6	Beta carotene	mcg	1

Extract from USDA National Nutrient Database for Standard Reference, Release 17 (2004)

***

Grain Milks

You may notice that some milk-making possibilities are missing from this book such as rice milk, spelt milk, millet milk, quinoa milk, amaranth milk, and others. Such milks are not included for the following reasons:

1. Grain milks generally have a poor taste that is bitter, particularly if made from raw, uncooked ingredients.

2. Grain milks made from fully cooked ingredients taste a little better, but the nutritional value is then mostly lost through the cooking process. Any kind of cooking creates substances that can lead to cancer. For this reason, and to preserve the nutritional value of the milk, none of the recipes in this book require cooking. The only exception is soy milk, as you cannot make the milk without cooking the soybeans.

3. All types of grains contain phytic acid which inhibits absorption of protein, minerals and trace elements. This is why the consumption of grain foods generally (whether raw or cooked) should be kept to a minimum. However, some whole-grain foods provide excellent sources of nutrition and should not be avoided even if they do contain phytic acid. It's a matter of choosing good quality food and eating in moderation.

For these reasons rice milk and other grain milks are not included and not recommended. However, if you do wish to make rice or other grain milks you may do this by simply following the soy milk recipe: for 'cooked soybeans' read 'cooked rice' or whatever grain you may wish to use.

If buying rice milk (or soy milk for that matter) be aware that some brands may contain high levels of sugar in the form of syrup, evaporated cane juice, or some other natural sweetener. Natural or not, most sweeteners put significant stress on your pancreas and liver. They also raise your insulin levels, which significantly increases your risk of suffering from unhealthy weight gain, high blood pressure, heart disease, premature aging, and several other negative side effects.

Another factor is that commercial rice milk and soy milk may contain added polyunsaturated vegetable oils which cause an imbalance between omega 6 and omega 3 fatty acids in the body. Such oils are unhealthy and a major cause of heart disease. Polyunsaturated oils should in general be avoided.

By making the milk recipes in this book *you* control the ingredients that go into the recipes, and as you will see, none of them require the addition of polyunsaturated oil or undesirable sweeteners.

***

Green Pea Milk

(For milk recipe please see *Part Three*)

The pea plant is a vine that can grow vertically to six feet tall, forming a dense mat of foliage. There are also low or bush varieties of peas which form a mound on the ground. The pea pods form at the leaf axils of the plant.

As most peas are a cool-weather crop, historians believe they mainly developed in middle Asia, the Near East, Afghanistan, Iran, and Ethiopia.

Today, more than a thousand varieties of peas are in existence, both green and yellow, but only a fraction of these are in widespread commercial use. Fresh or frozen peas can be purchased all over the world. Canada, the US, Europe, China, India, Russia and Australia lead the world in the production of peas.

Nutritional benefits

Green peas (fresh or frozen) are bursting with nutrients. They are high in protein and fibre, low in fat, and provide good amounts of 8 vitamins, 7 minerals, dietary fibre and protein. They are a very good source of vitamin K, which acts to anchor the calcium in your bones and prevent osteoporosis. Green peas are a rich source of folic acid and vitamin B. Here is a list of the main nutrients:

Note: The 'Value' column shows value per 100 grams of edible portion. Divide by six to work out approximate value per 100 grams of milk.

Peas, lightly boiled	Units	Value	Peas, lightly boiled	Units	Value
Calories	kcal	42	Vitamin C	mg	47.9
Protein	g	3.27	Thiamin	mg	0.128
Fat	g	0.23	Riboflavin	mg	0.076
Calcium	mg	42	Niacin	mg	0.539
Iron	mg	1.97	Pantothenic acid	mg	0.673
Magnesium	mg	26	Vitamin B-6	mg	0.144
Phosphorus	mg	55	Folate	mcg	29
Potassium	mg	240	Vitamin A	IU	1030
Zinc	mg	0.37	Vitamin E	mg	0.39
Copper	mg	0.077	Vitamin K	mcg	25.0
Manganese	mg	0.168	Beta Carotene	mcg	597
Selenium	mcg	0.7			

Extract from USDA National Nutrient Database for Standard Reference, Release 17 (2004)

***

Hazelnut Milk

(For milk recipe please see *Part Three*)

Also known as a *cobnut*, *filbert*, or *whole nut*, the hazelnut has been a favorite European treat for generations, and is gaining popularity in North America and other parts of the world. The name 'Hazel' comes from the Anglo-Saxon word for bonnet (Haesel). The term 'filbert' may have derived from 'full beard', descriptive of the long, leafy husk.

The cultivated hazelnut is native to Europe and Asia Minor, preferring regions with mild, moist winters and cool summers. For this reason, most production is located near large bodies of water at mid latitudes in the Northern Hemisphere (along the Black Sea in Turkey, the Atlantic coast in France and Spain, Sicily in Italy, and the Willamette Valley in Oregon, USA). All these regions are major exporters of hazelnuts.

The tree can grow to a height of about 15m (45ft) and commonly produces 20-25 lbs of hazelnuts over its lifetime. Its leaves are about three inches long and broadly ovate in shape with serrated edges.

Hazelnuts grow in clusters of up to twelve nuts and in appearance they resemble an oak acorn. Each hazelnut shell is surrounded by a green leafy husk. Inside the hard shell is the kernel itself, the hazelnut that we know. The shape, size and taste of hazelnuts can vary a little, depending on what part of the world they are grown in.

Storage

As with all nuts out of their shells, store in the refrigerator until used, or freeze for suture use. Hazelnuts in their shells stay fresh for several weeks if stored in a cool dry dark place.

Nutritional benefits

Hazelnuts are rich in thiamin (33% of RDA), calcium (26%), phosphorus (42%), iron (34%), and potassium (15%); plus small amounts of niacin. Because of the combination of calcium and phosphorus, hazelnuts are excellent for building and maintaining strong bones. Also, the high concentration of thiamin (vitamin B1) provides protection for the nervous system and heart muscles. Additionally, thiamin helps regulate appetite and burn energy more efficiently, thus helping you to stay slim.

In one cup of hazelnuts (not *hazelnut milk*) you get about 2g of protein because of the abundance of amino acids, and 3.5g of healthy mono-unsaturated fat, with just a trace of saturated and polyunsaturated fat. Hazelnut milk is not fattening and is a good choice in any weight loss regime. Here is a summary list of nutrients:

Note: The 'Value' column shows value per 100 grams of edible portion. Divide by six to work out approximate value per 100 grams of milk.

Unroasted hazelnuts	Units	Value	Unroasted hazelnuts	Units	Value
Calories	kcal	628	Selenium	mcg	2.4
Protein	g	14.95	Vitamin C	mg	6.3
Fat Sat. 4.464 Mono. 45.652 Poly. 7.920	g	58.036	Thiamin	mg	0.643
Calcium	mg	114	Riboflavin	mg	0.113
Iron	mg	4.70	Niacin	mg	1.800
Magnesium	mg	163	Pantothenic acid	mg	0.918
Phosphorus	mg	290	Vitamin B-6	mg	0.563
Potassium	mg	680	Folate	mcg	113
Zinc	mg	2.45	Vitamin A	IU	20
Copper	mg	1.725	Vitamin E	mg	15.03
Manganese	mg	6.175	Vitamin K	mcg	14.2

Extract from USDA National Nutrient Database for Standard Reference, Release 17 (2004)

***

Hemp Seed Milk

(For milk recipe please see *Part Three*)

Hemp seed milk is delicious and super nutritious. The hemp plant is not only one of the oldest cultivated plants, it is also one of the most versatile, valuable, and controversial plants known to man. The plant's stalks and seeds serve as raw materials for an extensive array of many diverse products. The plant's Latin name actually means "useful hemp" and it definitely measures up to its name!

The hemp plant should not be confused with the marijuana plant, which is its cousin. The appearance, planting patterns, and uses of the two plants are quite different.

The hemp plant is an annual belonging to the nettle family. It grows from 5 to 15 feet in height with rich dark-green leaves composed of 5 to 9 serrated, narrow, tapering leaflets that are pointed at the end and measure 2 to 5 inches in length and approximately one-sixth as wide. It is a tall, thin plant with most of its leaves concentrated at the top.

In contrast to the hemp plant, the marijuana plant is quite dense, leafier, shorter, bushier, and is planted in a different manner. Unfortunately, both plants have got mixed up in people's minds.

The use of hemp can be traced back to 8000 BC in the Middle East and China where the fibre was used for textiles, the oil for cosmetic purposes and the seeds for food.

The Pilgrims first brought hemp seeds to America in 1632 and by 1850 hemp was America's third largest crop. In fact, early American farmers were required to grow it. Two U.S. Presidents, Washington and Jefferson were hemp farmers when the U.S was formed and they signed the Bill of Rights. Both the Declaration of Independence and the Constitution were first drafted on hemp paper. Hemp was the world's largest single industry until the mid-1800's.

Hemp farming is legal in the United Kingdom, Canada, and most parts of the world. In the USA hemp can only be grown by obtaining a special government permit.

The hemp plant is used for an almost endless list of products: threads and yarn for cordage, rope, carpets, or knit or woven into a variety of durable high quality textiles which can be used for clothing, curtains, upholstery, shoes, backpacks, and towels. The variety of fabrics made from hemp range from those as tough as burlap and denim, to cotton-like fabrics, to those as fine as silk, or as intricate as lace. The original Levi's were made of hemp cloth and today designer Giorgio Armani, as well as other clothing manufacturers, are weaving hemp into clothes. Shoe companies are now using it in the manufacture of shoes.

Hemp seeds which have been sterilized can be legally imported into the USA. Such seeds do not lose their nutritional value, but cannot germinate and be grown. Also, new commercial varieties of hemp have been developed that contain virtually no tetrahydro cannabinol (the sticky resin used for making cannabis) and certainly not enough to perpetuate any psychoactivity. It is likely that the USA will allow these new varieties of hemp to be grown for industrial purposes. More information is available on this subject at: http://www.votehemp.com.

Caution

It should be clarified that hemp seeds (and therefore hemp seed milk) contain no drugs and no tetrahydro cannabinol (THC), and hence there is no danger of becoming addicted to hemp or cannabis. However, when you eat a plant food, just about any plant that you eat can be traced through appropriate professional blood tests (if carried out within a few hours). Therefore it is conceivable that a blood test carried out on a professional athlete might reveal traces of the hemp plant (even though it would have no effect on performance). People have been consuming hemp seeds for thousands of years with no ill effect. Here is a quote from 'Hemp Magazine' and Don Wirtshafter, Attorney at Law and Founder of www.hempoilcan.com:

Hemp Magazine: If hemp products cannot get you high, why is it that hemp products can affect drug testing?

Don Wirtshafter: THC is the active principle in marijuana (Cannabis Sativa). No hemp food contains anywhere near enough THC to have any psychoactive effect. The tests used for detection of drugs in your urine, hair or blood are amazingly sensitive. They measure their findings in parts per billion. The testing does not measure impairment. It does not even test for THC, but rather a metabolite of THC... Hemp is destined to be the power food of the century.

Hemp seed is technically not a seed but a nut. Therefore, people allergic to nuts might also be allergic to hemp seeds, although this is unusual. If giving hemp seed milk to a person known to be allergic to nuts, proceed with caution.

Storage

Out of their shells hemp seeds are slightly larger than sesame seeds. The hull of the seed consists mainly of dietary fibre and also contains small amounts of healthy chlorophyll. But it is the kernel that contains the powerful nutrients that are so beneficial. Hemp seeds can be purchased with or without their hulls. Either way, they should be refrigerated until used. Hulled seeds will keep fresh for about 2 months if refrigerated in air tight plastic bags or containers. Un-hulled seeds will keep fresh for about a 1-2 years if refrigerated in air tight bags. Hemp seeds can also be frozen for longer storage.

Nutritional benefits

The nutritional content of the hemp seed is impressive, offering 30% (Daily Recommended Allowance) of complete and highly digestible protein, and containing over 36% essential fatty acids, which is 16% more than flaxseed. It is the best source of Omega-3, Linolenic acid and Omega-6, Linoleic acid, as well as GLA, Gamma Linoleic acid (approximately 3%). Hemp seed contains protein, lipids, choline, inositol, enzymes, vitamins, minerals, phospholipids, phytosterols, and all eight essential amino acids. The amino acid profile is superior to soybean, human milk, *and cow's milk!*

The oil in hemp seeds comes in a well-balanced 3:1 ratio of Omega-6 to Omega-3. In his book, *Fats that Heal Fats that Kill,* Udo Erasmus states that 'hemp seed oil can be used in the long term to maintain a healthy *Essential Fatty Acid* balance without leading to either EFA deficiency or imbalance.'

This is so because hemp seeds provide the richest source of EFA's in the plant kingdom and contain a relatively low percentage of saturated fats. The EFA's in the oil and seeds promote cellular growth, healthy skin, hair, and eyes, aid in immune response, disease prevention, weight control, and even in cognitive functions. The human brain is 60% fat; therefore the EFA's are critically important to its proper function and good health. EFA's are also the raw material the body needs to produce hormones, the body's communication network for cellular activity.

Hemp seed milk supports the body's detoxification process due to the fact that the Linoleic Acid and Alpha – linolenic Acid in hemp seeds have the ability to carry toxic substances to the surface of the skin, intestinal tract, kidneys, and lungs where they can be eliminated from the body.

Here is a list of the main nutrients in hemp seeds:

Note: The 'Value' column shows value per 100 grams of edible portion. Divide by six to work out approximate value per 100 grams of milk.

Hemp seeds	Units	Value	Hemp seeds	Units	Value
Calories	kcal	567	Zinc	mg	11
Protein	g	33	Copper	mg	0.6
Fat Sat. 5.00 Mono. 5.00 Poly. 36.00	g	46.00	Manganese	mg	8
			Vitamin E	mg	27.50
Calcium	mg	80	Vitamin C	mg	1.0
Iron	mg	411	Thiamin	mg	1.4
Magnesium	mg	670	Riboflavin	mg	0.3
Phosphorus	mg	1500	Vitamin B-6	mg	0.1
Potassium	mg	1160	Vitamin A, IU	IU	4.0

***
Macadamia milk

(For milk recipe please see *Part Three*)

The macadamia nut (also known as *Australian nut* or *Queensland nut*) originates from southeastern Queensland in Australia. It spread to other parts of the world when it was introduced into Hawaii about 1881 where it was used as an ornament and for re-forestation – this led to the modern macadamia industry in Hawaii.

Macadamias are now grown in many parts of the world including Australia, Hawaii, California, New Zealand, South Africa, Malawi, Kenya, Costa Rica, Guatemala, Brazil, Thailand and China.

The macadamia tree thrives in mild, frost-free climates with abundant rainfall distributed throughout the year (roughly the same climate suitable for growing coffee). In the wild it typically grows along stream and river banks.

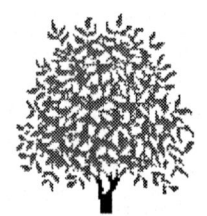

The macadamia tree is evergreen with beautiful small flowers, and it reaches a height of 10 - 13m (30 – 40ft). The bark is dark red when cut. Its roots have dense clusters of rootlets that form evenly around the tree for maximum moisture absorption. There are two species of macadamia tree, both quite similar. With one species the outer shell of the macadamia nut is rough & pebbled, with the other it is smooth.

The delicious macadamia nut is creamy white and can be eaten raw or roasted, salted or unsalted. Aboriginal Australians have been consuming macadamia nuts for thousands of years and today they are enjoyed all over the world.

Storage

Once out of their shells, they should be stored in airtight containers (whether or not roasted). They can be stored at room temperature for up to one year if unopened, or in the refrigerator for longer. Once opened, keep refrigerated. Macadamia nuts, the milk and okara are ideal for freezing.

Nutritional benefits

Macadamia nuts are full of valuable vitamins and minerals. In particular, they have a good combination of calcium, phosphorus, and magnesium, making them ideal for building and maintaining strong bones. Also, they are high in mono-unsaturated fats that promote good health, and relatively low in saturated fats (about a sixth of the fat is saturated). Macadamia milk provides an excellent source of nutrition, and can be consumed regularly as part of a balanced diet or as part of a weight loss regime.

Here is a summary list of nutrients:

Note: The 'Value' column shows value per 100 grams of edible portion. Divide by six to work out approximate value per 100 grams of milk.

Unroasted macadamia nuts	Units	Value	Unroasted macadamia nuts	Units	Value
Calories	kcal	718	Manganese	mg	4.131
Protein	g	7.91	Selenium	mcg	3.6
Fat Sat. 12.061 Mono. 58.877 Poly. 1.502	g	72.44	Vitamin C	mg	1.2
Calcium	mg	85	Thiamin	mg	1.195
Iron	mg	3.69	Riboflavin	mg	0.162
Magnesium	mg	130	Niacin	mg	2.473
Phosphorus	mg	188	Pantothenic acid	mg	0.758
Potassium	mg	368	Vitamin B-6	mg	0.275
Zinc	mg	1.30	Folate	mcg	11
Copper	mg	0.756	Vitamin E	mg	0.54

Extract from USDA National Nutrient Database for Standard Reference, Release 17 (2004)

***

Oat Milk

(For milk recipe please see *Part Three*)

The oat plant is a little like wheat, but smaller. It is cultivated as a grain, and sold in a variety of forms worldwide, particularly as breakfast cereals. Oats are chiefly a European and North American crop. Russia, Canada, the United States, Finland, and Poland are the leading oat producing countries.

Nutritional benefits

Oats contain more soluble fibre than any other grain, and a lot of this soluble fibre passes into oat milk The soluble fibre in oats is the kind that dissolves in water, so the body turns it into a super-healthy thick, viscous gel, which moves very slowly through your body. One of the benefits is that your stomach stays fuller longer, providing satiety. Soluble fibre also slows the absorption of glucose into the body, which prevents sugar highs and lows (a major cause of obesity).

Oats have been proven to help reduce cholesterol. The soluble fibre in oats (and oat milk) mixes with cholesterol-based bile acids in the digestive tract and prevents them from being absorbed. The oat fibre then carries them out of the body. In response, the liver pulls cholesterol out of the bloodstream to replace these bile acids. Cholesterol levels then drop.

Other research suggests that oats may help maintain healthy blood pressure levels and promote healthy blood flow. Researchers at *Yale University, USA*, found that eating a large bowl of porridge (oatmeal) may improve the harmful reduction in blood flow that may happen after eating a high-fat meal. (*Am. Journal of Preventive Medicine, Feb 2001*).

Oats are low in calories and contain valuable anti-oxidants that protect the heart, plus a big range of vitamins, minerals, and amino acids. Here is a list of the main nutrients:

Note: The 'Value' column shows value per 100 grams of edible portion. Divide by six to work out approximate value per 100 grams of milk.

Oats	Units	Value	Oats	Units	Value
Calories	kcal	389	Zinc	mg	3.97
Protein	g	16.89	Copper	mg	0.626
Fat Sat. 1.217 Mono. 2.178 Poly. 2.535	g	5.93	Manganese	mg	4.916
			Folate	mcg	56
Calcium	mg	54	Thiamin	mg	0.763
Iron	mg	4.72	Riboflavin	mg	0.139
Magnesium	mg	177	Niacin	mg	0.961
Phosphorus	mg	523	Pantothenic acid	mg	1.349
Potassium	mg	429	Vitamin B-6	mg	0.119

Extract from USDA National Nutrient Database for Standard Reference, Release 17 (2004)

***

Peanut Milk

(For milk recipe please see *Part Three*)

The peanut is not a nut at all – it is part of the legume family, and it grows into a green oval-leafed plant about 18 inches tall. Unlike most plants, it flowers above the ground, but fruits below ground. Yellow flowers appear about 40 days after planting. Once the flowers pollinate themselves, the petals fall off as the peanut ovary begins to form. This budding ovary, called a 'peg,' grows away from the plant on a vine and penetrates the soil.

Some other names for peanuts are goobers, pinders, earthnuts, ground peas, guinea seeds, groundnuts and monkey nuts. Peanuts have been around for 3500 years. Its original home is believed to originate on the slopes of the Andes in Brazil and in Peru. Portuguese traders, explorers and missionaries transported the peanut to Africa and Spain. From Africa they traveled by ship to 'The New World', and were planted throughout southern USA. Peanuts were an excellent food source aboard ships because they were inexpensive and nutritious.

Peanuts grow best in tropical and sub-tropical climates, and the USA is the third-largest peanut producing country in the world behind India and China. However, the US is the largest producer and exporter of edible grade peanuts in the world - most other countries crush their peanuts for oil.

Storage

Peanuts should be sealed in a plastic bag or air-tight container and stored in a cool, dry place. Alternatively, they can be stored in the refrigerator. If purchased in vacuum-sealed cans, peanuts can be stored for up to 9 months. Raw peanuts (whether shelled or unshelled) will store almost indefinitely if sealed from the air and kept in a cool dry place (or if frozen).

Nutritional benefits

Peanuts are very high in good quality protein, an essential building block of all life. Relative to other protein-rich foods, peanuts are not 'fattening' because most of the fat is monounsaturated oil, vital for good health and for keeping arteries clear.

The big range of nutrients in peanuts (13 vitamins and 26 minerals) means that they offer an almost 'complete food' with only vitamin C missing. Peanuts also possess a natural **high folate** content, along with vital **antioxidants**. Nutritionists now recognize that both of these make a vital contribution to human well-being and that antioxidants also tend to slow down the aging process.

As if that was not enough, peanuts are high in sterols. As mentioned in the chapter titled **'Non-dairy milk'** sterols play a vital part in human health, and the latest research shows that they inhibit cancer growth, protect against heart disease, and may help against colon, prostate and breast cancer.

Here is a list of the main nutrients in peanuts:

Note: The 'Value' column shows value per 100 grams of edible portion. Divide by six to work out approximate value per 100 grams of milk.

Peanuts, all types, raw	Units	Value	Peanuts, all types, raw	Units	Value

Calories	kcal	567	Manganese	mg	1.934
Protein	g	25.80	Selenium	mcg	7.2
Fat Sat. 6.834 Mono. 24.429 Poly. 15.555	g	46.818	Thiamin	mg	0.640
Calcium	mg	92	Riboflavin	mg	0.135
Iron	mg	4.58	Niacin	mg	12.066
Magnesium	mg	168	Pantothenic acid	mg	1.767
Phosphorus	mg	376	Vitamin B-6	mg	0.348
Potassium	mg	705	Folate	mcg	240
Zinc	mg	3.27	Vitamin E	mg	8.33
Copper	mg	1.144	Sterols	mg	220

Extract from USDA National Nutrient Database for Standard Reference, Release 17 (2004)

***

Pecan Nut Milk

(For milk recipe please see *Part Three*)

The pecan nut is the delicious fruit of the pecan tree which originates from the northeastern United States. The tree can grow to more than 10 m high and 6 m wide. Pecan nuts are oblong and thin shelled, and are eaten fresh or used in confectionery, pies and cakes. Pecan fossil remains show that the pecan tree and nut were prehistoric and pre-dated the first arrival of any human on the North American Continent.

It is undoubtedly the most important nut tree native to North America. The pecan served the North American Indians as a dietary staple long before the arrival of Europeans. Later the Indians traded pecans to the settlers for furs, trinkets and tobacco. Before the early sixteenth century, no European had ever seen a pecan.

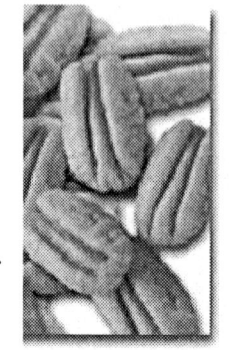

In the 1970's pecans were selected as the first and only fresh food to nourish American astronauts to the Moon and back on Apollo 13 and Apollo 14.

Today there are more than 500 improved varieties of pecan nuts, many with thinner shells, making them easier to crack. Annual production of pecan nuts is about one pound in weight for every citizen of the United States. The U.S. produces 80 percent of the world's pecan output.

Storage

Pecan nut oil is the very finest, and if the nuts are not stored properly they can go rancid. They must be sealed in airtight containers or plastic bags and be kept in a cool dark place. Pecans can be refrigerated, shelled or unshelled, for up to 9 months. Refrigeration is preferred for retaining the best possible flavor.

They can also be frozen shelled or unshelled for up to 2 years. They can be thawed and refrozen repeatedly without loss of flavor or texture. After removal from cold storage, pecans will stay fresh for about 2 months. When a pecan nut is fresh it will 'snap' when broken in half.

Nutritional benefits

Pecans are high in fat, but 90% is monounsaturated and polyunsaturated fat. The oils in pecans have a protective effect on the blood, lowering total blood cholesterol and preserving the HDL's that help combat heart disease. And in addition, pecans are believed to be helpful in fighting some cancers.

Loma Linda University researchers have determined that the oils in pecans are similar to olive oil, i.e. they are an excellent source of oleic acid, a fatty acid that combats cancer. Researchers have also found that eating one-third cup of pecans a day lowers the bad LDL cholesterol by 10% after four weeks. *'Pecan nuts can be part of a healthy diet'*, says Wanda Morgan, a nutritional scientist with the Agricultural Experiment Station at New Mexico State University.

Pecans are exceptionally high in Gamma-tocopherol, a compound that helps to slow down or stop the growth of prostate and lung cancer cells. ***'This is the first time gamma-tocopherol has been shown to induce death in laboratory-grown human cancer cells while leaving healthy cells alone.'*** [82]

Also, pecans have high levels of zinc, believed to be beneficial to the body's immune rejuvenation system; high levels of magnesium, beneficial in fighting heart disease and osteoporosis; and selenium, an antioxidant that fights stomach cancer. Pecans also contain vitamin E that helps prevent heart disease, some cancers, Parkinson's disease and cataracts.

Pecans are high in vitamin A, thiamin, and riboflavin (which are good for the eyes, the nervous system, and the skin). Pecan milk is delicious and provides an excellent source of nutrition. Consumed regularly, it is ideal as part of a balanced diet or a weight-loss regime.

Here is a summary list of the nutrients in pecan nuts:

Note: The 'Value' column shows value per 100 grams of edible portion. Divide by six to work out approximate value per 100 grams of milk.

Un-roasted pecan nuts	Units	Value	Un-roasted pecan nuts	Units	Value

Calories	kcal	691	Vitamin C	mg	1.1
Protein	g	9.17	Thiamin	mg	0.660
Fat Sat. 6.180 Mono. 40.801 Poly. 21.614	g	68.599	Riboflavin	mg	0.130
Calcium	mg	70	Niacin	mg	1.167
Iron	mg	2.53	Pantothenic acid	mg	0.863
Magnesium	mg	121	Vitamin B-6	mg	0.210
Phosphorus	mg	277	Folate	mcg	22
Potassium	mg	410	Vitamin A	IU	56
Zinc	mg	4.53	Vitamin E	mg	1.40
Copper	mg	1.200	Vitamin K	mcg	3.5
Manganese	mg	4.500	Gamma-tocopherol	mg	24.44
Selenium	mcg	3.8	Beta carotene	mcg	29

Extract from USDA National Nutrient Database for Standard Reference, Release 17 (2004)

***

Pine nut milk

(For milk recipe please see *Part Three*)

Pine nuts are seeds produced by pine trees (also known as *Pinon* or *Pynon* trees). They have been used as a food source for thousands of years, wherever pine trees grow. But only some species of pine trees produce edible pine nuts, and evidence of harvesting pine nuts goes back to before the time of ancient Rome and Greece.

Pine nuts have been a staple in the diet of native North American Indians, and the indigenous peoples of Siberia and the Russian Far East. Today pine nuts continue to be harvested in many regions of the Northern hemisphere and are marketed as a gourmet product because of their scarcity.

Pine trees that produce edible nuts vary in size from shrubs to 30m trees, depending on the species. They are adapted to a variety of conditions, from the extremely harsh and cold climate Siberia to the hot dry deserts of Nevada and Mexico. They also vary greatly in terms of pine nut productivity. Today the most important pine nut producers are located in Siberia, China, Korea, Italy, USA, and Mexico.

Apart from cooking and medicine, pine nut oil is used in cosmetics, beauty products, and as a high-end massage oil. It also has a variety of specialty uses such as a wood finish, paint base for paintings and treatment of fine skins in the leather industry.

The market for pine nuts and pine nut products is greatly underdeveloped, mainly because world pine nut production is so small. As a result demand for pine nuts is significantly greater than the available supply.

Efforts are being made to develop pine trees specifically for harvesting pine nuts – trees that can grow quickly, and produce lots of nuts that can be collected with machinery. Labour costs are particularly important given that pine nut collection and processing is very labour intensive.

Storage

Pine nuts are high in oil and if not stored properly they can go rancid. They must be sealed in airtight containers or plastic bags and may be kept in a cool dark place for up to two weeks if not refrigerated. Ideally, keep pine nuts refrigerated at all times.

Nutritional benefits

Pine nuts are rich in good quality protein as they are packed with all the 20 amino acids that make up protein, putting them on a par with soybeans in this respect. They are also high in vitamin A, thiamin, potassium, magnesium, niacin, and folate.

The fats in pine nuts are high quality, containing a healthy mix of monounsaturated polyunsaturated oils, characterized by high levels of both oleic and linoleic acids. Pine nuts also contain a small amount of saturated fat (about 16%). Here is a list of nutrients:

Note: The 'Value' column shows value per 100 grams of edible portion. Divide by six to work out approximate value per 100 grams of milk.

Raw pine nuts	Units	Value	Raw pine nuts	Units	Value
Calories	kcal	629	Copper	mg	1.035
Protein	g	11.57	Manganese	mg	4.333
Fat Sat. 9.377 Mono. 22.942 Poly. 25.668	g	57.987	Vitamin C	mg	2.0
Calcium	mg	8	Thiamin	mg	1.243
Iron	mg	3.06	Riboflavin	mg	0.223
Magnesium	mg	234	Niacin	mg	4.370
Phosphorus	mg	35	Pantothenic acid	mg	0.210
Potassium	mg	628	Vitamin B-6	mg	0.111
Sodium	mg	72	Folate	mcg	58

| Zinc | mg | 4.28 | Vitamin A | IU | 29 |

Extract from USDA National Nutrient Database for Standard Reference, Release 17 (2004)

***

Pumpkin Seed Milk

(For milk recipe please see *Part Three*)

Pumpkin seeds (also known as *pepitas*) are regarded by many as the most nutritious and delicious of all seeds. Their subtly sweet and nutty flavour is second to none, and they can be eaten raw or lightly roasted. People allergic to nuts can usually eat pumpkin seeds without any problems.

The flat, dark green pumpkin seeds are harvested from pumpkins that grow on the ground like melons. The seeds of all varieties of pumpkins are edible and today they are used all over the world in salads, soups, baked goods, casseroles, fish and meat dishes, and as snacks.

Pumpkin seeds also make excellent butters and oils, and of course, they make delicious milk (see recipe below). The dark green oil from pumpkin seeds can be purchased cold-pressed from health food stores – it is highly valued for its health promoting Omega-3 and Omega-9 fatty acids.

Demand for pumpkin seeds and oils has increased dramatically in recent years, approaching around US $200 million per year worldwide. Today, the leading commercial producers of pumpkins include the United States, Mexico, India and China.

Storage

The oil in pumpkin seeds can easily deteriorate, so they should be stored in an airtight container in the refrigerator. While they may stay edible for several months, they tend to lose their peak freshness after about two months of refrigeration. For longer storage, keep them in the freezer.

Nutritional benefits

The US Dept. of Agriculture says: *'Pumpkin seeds are loaded with vitamins and minerals. The seeds are rich in protein and unsaturated oil and contain significant zinc, potassium, and phosphorus.'* In a study, the USDA also concluded that diets high in pumpkin tended to curb the appetite yet provided more food for the same calorie count. The subjects in the study also absorbed less fat and calories from their food generally, making them less likely to become overweight.

Increasing incidence of prostate enlargement in U.S. men has catapulted pumpkin seeds into the health spotlight. The seeds contain chemical substances called *cucurbitacins* that can prevent the body from converting testosterone into a much more potent form of this hormone called *dihydrotestosterone*. Without *dihydrotestosterone*, it is more difficult for the body to produce more prostate cells, and therefore more difficult for the prostate to keep enlarging. The fact that pumpkin seeds serve as a good source of zinc makes them doubly well-suited for this role as a prostate protector, since zinc is a mineral also used by healthcare practitioners to help reduce prostate size.

In addition to a good range of minerals, pumpkin seeds provide significant amounts of vitamin A, E, and K.

Also, the high quality *essential fatty acids* in pumpkin seeds (Omega-6 and Omega-3 oils) help children grow well, and help adults prevent strokes and heart attacks. These fatty acids, also present in pumpkin seed milk, provide valuable nutrition for people of all ages.

Pumpkin seeds contain as much protein as meat, and a handful of pumpkin seeds provides nearly half the *Recommended Daily Allowance* for protein. The healing properties of pumpkin seeds have been investigated with respect to arthritis. Here is a list of the main nutrients in pumpkin seeds:

Note: The 'Value' column shows value per 100 grams of edible portion. Divide by six to work out approximate value per 100 grams of milk.

Raw pumpkin seeds	Units	Value	Raw pumpkin seeds	Units	Value
Calories	kcal	541	Selenium	mcg	5.6
Protein	g	24.54	Vitamin C	mg	1.9
Fat Sat. 8.674 Mono. 14.258 Poly. 20.702	g	43.634	Thiamin	mg	0.210
Calcium	mg	43	Riboflavin	mg	0.320
Iron	mg	14.97	Niacin	mg	1.745
Magnesium	mg	535	Pantothenic acid	mg	0.339
Phosphorus	mg	1174	Vitamin B-6	mg	0.224
Potassium	mg	807	Folate	mcg	58
Zinc	mg	7.46	Vitamin A	IU	380
Copper	mg	1.387	Vitamin K	mcg	51.4
Manganese	mg	3.021	Beta Carotene	mcg	228

Extract from USDA National Nutrient Database for Standard Reference, Release 17 (2004)

***

Sesame Seed Milk

(For milk recipe please see *Part Three*)

The exact origins of the sesame seed are unknown, though some claim it was the East Indies where it is also native. Now it is found growing in most tropical, subtropical, and southern temperate areas of the world. Most of today's commercially produced sesame seeds are grown throughout Central America, Mexico, and China, with India and Africa a close second.

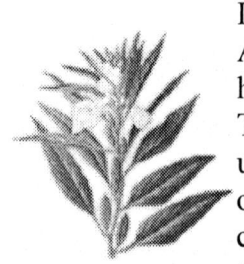

In the United States, sesame seeds are grown mainly in Arizona and Texas. Sesame seeds grow on a plant that has a hairy single stalk, though some do have branches. The average plant grows two to four feet high, some even up to 9 feet in high. The plant blossoms with white, pink or purplish flowers that develop into elongated pods containing numerous seeds stacked horizontally, one on top of the other, within the pod. The pear-shaped seed itself is encased in a fibrous hull that offers a range of colour from light tan to red, brown, and even black. Hulled seeds, those with the hulls removed, are an ivory white.

It is surprising that the tiny sesame seeds can be endowed with such depth of flavor. They are delicately sweet and nutty, and are delicious raw or toasted. Sesame seed oil and wine are highly prized.

The Europeans encountered sesame seeds when they were imported from India during the 1st century AD. They arrived in the United States with West African slaves during the 17th and 18th centuries. Today sesame seeds and their oils are used all over the world, and by all cultures and religions. Apart from food, sesame oil is used for many medicinal purposes, in cosmetics, and even in a variety of industrial processes.

Storage: Sesame seeds may be stored in an airtight container in a cool, dry place for up to three months, refrigerated up to six months or frozen up to one year.

Nutritional benefits

Sesame seeds are 25 percent protein and are rich in methionine and tryptophan, often lacking in adequate quantities in many plant proteins. One ounce of sesame seeds contains 6 grams of protein, 3.7 grams of fibre, and 14 grams of total fat. When toasted they lose nutrients, scoring 4.8 grams of protein and gaining a little fibre at 4.8 grams.

The fat in sesame seeds is truly super-healthy: 38% monounsaturated and 44% polyunsaturated, which equals ***82% unsaturated fatty acids.*** They are high in oleic and linoleic fatty acids and other health promoting oils. Also, unlike other oil-rich seeds, sesame seeds contain sesamol, a natural preservative that stops the seeds from going rancid too soon

Weight for weight, sesame seeds contain more than four times the amount of calcium compared to dairy milk. They also contain healthy amounts of the B vitamins riboflavin, thiamine, and niacin. With natural seeds scoring 8.7 mcg of folic acid for 1 tablespoon and plenty of vitamin B6, you can count on sesame seeds for excellent nourishment.

Sesame seeds, like pecan nuts, are exceptionally high in Gamma-tocopherol, a compound that helps to slow down or stop the growth of prostate and lung cancer cells. *'This is the first time gamma-tocopherol has been shown to induce death in laboratory-grown human cancer cells while leaving healthy cells alone.'* [82]

When it comes to minerals, sesame seeds are rich in iron, containing more than any meat, weight for weight. The high content of phosphorus in sesame seeds is counter-balanced by the high amounts of calcium and magnesium, ensuring good assimilation for strong bones and teeth. They also have good amounts of potassium, zinc, copper, manganese, and other health promoting nutrients.

All the goodness of sesame seeds is passed into the sesame milk and okara, giving everybody in your household a truly delicious and nutritious treat. Here is a list of the main nutrients in sesame seeds:

Note: The 'Value' column shows value per 100 grams of edible portion. Divide by six to work out approximate value per 100 grams of milk.

Raw sesame seeds	Units	Value	Raw sesame seeds	Units	Value
Calories	kcal	592	Manganese	mg	1.430
Protein	g	20.33	Selenium	mcg	1.7
Fat Sat. 7.672 Mono. 20.687 Poly. 24.011	g	52.37	Thiamin	mg	0.722
Calcium	mg	131	Riboflavin	mg	0.085
Iron	mg	7.80	Niacin	mg	4.682
Magnesium	mg	347	Pantothenic acid	mg	0.681
Phosphorus	mg	776	Vitamin B-6	mg	0.146
Potassium	mg	407	Folate	mcg	96
Sodium	mg	40	Vitamin A	IU	66
Zinc	mg	10.25	Vitamin E	mg	0.25

| Copper | mg | 1.460 | Beta Carotene | mcg | 40 |

Extract from USDA National Nutrient Database for Standard Reference, Release 17 (2004)

***

Soy milk

(For milk recipe please see *Part Three*)

The first written record of soybean (or soya bean) cultivation is from China in 2838 BCE. In 2853 BCE, Emperor Sheng-Nung of China named five sacred plants – soybeans, rice, wheat, barley, and millet. The Chinese farmers who grew soy fed it to their families as well as to their livestock.

Soybean plants were domesticated between 17th and 11th century BC in eastern China where they were cultivated into a regular food crop. Soybean cultivation spread to many parts of the world through the establishment of sea and land trade routes.

Soybean cultivation was introduced into Europe in 1712, and their cultivation became widespread in America in the 1900's. The US produced 75 million metric tons of soybeans in 2000 of which more than one-third was exported. Other leading producers of soybeans are Argentina, Brazil, China and India. Much of the US production is either fed to animals or exported, though US human consumption has been increasing. Brazil became the world's biggest soybean exporter in 2004, displacing the United States from the top seat. Today, the soybean is the world's foremost provider of protein and edible oil.

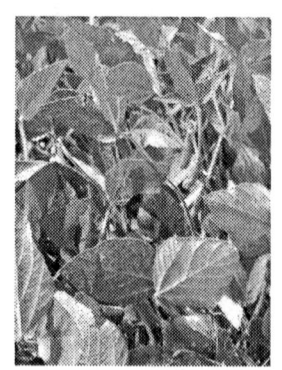

The soybean plant is like a small bush – it branches out in all directions and produces many leaves. The stems, leaves and pods are covered with short, fine hairs. Small white or purple flowers grow where the leaf joins the stem. These flowers then become pods of soybeans.

Soybeans can be found in a wide variety of products, ranging from tofu, soy milk and soy sauce to plywood, particle board, soy crayons, soy diesel, candles, printing inks, soap, candy products, cosmetics, and antibiotics.

Storage

Like all dried beans, soybeans are best stored in airtight containers or sealed in plastic bags, and kept in a cool, dark, day place. Under these conditions, soybeans will keep fresh for over a year. Do not store dried beans in the refrigerator. If storing for longer than a year freeze at the outset and use whenever thawed. Cooked soybeans should be consumed within 5 days if refrigerated, or within a year if deep frozen.

Nutritional benefits

Soybeans contain all three of the macro-nutrients required for good nutrition: complete protein, carbohydrate and fat, as well as being an excellent source of B vitamins, calcium, folic acid and iron.

Extensive research shows soybeans to have many anti-carcinogenic properties related to the unique benefits of soy isoflavones – these are phytochemicals which exert biological effects in humans and animals.

As mentioned in *Part One*, it may not be healthy to consume soy foods with high concentrations of isoflavones because of the high concentration of estrogen. But the consumption of soy foods made from *soy beans*, rather than soy protein powder, is known to be safe and healthy in moderation. In addition to fighting cancer, other scientific studies show that soybeans may help heart disease and diabetes.

Apart from quinoa, the soybean is the only common plant food that contains complete protein. Soybean protein provides all the essential amino acids in the amounts needed for human health. The amino acid profile of soy protein is better than most other protein foods, providing a high quality protein without the associated cholesterol or saturated fat.

Healthy fat

The fat in soybean is 61% polyunsaturated and 24% monounsaturated which is comparable to the total unsaturated fat content of many other vegetable oils. It is rich in two essential fatty acids, linoleic and linolenic, that are not produced in the body. Linoleic and linolenic acids help the body to absorb vital nutrients and are required for good health. These two essential acids are also precursors to hormones that regulate smooth muscle contraction, blood pressure, and the growth of healthy cells.

Pure soybean oil is about 50% linoleic acid and 8% linolenic acid. The small amount of saturated fat in soybeans is about 15% of total fat, which is similar to most vegetable oils.

Essential fibre

Soybeans contain both soluble and insoluble fibre, both essential for good health. In the soy milk recipe the soluble fibre is present in the milk, and the insoluble fibre is present in the leftover okara – so nothing is lost. Soluble fibre helps lower serum cholesterol and control blood sugar. Insoluble fibre increases stool bulk, prevents colon cancer, and can help relieve symptoms of several digestive disorders.

Here is a list of nutrients in soybeans:

Note: The 'Value' column shows value per 100 grams of edible portion. Divide by six to work out approximate value per 100 grams of milk.

Soybeans, cooked	Units	Value	Soybeans, cooked	Units	Value
Calories	kcal	173	Selenium	mcg	7.3
Protein	g	16.64	Vitamin C	mg	1.7
Fat Sat. 1.297 Mono. 1.981 Poly. 5.64	g	8.342	Thiamin	mg	0.155
			Riboflavin	mg	0.285
Calcium	mg	102	Niacin	mg	0.399
Iron	mg	5.14	Pantothenic acid	mg	0.179
Magnesium	mg	86	Vitamin B-6	mg	0.234
Phosphorus	mg	245	Folate	mcg	54
Potassium	mg	515	Vitamin A	IU	9
Zinc	mg	1.15	Vitamin E	mg	0.35
Copper	mg	0.407	Vitamin K	mcg	19.2
Manganese	mg	0.824	Beta Carotene	mcg	5

Extract from USDA National Nutrient Database for Standard Reference, Release 17 (2004)

***

Sprouted Seed Milk

(For milk recipe please see *Part Three*)

Whole books have been written on the wonders of sprouted seeds, their nutritional value, how to grow them, store them, etc. Here we are talking about baby plants that sprout from a variety of seeds. Common varieties include the seeds of nuts, grains, vegetables, grasses, and beans. Some of these sprouted seeds are suitable for making wonderful and nutritious milk.

When a tiny plant springs from a seed it is packed full of nutrients and valuable enzymes that are often lacking in the human diet. As a result of sprouting, the baby plant, weight for weight, contains an amazing 5 to 20 times more nutrients than a similar unsprouted seed. Virtually all sprouted seeds contain a healthy mix of digestible proteins, vitamins, minerals, trace minerals, antioxidants, chlorophyll pigments and enzymes, and generally have more nutritional value than any other kind of raw food.

A book on this subject noted that plant enzymes maintain digestion, detoxification, immunity and all other metabolic and regenerative processes. In addition to digesting food, enzymes destroy toxins, break down fats and cellulose, and metabolize starch and proteins. Enzymes are involved in every biochemical and physiological function of the body. [164]

In a major study of 120,000 people eating sprouted seeds over 33 years it was concluded that the health benefits of people who eat sprouted seeds were unsurpassed compared to a control group (those who didn't). [165]

In fact, it is known that by just eating two or three varieties of sprouted seeds you will get virtually every nutrient needed for good health, with nothing lacking. An examination of sprouted seeds and their nutritional benefits is beyond the scope of this book, and in any event the lists of nutrients for all varieties would be too long to publish. However, here are a few bullet points:

- **Where to buy sprouted seeds.** Sprouted seeds *ready for eating* are widely available from health food stores and many supermarkets. They can also be purchased by mail order or over internet, for postal or special delivery.

- **Where to buy seeds for sprouting.** Seeds for sprouting are also widely available from health food stores, specialist retailers, and gardening centres. Be sure to get seeds packaged especially for sprouting. Do not sprout seeds that have been treated for *outdoor* planting: they are not intended for human consumption and have been treated with pesticides.

- **Common sprouted seeds.** Some of the more common sprouted seeds include alfalfa, mung, radish, clover, adzuki, garbanzo (chickpea), lentil, soybean, sunflower, millet, quinoa, buckwheat, fenugreek, wheat, barley, corn, oats, green peas, and lima.

- **Out of sunlight.** Sprouted seeds develop best and are sweetest when grown indoors in the dark (sunlight is best avoided at all times). Sprouts will grow from the seeds very quickly and will be ready to eat within two to five days, depending on variety. All they require is clean water (no soil). Once ready to eat, they are best kept fresh in the refrigerator. Do not expose to sunlight. If exposed to sunlight they age more quickly, lose their nutritional value, and turn greener. The whiter the sprouts the better, particularly for making milk.

- **Wash & rinse.** Whether purchased or grown at home, always wash sprouted seeds before consumption or before making milk. Some kinds of sprouted seeds contain small amounts of natural toxins which act as deterrents to other plants and insects that may encroach. Simply immerse the sprouts in water and give a thorough rinse. Use cold water only.

- **All about sprouted seeds.** An excellent website with lots of good information about sprouted seeds is www.sproutpeople.com, based in the USA. To find a source of sprouted seeds or a website in your country simply enter 'sprouted seeds' in a search engine like Google and check the results. You can also find health books on Amazon.com that have sections relating to sprouted seeds. Fortunately, sprouted seeds store well in the refrigerator. A golden rule is to store the sprouts in as dry a condition as possible, using *airtight* containers or plastic bags. If stored correctly, most sprouted seeds can be refrigerated for several weeks and still stay fresh.

- **How much to consume.** As you become accustomed to consuming sprouts and *sprouted seed milk* you will find that you eat fewer unhealthy foods. Since the body is receiving a healthy daily dose of nutrients, the brain lessens the body's cravings for excessive eating. Sprouts are generally associated with healthy weight loss for those who are overweight. Most regular consumers of sprouted seeds typically eat 1 to 2 cupfuls in volume every day. Sprouted seed milk provides an ideal and convenient way of benefiting from their nutrients. Also, it provides an easy source of excellent nutrition for children.

- **Types of seeds to sprout.** In general, most nuts are not recommended for sprouting because they take weeks to germinate and may not taste very good when sprouted. Large beans such as black, red, navy, lima, pinto, and kidney beans will all sprout but don't taste very good in the raw sprouted form because they are so high in starch. Some grains are good sprouters. Hard and soft wheat, rye, and triticale all sprout well. Oats, barley, millet and brown rice will sprout, but are not very flavorful. Rice is impractical because it has such a long germination period.

- **Phytic acid.** In the chapter **Grain Milks** it was stated that grains should be eaten sparingly because they contain phytic acid which inhibits absorption of protein, minerals and trace elements. This does not apply to sprouted seeds from grains. In fact, grain sprouts are among the most nutritious and delicious of all sprouts.

- **Best sprouts for milk.** Whether you buy them ready-sprouted, or sprout them yourself, the following sprouted seeds make the best kinds of milk (listed in order of sweetness): Wheat, rye, triticale, spelt, kamut, sesame, amaranth, millet, quinoa, clover, mung bean, oats, alfafa. However, taste is very subjective and you may differ. Try starting with wheat, rye or triticale sprouted seeds and take it from there.

- **How to make sprouted seed milk.** Simply obtain enough sprouted seeds to fill one tightly packed cupful (8 fl ozs). Choose from one of the following: Wheat, rye, triticale, spelt, kamut, sesame, amaranth, millet, quinoa, clover, mung bean, oats, alfafa. Then refer to **Part Three** of the book where you will find **Table A** which shows how to prepare the sprouted seeds for making milk. Then follow the **Master Recipe** (see last page of book). As flavours of sprouted seeds vary, and as human tastes vary, you may have to adjust the finished flavour more to your liking. You may wish to use a different sweetener or add more salt, or more oil, or make the milk thicker/thinner. Ideally, you want to achieve a smooth milky flavour that has just a hint of sweetness. To get further ideas for tweaking the milk to your liking see the chapter 'Blended Milks' in **Part Three**. With flexibility and a degree of experimentation you will soon know exactly how to make sprouted seed milk just the way you like it. **Note:** in case you have jumped straight to this paragraph, please realize that we are talking about making milk out of the baby plants that grow out of the seeds, not the seeds themselves. For example, in the case of oats, you would be using the plants that grow out of the oat seeds.

***

Sunflower Seed Milk

(For milk recipe please see *Part Three*)

Sunflowers are native to both North and South America where indigenous people were first to cultivate them. The natives, following a 4,000-year-old practice, chose the largest seeds from the biggest heads year after year, developing the largest sunflowers that, in turn, produced the largest seeds.

Sunflower seeds were an important staple for Native Americans as early as 2300 BCE, and the Aztecs in Mexico were growing sunflowers and eating the seeds well before the white man arrived.

Spanish explorers and colonists introduced sunflower seeds to Europe in the 1500's from where they spread to Russia in the 1700's. During the 1800's sunflower seeds became popular in the USA and today they are mostly produced in the USA, Russia and Argentina.

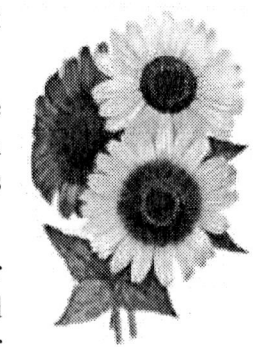

Storage: They are best stored in airtight containers or plastic bags in a cool dark place for up to four weeks if not refrigerated. Ideally, keep sunflower seeds refrigerated at all times. They can also be frozen.

Nutritional benefits

Sunflower seeds are rich in vitamin E, magnesium and selenium. Vitamin E helps protect the body from wear and tear by combating harmful free radicals. Magnesium is good for building and maintaining strong bones, and selenium helps protect against disease.

One ounce (28 grams) of raw seeds contains 160 calories and only 6 grams of carbohydrates. This, combined with the healthy non-fattening oils in the seeds make them an ideal snack in any weight-loss regime.

Excellent source of protein

Sunflower seeds are one of the richest sources of easily digested protein, containing all the essential amino acids. About 90% of the fat in sunflower seeds is unsaturated, providing valuable oils that the body can use for nutrition or for energy.

Here is a list of the main nutrients in sunflower seeds:

Note: The 'Value' column shows value per 100 grams of edible portion. Divide by six to work out approximate value per 100 grams of milk.

Raw sunflower seeds	Units	Value	Raw sunflower seeds	Units	Value
Calories	kcal	570	Selenium	mcg	59.5
Protein	g	22.78	Vitamin C	mg	1.4
Fat Sat. 5.195 Mono. 9.462 Poly. 32.735	g	47.392	Thiamin	mg	2.290
			Riboflavin	mg	0.250
Calcium	mg	116	Niacin	mg	4.500
Iron	mg	6.77	Pantothenic acid	mg	6.745
Magnesium	mg	354	Vitamin B-6	mg	0.770
Phosphorus	mg	705	Folate	mcg	227
Potassium	mg	689	Vitamin A, IU	IU	50
Zinc	mg	5.06	Vitamin E	mg	34.50
Copper	mg	1.752	Vitamin K	mcg	2.7
Manganese	mg	2.020	B-Carotene	mcg	30

Extract from USDA National Nutrient Database for Standard Reference, Release 17 (2004)

***

Tiger Nut Milk

(For milk recipe please see *Part Three*)

Tiger nut milk is one of my favourite non-dairy milks. It is delicious and refreshing, and can be used as a perfect substitute for dairy milk in just about any situation. The mis-named 'tiger nut' is not a nut – it is the root of the 'chufa' plant, hence tiger nuts are sometimes referred to as 'chufa tubers'. The plant itself looks like luscious long grass reaching about 45 cm (18 inches) in length – see picture.

The chufa plant is a perennial which, like the potato plant, sends out underground runners. When these long tubular roots are cut into one-inch sections they dry up into small acorn-size balls known as tiger nuts.

This plant has its origin in ancient Egypt, as the chufa is one of the earliest domesticated crops known to man. Pictures of the chufa plant can be seen on ancient vases, and chufa remains have been found in the tombs of the Egyptian pharaohs.

Tiger nuts are cultivated mainly in North Africa and Spain, and tiger nut milk is becoming increasingly popular, particularly in the Americas and in Europe.

Tiger nut milk has an almost almond-like flavor and is used as a flavoring agent for nut roasting, ice cream and biscuits/cookies. Consumers in Spain enjoy tiger nut milk as a popular beverage that is widely served in restaurants and cafes.

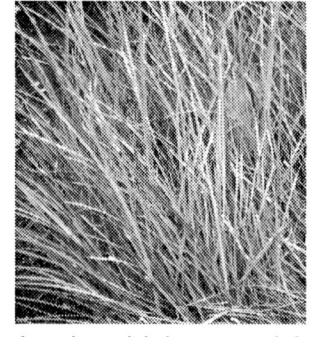

The tiger nut plant is also produced in Florida, USA, as food or fodder for livestock, hogs, deer, turkey, and waterfowl. Tiger nut oil, considered to be superior to olive oil, is used in many beauty products, and industrial processes such as the waterproofing of textile fibers. When trying to buy tiger nuts you may discover they are sold as bait for fishing – do not let this put you off as tiger nuts make a delicious, healthy, and super nutritious non-dairy milk that is second to none!

Storage: Store in an air tight bag or container, in a cool dark place.

Nutritional benefits

Tiger nuts are rich in nutrients as summarized below.

Oils. The high amount of unsaturated fatty acids (83.8%) and especially the high percentage of oleic acid (70%) is similar to that of olives and hazelnuts. Here are some of the health benefits:

- Reduces bad/LDL cholesterol and increases good/HDL cholesterol by reducing levels of triglycerides in the blood.
- Reduces risk of formation of blood clots and produces dilatation in veins, preventing arteriosclerosis.
- Positive effects on digestive secretions (gastric, pancreatic and biliar), due to high content of oleic acid, the most powerful stimulator of production of colecistokine (responsible for digestive secretions).

Vitamins. The excellent amount of vitamin E makes tiger nuts ideal for infants and the elderly because of the antioxidant effect on cell membranes. For fertility vitamin E helps to fix the embryo in the uterus and increases fertility of men and women. Also, vitamin E helps keep the skin healthy. Tiger nuts are also high in vitamin A, important for vision, reproduction, body cell growth, healthy skin, and a stronger immune system.

Prevention of cancer

'Scientists have discovered why eating a Mediterranean diet rich in fruits, vegetables and particularly olive oil can help to protect women from developing breast cancer. The key is oleic acid, the main component of olive oil [and tiger nuts]. Oleic acid blocks the action of a cancer-causing oncogene called HER-2/neu which is found in about 30 percent of breast cancer patients.' **Source:** study by Northwestern University Feinberg School of Medicine (Dr Javier Menendez), Chicago, USA, January 2005.

'According to several studies, tiger nuts have been shown to reduce the risk of colon cancer, they are suitable for diabetic persons, and they help you lose surplus body fat.' **Source:** study by University of Valencia, Facultad de Medicina (Valls, Bixquert, Farre), Spain, 2003.

Minerals. Tiger nuts have good amounts of calcium and magnesium. They also provide small amounts of manganese, iron, zinc, and copper.

Folic acid. Folic acid helps the body make new cells for general good health, making tiger nut milk a super healthy option (just one cup provides more than half the Recommended Daily Allowance). Tiger nut milk is ideal for any woman contemplating pregnancy as folic acid helps prevent birth defects. Some studies show that folic acid helps protect women and men from heart disease, cervical and colon cancer and possibly breast cancer.

Here is a list of the main nutrients in tiger nuts:

Note: The 'Value' column shows value per 100 grams of edible portion. Divide by six to work out approximate value per 100 grams of milk.

Tiger nuts	Units	Value	Tiger nuts	Units	Value
Calories	kcal	266	Zinc	mg	16.66
Protein	g	7.5	Copper	mg	4.915
Fat Sat. 4.165 Mono. 11.66 Poly. 2.5	g	18.325	Manganese	mg	4.082
			Thiamin	mg	0.167
Calcium	mg	14.161	Riboflavin	mg	trace
Iron	mg	23.32	Vitamin D	mg	2.416

Magnesium	mg	42.48	Vitamin E	mg	4.165
Phosphorus	mg	372.35	Folic acid	mcg	47.48
Potassium	mg	0.158	Vitamin A	IU	24.157

***

Walnut Milk

(For milk recipe please see *Part Three*)

Walnuts are an ancient human food as evidenced by walnut shells dating back more than 8,000 years found in France.

Around 2,000 BC in Mesopotamia, the Chaldeans left inscriptions on clay tablets revealing the existence of walnut groves within the famed Hanging Gardens of Babylon. Other evidence shows that walnuts and walnut oil have been used since ancient times.

USA Walnuts

The first commercial plantings of walnuts in the USA began in 1867 when Joseph Sexton planted *English walnuts*. (The name English walnut came from transport of walnuts from Asia Minor to England aboard English boats).

California, USA, is now a major walnut growing region. Its mild climate and deep fertile soils provide ideal growing conditions for the California walnut which accounts for 99 percent of the commercial US supply and about a fifth of world supply.

Walnuts are produced commercially in about 49 countries, the biggest production being in China, followed by the USA, Iran, Turkey, and Ukraine. Black walnuts, a much sought after variety, are grown in the USA.

Apart from the nut kernels, walnuts are used in many other ways: the leaves of walnut trees are being studied for use as a cancer therapy drug among other things. Walnut shells are ground and used as anti-skid agents for tires, blasting grit, activated carbon, and sometimes as an adulterant of spices. The husk yields a valuable oil and a yellow dye when pressed. Walnut oil is used in soaps, paints, and dyes. The oil from walnut kernels is high in unsaturated fats and can be used in cooking. The wood from walnut trees is highly prized and is used mostly for top quality furniture and gun making.

Storage

Walnuts go rancid more quickly than most nuts because of their high quality oil. Therefore, walnuts out of their shells should be kept refrigerated in an air tight plastic bag where they will stay fresh for about 4-6 months.

Walnuts in their shells do not have to be refrigerated: they will stay fresh for about 4-6 months if stored in a cool dry place, in airtight plastic bags or containers. Walnuts can be frozen (shelled or unshelled) for 12 – 18 months, so long as used as soon as thawed. *Never use walnuts for making milk if they are beginning to taste rancid.*

Nutritional benefits

Walnuts contain a wide variety of nutrients including numerous vitamins and minerals, such as vitamin E, thiamin, vitamin B6, folate, magnesium, copper and zinc. They are also a good source of protein. Walnuts are one of the few good plant sources of Omega-3 oil. Just one ounce of walnuts contains 2.57 grams (many times higher than any other kind of nut). This means it is an excellent source of alpha-linolenic acid, an essential fatty acid that is good for the brain and general good health. Most of the fats in walnuts are unsaturated, with only about ten percent saturated, making walnuts a healthy and non-fattening addition to the diet.

Good for combating diabetes & heart disease

The Walnut Marketing Board in the USA recommends eating about 8 walnut halves a day to fully benefit from walnut nutrition. A study in Australia shows that for patients with type 2 diabetes, a *whole-foods-diet* including walnuts can reduce LDL 'bad' cholesterol by 10%. [92]

The US FDA states that *walnuts can aid in reducing cholesterol levels.* Walnuts are also noted for reducing the risk of heart disease and inflammation. Here is a list of the main nutrients in walnuts:

Note: 'Value' column shows value per 100 grams of edible portion. Divide by six to work out approximate value per 100 grams of milk

Unroasted walnuts	Units	Value	Unroasted walnuts	Units	Value
Calories	kcal	654	Vitamin C	mg	1.3
Protein	g	15.23	Thiamin	mg	0.341
Fat Sat. 6.126 Mono. 8.933 Poly. 47.174	g	62.23	Riboflavin	mg	0.150
			Selenium	mcg	4.9
Calcium	mg	98	Niacin	mg	1.125
Iron	mg	2.91	Pantothenic acid	mg	0.570

Magnesium	mg	158	Vitamin B-6	mg	0.537
Phosphorus	mg	346	Folate	mcg	98
Potassium	mg	441	Vitamin A, IU	IU	20
Sodium	mg	2	Vitamin E	mg	0.70
Zinc	mg	3.09	Gamma Tocopherol	mg	20.83
Copper	mg	1.586	Vitamin K	mcg	2.7
Manganese	mg	3.414	Beta Carotene	mcg	12

Extract from USDA National Nutrient Database for Standard Reference, Release 17 (2004)

PART THREE: NON-DAIRY MILK RECIPES

All milk recipes are given in the chapter titled:
The Master Recipe.
Milk recipes can also be located by checking the index at the end of this book.

***

Recipe Tips & Tricks

Important note: No milk of any kind (dairy or non-dairy) should be given to a child under one, except mother's breast milk or infant formula. If giving non-dairy milk to a child under four please see the chapter Dairy Milk Effect on Young People in Part One.

The information that follows will save you time and make the recipes easy to make.

1. Measurements. The volume for every recipe will give you at least 1 litre (2 pints or 1 US quart) of liquid milk, plus the leftover residue. In the recipes, no distinction is made between British and American sizes for cups, fluid ounces, and spoons because the differences are too small to matter for the amount of milk being made. In case you are wondering how they compare, Fig. 1 gives a comparison.

Fig. 1
British & American Measurements

British Standard	American Standard
1 cup = 0.227 litres (liters)	1 cup = 0.236 litres (liters)
1 pint = 0.568 litres (liters)	1 pint = 0.473 litres (liters)
1 fluid ounce = 0.0284 litres (liters)	1 fluid ounce = 0.0295 litres (liters)
1 tablespoon = 18 ml.	1 tablespoon = 15 ml.

| 1 teaspoon = 6 ml. | 1 teaspoon = 5 ml. |

As you can see, compared to British measurements, American cup measurements are slightly larger but the spoon measurements are slightly smaller, but not enough to matter. Whether you are using British or American measurements, the main thing to remember is that 1 cup equals 8 fluid ounces.

To make a different volume simply increase or reduce the ingredients proportionally. Afterwards, the milk can be made thinner at any time by just adding water. Always use the cleanest drinking-quality water available when making milk. ***Important: if you only have tap water available, boil the water and let cool before use. This will stop the milk deteriorating while stored for several days in the refrigerator.***

Throughout the recipes in this book, a *cup measurement* of the basic ingredient refers to the raw, uncooked, non-soaked ingredient. Regarding nuts, a cup measurement refers to non-soaked nuts without their shells.

2. Straining. A large strainer (sieve) may be used by pressing the okara (the leftover residue) into the strainer with the back of a large spoon. ***Always use a large bowl.*** Alternatively a cheese cloth or 'jelly strainer' (from Wallmart) may be used but the cloth mesh may be too tight for easy straining. A good method is to use a nylon stocking. Use a new white-coloured knee-high nylon stocking, and squeeze with your hand to get the last of the milk through the nylon. It's a good idea to re-cycle the okara through the strainer or cloth a *second time* to extract the maximum amount of milk form the okara (use less water the first time). Simply put the okara back into the blender and briefly blend with more water, then strain again.

Tip
When pouring the recipe-mixture into nylon stoking, use a funnel. Hold funnel inside the top of the stocking. To make a funnel use a pair of scissors to cut off the bottom of an empty yogurt container. Add this item to your milk-making kit.

---

3. Cleaning the straining cloth. After making milk, rinse out the nylon stocking (or cheese cloth) and boil or microwave the item *immersed in water* for 3-5 minutes to sterilize for future milk-making. **Do not put the item in the laundry or wash with any soap powders** as traces of detergents will get into the cloth. **Note:** if using for the first time (whether new or not) boil the cloth or nylon stocking *twice* (and discard water in between boils) before using. This will remove any harmful chemicals and detergents in the fabric.

4. Refrigeration. Keep home-made milk refrigerated in a jug or container *with a lid*. Use within 4 – 5 days maximum. Mix or shake milk whenever serving. Some non-dairy milks stay better mixed than others, but they are all just as good! The milk may also be frozen for future use, using either freezer bags or air-tight freezer containers. When freezing, always divide milk into smaller serving portions of, say, 1 or 2 cups. That way, the milk will be fresher when used. The same goes for the okara.

5. Okara. The leftover okara for many of the recipes is super-nutritious and full of valuable easy-to-digest fibre. It also contains the same kind of vitamins and minerals as in the original ingredients for the milk. Use the okara to add flavour, fibre, and nutrition to just about any dish you are making.

You will find that okara 'gets lost' into whatever you are making as it absorbs the taste of the dish. Think of it as a neutral, but nutritious bulking agent. Okara is easily frozen for future use – best to freeze in 1 cup portions. Do not keep okara in the fridge unless using within 1 – 3 days.

The golden rule is: whenever cooking, think OKARA. Here are some ideas for using okara:

- Add it to soups, casseroles, lasagna, baked dishes, or just about any savoury dish you can think of.
- Add it to steamed or fried food by simply mixing it in as you cook.
- Add it to desserts, home made ice-creams, home-made cookies, bread, cakes, trifles, and just about any kind of cooked dessert.
- Add it to any kind of fruit smoothie or ice-cream to give it valuable fibre, and make it super-nutritious.

6. Sweetening agent. The milk recipes include a 'sweetening agent.' The amount of sweetness is entirely optional as personal tastes vary, and the natural sweetness of the different kinds of milk will vary. Here is a list of possible sweetening agents – ***use just one of them at a time***, and feel free to increase or reduce the amounts according to taste:

- 4 dates or 4 prunes, soaked in water until soft.
- 4 teaspoons maple syrup or agave syrup.
- 4 teaspoons treacle (black strap molasses).
- 4 table-spoons of any kind of berries (frozen or fresh): strawberries, blackberries, blueberries, cranberries, or raspberries. It does not matter at all if this causes the milk to become slightly fruit-coloured, but you may have to explain it to your guests!
- Half a teaspoon or less of stevia (a natural sweetener).
- 4 table-spoons of pure apple juice (less if concentrated).

It is best to avoid sugar and artificial sweeteners as they contain empty calories and are not good for health. Also, honey is best avoided because of the risk of infant botulism and its high glycaemic index rating (83). If you want to know the blunt facts about honey go to:

http://www.sammonsays.com/artman/publish/printer_truth-about-honey-article.shtml (but you may not like what you read).

7. Nutritional content. *Part Two* of this book gives nutritional tables for non-dairy milk. To calculate the approximate nutritional content of the derived milk, divide the figure in the third column of the nutritional table (value per 100 grams) by **SIX**. This will give you the approximate value per 100 grams of liquid milk. This is, of course, only a rough & ready calculation that assumes the nutrients are spread over 5 parts of water and 1 part of left-over okara.

8. Enjoy a different taste. Please do not expect any kind of non-dairy milk to taste like cow's milk. Every non-dairy milk (whether home-made or commercial) has a unique taste that is quite different to the dairy milk you may be used to.

Some non-dairy milks will be an acquired taste (please be patient and give them a chance), and some will be instantly gratifying. Some non-dairy milks will separate more easily than others while stored in the fridge. This is quite normal – just mix the milk each time before serving. Also, the colour and even the texture of some non-dairy milks will vary from one making to another.

Think of each batch of home-made milk as a unique product with its own special characteristics rather than as a substitute for dairy milk. When offering it to other people (family or guests) get into the habit of referring to any kind of non-dairy milk by its full name, e.g. *almond milk*. This avoids the danger that somebody who is allergic to nuts might inadvertently consume it. Always be aware that some people are allergic to nuts (and this includes milk made from nuts).

***

The Master Recipe

Note: For background and nutritional information to the recipes please see *Part Two* of book.

Instead of giving a separate recipe for each kind of non-dairy milk, there is just *one master recipe* to follow. This makes it much easier to remember how to make milk. It is strongly recommended that you start by making a nut or seed-based milk such as *almond milk* – this kind of milk is delicious and it will encourage you to keep making milk.

Step one: Prepare the basic ingredient as indicated in Table A below. For example, if you want to make chestnut milk, Table A shows how to prepare the chestnuts before following the *master recipe* in step two.

Step two: Follow the master recipe given at the end of this chapter. For quick reference, a summary of the master recipe is also given on the last page of this book.

> *You can make any recipe in this book in under ten minutes once you have prepared the basic ingredient as explained in Table A*

Table A starts on the next page ▶

Table A

Preparation of basic ingredient
(See notes at the end of Table A)

Basic ingredient	Okara *Left-over residue*	Preparation *For basic ingredient measure 1 cup of raw product before grinding/soaking/cooking, etc.*
Almonds (dry almonds)	Good to use	Grind dry almonds into powder using grain mill. Raw unsalted nuts are best. Put into blender.
Almonds (soaked almonds)	Good to use	Soak raw almonds in large bowl, overnight or minimum 6 hours. After soaking, rinse and discard water. Put soaked almonds in blender. This method produces a slightly richer and more nutritious milk than using dry almonds.
Brazil nuts	Good to use	Grind brazil nuts into powder using grain mill. Raw unsalted nuts are best. Put into blender.
Cashew nuts	Good to use	Grind cashew nuts into powder using grain mill. Fresh unsalted nuts are best. Put into blender.

Basic ingredient	Okara *Left-over residue*	Preparation *For basic ingredient measure 1 cup of raw product before grinding/soaking/cooking, etc.*
Chestnuts	Good to use	1. There is no need to cook the chestnuts except for the purpose of removing skins. Use fresh or frozen peeled chestnuts. To remove skins cut the skin three quarters of the way around using a sharp or serrated knife. Boil or bake for 5 - 10 minutes for purpose of removing skins. If defrosting peeled chestnuts, wash and dry before grinding. Check to make sure there are no remaining bits of skin on the chestnuts. Also check for signs of mould, and either discard the chestnut or cut off the affected part. Burn marks caused by the mechanized chestnut peeling-process do not matter as they only affect the surface. Mould marks go into the chestnut, so if necessary cut open and check. 2. Grind chestnuts into powder using grain mill. If any chestnut bits fail to grind into powder, chop into crumbs instead. Put into blender. Also add 2 spoonfuls of olive oil or any good quality monounsaturated oil.
Coconut	Not suitable	1. Drain and strain coconut juice and put into blender. To check that coconut is edible and fresh, coconut juice should be sweet tasting. If bitter, discard coconut. 2. To remove coconut flesh from shell: wrap coconut in towel/cloth and smash coconut with hammer, on a flat hard/concrete floor. There is no need to take brown skin off the flesh unless you intend to use the left-over okara for other recipes. Wash coconut flesh to remove debris, and cut into 1-2 inch pieces. Be careful to remove all pieces of coconut shell so that blender blades do not get damaged. Put coconut pieces into blender.

Basic ingredient	Okara *Left-over residue*	Preparation *For basic ingredient measure 1 cup of raw product before grinding/soaking/cooking, etc.*
Corn, fresh off the cob. **Note:** Must be freshly picked cobs with sweet, juicy corn (known as *sweet corn*, not *field corn*),	Good to use	Blanch for 1 minute (see **Part Two** if unsure). Then remove corn kernels and put into blender. Also add to blender: • 2 heaped tablespoons of sesame seeds or pine kernels, ***ground into powder***. • 1/4 teaspoon almond, vanilla, or coconut extract (do not overdo). • 1/8 tsp. ground cinnamon. • 2 tablespoons (4 teaspoons) olive oil, or any good-quality monounsaturated oil. For added flavour, blend finished milk with a nut or seed based milk.
Green peas (frozen or fresh)	Not suitable	Steep for 15 min. or simmer for 2 min. Then put peas *and water* into blender. Also add to blender: • 2 heaped tablespoons of sesame seeds or pine kernels, *ground into powder*. • 1/4 teaspoon almond, vanilla, or coconut extract (do not overdo). • 1/8 tsp. ground cinnamon. • 2 tablespoons (4 teaspoons) olive oil, or any good-quality monounsaturated oil. For added flavour, blend finished milk with a nut or seed based milk.
Hazelnuts (dry hazelnuts)	Good to use	Grind dry hazelnuts into powder using grain mill. Raw unsalted nuts are best. Put into blender.
Hazelnuts (soaked hazelnuts)	Good to use	Soak raw hazelnuts overnight or minimum 6 hours. After soaking, rinse and discard water. Put soaked hazelnuts in blender. This method produces a slightly richer and more nutritious milk than using ground dry hazelnuts.

Basic ingredient	Okara *Left-over residue*	Preparation *For basic ingredient measure 1 cup of raw product before grinding/soaking/cooking, etc.*
Hemp seeds	Not suitable	1. Depending on the country, hemp seeds in their hulls may be purchased as *sterilized* or *unsterilized*, the latter being better for milk making. Hemp seeds may be purchased over Internet if not available locally (do a search for 'hemp seeds'). In the USA and North America there are several suppliers, among them www.hempoilcan.com, Canada, T 204-275-7616. In the UK unsterilized hemp seeds in their hulls can be purchased from most health food stores. 2. It is best to use and grind hemp seeds *in their hulls* for making nutritious milk. Hemp seeds without hulls can also be purchased and used but the milk will be a little less tasty and nutritious. 3. Grind hemp seeds into powder using grain mill. Put into blender
Macadamia nuts	Good to use	Grind macadamia nuts into powder using grain mill. Raw unsalted nuts are best. Put into blender.
Oats, use one of following: • Old fashioned oats • Rolled oats • Quick oats (not 'instant') • Steel cut oats • Porridge oats	Not suitable	Grind into powder (no hot water or cooking). Then put ground oats into blender. Also add to blender: • 2 heaped tablespoons of sesame seeds or pine kernels, *ground into powder*. • 1/4 teaspoon almond, vanilla, or coconut extract (do not overdo). • 1/8 tsp. ground cinnamon. • 2 tablespoons (4 teaspoons) olive oil, or any good-quality monounsaturated oil. For added flavour, blend finished milk with a nut or seed based milk. *Note: Do not use warm or hot water at any stage of making recipe*

Basic ingredient	Okara *Left-over residue*	**Preparation** *For basic ingredient measure 1 cup of raw product before grinding/soaking/cooking, etc.*
Pea milk	→	See under '**Green peas**'
Peanuts	Good to use	Grind peanuts into powder using grain mill. Raw unsalted nuts are best. Put into blender.
Pecan nuts	Good to use	Grind pecan nuts into powder using grain mill. Raw unsalted nuts are best. Put into blender.
Pine nuts	Good to use	Grind pine nuts into powder using grain mill. Raw unsalted nuts are best. Put into blender.
Pumpkin seeds	Good to use	Grind pumpkin seeds into powder using grain mill. Raw unsalted seeds are best. Put into blender. Note: pumpkin seed milk may look a little green – it is perfectly normal and perfectly delicious!
Sesame seeds	Good to use	Grind sesame seeds into powder using grain mill. Put into blender.
Soybeans (Soya beans)	Good to use	1. Thoroughly wash and rinse soybeans. Then soak soybeans overnight (minimum eight hours) in plenty of water. Soybeans swell to at least three times their size. After soaking, throw away soaked water and rinse beans again. 2. Boil soybeans until tender enough to eat (30 – 60 minutes or longer). Do not over-boil. Do not add any salt or fat to cooking process. Discard boiled water as this gets rid of the *trypsin inhibitor*, a natural substance that inhibits digestion of soy protein. Then put cooked soybeans into blender. 3. Add to blender 1/8 tsp. vanilla or coconut extract and 2 tablespoons olive oil (or any good quality monounsaturated oil).

Basic ingredient	Okara *Left-over residue*	Preparation *For basic ingredient measure 1 cup of raw product before grinding/soaking/cooking, etc.*
Sprouted seeds **Note:** The best tasting sprouted seeds for making milk are given in the chapter 'Sprouted Seed Milk' in *Part Two*.	Good to use	1. Measure one tightly packed cupful of sprouted seeds. Then Wash and rinse sprouts and put into blender. 2. Also add to blender: • 2 heaped tablespoons from one of the following: sesame seeds, pine kernels, brazil nuts, or macadamia nuts (but first they must be ***ground into powder***). • 1/4 teaspoon almond, vanilla, or coconut extract (do not overdo). • 1/8 tsp. ground cinnamon. • 2 tablespoons (4-6 teaspoons) olive oil, or any good-quality monounsaturated oil. 3. For added flavour, blend finished milk with a nut or seed based milk.
Sunflower seeds	Good to use	Grind sunflower seeds into powder using grain mill. Raw unsalted seeds are best. Put into blender. Note: For a better result, soak the seeds overnight, wash and blend.

Basic ingredient	Okara *Left-over residue*	Preparation *For basic ingredient measure 1 cup of raw product before grinding/soaking/cooking, etc.*
Tiger nuts **Note:** Tiger nuts are not nuts, they are the roots of a plant.	Not suitable	1. Tiger nuts are generally available from health food stores or fishing tackle stores (do not let this put you off). Alternatively, contact a major grain wholesaler or do a search on Internet. To find out where to buy tiger nuts in the UK contact *Community Foods Ltd*, tel. 0208 2082966, www.communityfoods.co.uk. 2. Thoroughly wash/rinse tiger nuts to remove any debris. Then soak overnight or for a minimum of 12 hours. After soaking, discard soaked water, rinse again, and dry the nuts in a cloth before grinding. **Soaking the tiger nuts is essential** because it softens them and this helps the grinding and blending process. 3. Grind tiger nuts into powder using grain mill and put into blender. Also add 1/8 teaspoon cinnamon and 2 spoonfuls of olive oil, or any good quality monounsaturated oil. 4. For added flavour, blend finished milk with a nut or seed based milk.
Walnuts	Good to use	Carefully check that all pieces of walnut shell have been removed. Then grind walnuts into powder using grain mill. Raw unsalted nuts are best. Put into blender.

Notes relating to Table A:

1. **Remove debris:** Carefully check basic ingredient to make sure it is clean and free from debris before starting any recipe.

2. **Approximate conversions:**

    1 litre (liter) = 2 pints = 4 cups = 32 fl. ounces = 1 US quart

3. **Tips & tricks:** Please see 'Recipe Tips & Tricks' chapter before making milk as this will save you time.

4. **Nut allergy:** Always be aware that some people may be allergic to nuts and nut-based milks.

5. **To steep:** Pour boiling water over the basic ingredient until fully immersed. Cover and let stand until ingredient is tender enough to bite into (steep for 10 to 60 minutes, depending on ingredient).

6. **Water measurement:** Mark your blender at the six-cup point (48 fl oz, 1420 ml) – use a dab of nail varnish or tippex to mark point. This saves having to measure each cup of water. Simply add the ingredients to the blender. Then blend the ingredients by gradually adding water until you reach the 6-cup point.

7. **Okara:** 'Good to use' means it can be used successfully in other recipes and is therefore worth keeping. 'Not suitable' means it is not practical to use and should be discarded or recycled in the garden.

The Master Recipe

(A summary of this master recipe is also given on last page of book)

Makes approximate volume: 1 litre/2 pints/1 quart

1 CUP = 8 FL OZS = 1/2 PINT = 237ML

You will need:

A. Blender.
B. Grinder or grain mill (required for some of the recipes).
C. Knee-length nylon stocking (or strainer/sieve/cheesecloth) for separating the milk from the okara.
D. Drinking-quality water (at least 5 cups, depending on preparation of basic ingredient).
E. 1 cup **basic ingredient**, i.e. raw ingredient, before being prepared/ground/soaked/cooked.
F. 1/8 tsp. salt.
G. Sweetening agent (see chapter titled **Recipe Tips & Tricks** for sweetener suggestions).

Method:

1. **First blend:** Put all ingredients that apply into the blender, i.e. the ingredients listed above plus the ingredients mentioned in Table A. Also add enough water (as little as possible) for blender to work and mix the ingredients. Use warm or hot water, but not too hot to touch. Blend until smooth.

2. **Adding water:** Gradually add further *cold* water until you reach the 6 cup mark (48 fl. oz or 1420 ml) on your blender. Blend for 1 to 3 minutes until you think the mixture is smooth.

3. **Straining:** Strain the mixture to get as much milk as possible. If using a nylon stocking, knead and squeeze the filled-up stocking over a large bowl to extract as much liquid as possible. This will only take 1 or 2

minutes using your hands. Alternatively, use a large strainer and the back of serving spoon to press out as much liquid as possible. You may have to do this in two stages: half first, then remove the okara (left-over residue) to do the second half.

4. **Extra bonus:** You may wish to squeeze extra milk out of the recipe by putting the okara back into the blender and briefly blending with a little more water. This works particularly well with coconut and other nut-based milks.

5. **Tweaking the milk:** If after straining, the result is too thick, simply mix in a little extra water. If the taste is not sweet enough, add extra sweetener. With any recipe there is a degree of 'trial and error' as human tastes and ingredients vary, but you will soon get to make milk exactly how you like it. Always remember that when left standing, some of the milks will separate (from the water) more than others. This is perfectly natural – simply shake or stir before serving!

6. **Refrigeration:** It is essential to keep the milk refrigerated at all times, and use up within five days maximum. Alternatively, freeze some of the milk for future use.

7. **Okara:** Either keep/freeze the left-over okara for use in other cooking recipes or discard. Some recipes do not produce okara that can be used (or enough of it), depending on the ingredient – see Table A for guidance.

***

Blended Milks

This book gives recipes for a big selection of non-dairy milks, and some recipes will no doubt become your favourites. It's useful to know, however, that there are several things you can do to add variety and zest to home-made milk. Also, you can mix or blend different milks for exciting new tastes. An added advantage of blending milk is that you get a greater range of nutrients in a single helping.

Before proceeding we recommend that you first become familiar with at least two or three milk recipes given in this book, and then come back to this chapter whenever you wish to experiment with other milk-making possibilities.

Adding variety to your milk

For added variety, here are some things you can do to 'tweak' the milk:

- Add a condiment to the recipe. Chose one of the following:
  - **Cinnamon.** Add 1/8 teaspoon of ground cinnamon to ingredients. This will give a very light sense of cinnamon without being overbearing. Be careful to not overdo the amount.
  - **Cardamom.** Add 1/8 teaspoon of ground up cardamom to ingredients. This condiment goes well with home-made milk, particularly the recipes that do not include nuts. Be careful to not overdo the amount.
  - **Nutmeg.** Add 1/8 teaspoon of ground nutmeg to ingredients. This condiment is a good alternative to cinnamon or cardamom, giving home-made milk a lovely aroma. Recommended for recipes that do not include nuts. Be careful to not overdo the amount.

- **Almond & coconut extract.** If a recipe calls for vanilla extract, change this for almond or coconut extract to give variety. Do not fall into the trap of adding vanilla extract to every milk recipe, or over-doing the amount – you may get fed-up with it!

- **Sweetener.** Change the sweetener (or the amount) that you have been using so as to give a different taste. Concentrated apple juice goes well with just about any milk recipe, and this is often used by commercial producers of non-dairy milk. Or try different kinds of dried fruit (soaked overnight in water).

- **Lecithin.** Add a heaped tablespoon of lecithin granules to the recipe. I do this whatever kind of milk I am making. Lecithin granules (made from soybeans) are widely available from health food stores all over the world. Lecithin is also made by the body as it plays an important role in protecting the nervous system, the liver, the avoidance of gallstones, and the breakdown and efficient use of dietary fat. Lecithin is often recommended for people on low fat diets. By adding a spoonful of lecithin granules to a milk recipe the fat and the water in the milk will mix better, giving you a thicker, better tasting milk (and more nutritious!).

- **Salt.** Many recipes include salt (1/8 teaspoon) in the ingredients. This is a tiny amount. If you wish, you may try increasing this to say ¼ teaspoon, to see if you like this better – this is still not very much when diluted with at least 5 cups of liquid. Equally, if you are keen to reduce salt in your diet, you can completely avoid adding any salt to the recipe. Let's remember that all kinds of non-dairy milk contain low amounts of salt (i.e. sodium), as found naturally in all plant foods. Even *dairy* milk contains salt (about a twentieth of a teaspoon per pint).

- **Fruit.** If making milk that is likely to be consumed within a day or so, be daring and add a ripe banana to the recipe. Other possibilities can include ripe pear, ripe melon, or just about any kind of fruit that is ripe and whitish in colour. This will certainly give the milk a unique flavour, and is well worth doing as an occasional treat. Add the fruit while blending the milk so that any hard bits of fruit are taken out with the straining.

- **Flavourings.** The same flavourings that are commercially available for dairy milk can also be used for non-dairy milk, and these are particularly liked by children. For example, the chocolate or strawberry malt flavourings widely available for dairy milk can equally be used with non-dairy milk. Usually, you would use such flavourings for adding to a *serving* of milk rather than adding to the recipe.

- **Carob powder.** Roasted carob powder is widely available from health food stores, and is ideal for adding to a glass of nut-based milk for a satisfying treat. The same goes for cocoa powder. This provides a nutritious and delicious-tasting drink which can be consumed ice-cold or as a hot drink.

Blending milk

You will have noticed that many recipes in this book are similar in execution, with only the ingredients being different. It is therefore perfectly practical to blend different milks together.

By 'blend' we simply mean mixing two milks together *after they have been made*. Alternatively, two different recipes can be made simultaneously by mixing the ingredients *as you make it* (although some creativity in execution may be required!). I often like to soak half a cup of almonds mixed with half a cup of hazelnuts, and then make milk out of that – it provides a delicious nutty flavour that's neutral enough to use with anything or drink on its own (perfect for making coffee!).

To blend ready-made milk here's a way you might proceed:

Make *milk B* on a day when you only have about 2 cups left of *milk A*. Then take 2 cups of each milk and mix together. This becomes your blended milk, to be consumed *before* starting on *milk B*.

Four golden rules for blending milk

You are, of course, free to blend milk in any way you wish, but here are four golden rules:

1. It is best to avoid blending a non-nut milk with another type of non-nut milk. (Note that about half the milks recipes are nut-based). Blend a nut milk with a nut milk, or a nut milk with a non-nut milk. Of course, if you have a child who is allergic to nuts, this rule goes out of the window.

2. The blending proportions are best when they are two equal parts.

3. Always consume blended milk first.

4. Never blend two different batches of milk made from the *same recipe*. This avoids the danger of mixing milk that gets older and older with freshly made milk.

By blending milk you will get some wonderful and unique new flavours. Another major advantage is that you get a wider spectrum of nutrients which is always a good thing.

Fig. 2 below gives some examples of blended milks you may wish to try, but feel free to blend any two milks you fancy. You can also combine a blended milk with any of the above methods for **adding variety**. Any ideas from readers for improving or changing the milk recipes will be gratefully received by the author, and may be included in a future edition of this book. Please send all comments to: milkimperative@milkimperative.com.

Note that it is not necessary to combine different milks to get the full nutritional benefits. So called 'food combining' has been proved to be unnecessary because the body does this very successfully by creating a pool of nutrients to serve its needs. The purpose of blending milks is two-fold: to provide exciting new tastes, and to give the body a greater *range* of nutrients consumed.

Fig. 2
Examples of Blended Milks

Blending of two milks: milk A + milk B				
Milk A	**Milk B**		**Milk A**	**Milk B**
Almond	Hazelnut		Pecan	Quinoa
Pecan	Chestnut		Oats	Almond
Brazil	Macadamia		Spelt	Coconut
Pumpkin	Coconut		Rice	Hazelnut
Rice	Sesame		Macadamia	Sunflower
Soy	Walnut		Millet	Coconut
Pine	Hemp		Pecan	Tiger Nut
Millet	Peanut		Pumpkin	Hemp
Pea	Brazil		Pea	Almond

***

Non-Dairy Smoothies & Ice-Cream

Delicious and nutritious smoothies can be made using non-dairy milk and the left-over okara. The following chart shows which non-dairy milks and okara are best for making wonderful smoothies:

Smoothie Chart
Shows which milks/okaras are best for making smoothies

Almond Milk	Pecan Nut Milk
Brazil Nut Milk	Pine Nut Milk
Cashew Nut Milk	Pumpkin Seed Milk
Chestnut Milk	Sesame Seed Milk
Coconut Milk*	Soybean Milk
Hazelnut Milk	Sunflower Seed Milk
Hemp Seed Milk*	Tiger Nut Milk*
Macadamia Milk	Walnut Milk
Peanut Milk	Blended Milk

* Okara not suitable for making smoothies

Examples: Make a delicious smoothie using pumpkin seed milk and pumpkin seed okara. Alternatively, you can mix any of the above milks with any okara to make a smoothie. You can even mix two different okaras into the same smoothie recipe.

For example, you can use Coconut milk with soybean okara. Clearly, if you have recently made milk, it will be more practical to use the fresh milk and okara that is available, rather than defrosting another batch of milk or okara. To make a smoothie that is more creamy, try adding 'soy dream' (cream made from soy beans). Alternatively, adding a spoonful of lecithin granules will help to make the smoothie thicker and more creamy.

Smoothies made from non-dairy milk provide an ideal and healthy snack at any time of the day, or as a dessert for both children and grown-ups. Alternatively, put the same smoothie ingredients into an ice-cream maker instead of a smoothie blender, and make ice-cream!

If making ice-cream and freezing, make sure you freeze several small portions instead of freezing one big portion. That way it stays fresher as gradually used up.

The health benefits of smoothies

- **Non-fattening:** Smoothies are low-fat, low carbohydrate, and have no added sugar (unless you add it!).
- **Nutritious:** Smoothies are super-nutritious because you get the goodness of the non-dairy milk and okara combined with the highly nutritious berries used in the recipe. Berries of all kinds are packed with a wide variety of vitamins, minerals, sterols, enzymes, fibre, and other health-promoting properties.
- **Healthy fibre:** Soluble and non-soluble fibre are both essential for good health. The okara and berries provide plenty of both.
- **Variety:** By combining different milks with different okaras, or by making smoothies using a different milk each time, you get a varied diet which is important for good health.

The recipe

Notes: (i) Do not give any kind of nuts or foods made from nuts to people allergic to nuts. (ii) This recipe makes about 1 litre or 2 pints. (iii) If serving smoothie straight away, use frozen berries and refrigerated milk/water.

You will need:

A. 1 cup of okara (if not enough fresh okara, either reduce proportions of all ingredients, defrost further okara if available, or supplement with your favourite breakfast cereal (suitably ground up).

B. 2 cups non-dairy milk (choose from the above chart).

C. 2 cups drinking-quality water. Alternatively, use a total of 3 cups non-dairy milk and 1 cup water.

D. 12 ounces (340 grams) or fresh or frozen berries. This can be any mix and match of berries, or use just one kind of berry. Choose from raspberries, strawberries, blackberries, blueberries, cranberries, elderberries, gooseberries, in fact any edible berry that is sweet-tasting. Try starting by just using raspberries or strawberries.

E. 2 medium size bananas, cut into chunks.

F. 2–3 tablespoons of maple syrup or treacle (black strap molasses).

G. 1/2 teaspoon almond or vanilla extract (or a ¼ teaspoon of each).

H. Optional extras: 'Soy dream' or lecithin granules can make a smoothie more creamy. As a sweetener, try using stevia, or prunes soaked overnight, instead of maple syrup.

Method:

Add ingredients to blender (or smoothie machine). Process at low speed for 1 minute, and then 3 minutes at high speed or until smooth. Pour into tall glasses and serve while cold, or put in freezer for ten minutes before serving.

If making ice-cream, pour contents of blender into an ice-cream maker and enjoy healthy ice-cream.

Bibliography & Notes

1. Nathaniel Mead, M.D., Natural Health, July 1994.
2. Pediatric-Allergy-Immunology, August, 1994, 5(3).
3. Robert Cohen, Milk A-Z, 2001, Argus Publishing, ISBN 0965919684.
4. Science, vol. 249, august 24, 1990.
5. Journal of the National Institute of Health, 1991,3.
6. Abelow BJ, Holford TR, Insogna KL. Cross-cultural association between dietary animal protein and hip fracture: a hypothesis. Calcif Tissue Int 1992;50:14-8.
7. Sellmeyer DE, Stone KL, Sebastian A, Cummings SR. A high ratio of dietary animal to vegetable protein increases the rate of bone loss and the risk of fracture in postmenopausal women. Am J Clin Nutr 2001;73:118-22.
8. Remer T, Manz F. Estimation of the renal net acid excretion by adults consuming diets containing variable amounts of protein. Am J Clin Nutr 1994;59:1356-61.
9. Julian Whiaker, M.D. Health & Healing, October, 1998, Volume 8, No. 10.
10. Acta Otolaryngol 1999: 119(8).
11. William Northrup, M.D., Natural Health, July 1994.
12. Journal of Pediatrics, 1990, 116.
13. Acta Paediatrica, 1999 Dec, 88:12
14. Journal of Pediatric Surgery, 1999 Oct, 34:10
15. West Virginia Medical Journal, 1999 Sep-Oct; 95(5).
16. Townsend Medical Letter, May, 1995.
17. Mulhall and Hansen, The Calcium Bomb, The Writers Collective, 2005, ISBN 1594111014.
18. Robert M. Kradjian, M.D., Breast Surgery, Chief Division of General Surgery, Seton Medical Centre, Daly City, CA 94015 USA, website: www.afpafitness.com/articles/MILKDOC.HTM.
19. Nurses Health study, USA, Feskanich et al. (1999).
20. Weber, P. *Nutrition.* 2001 Oct; 17(10):880-7.
21. PDR for Nutritional Supplements, 1st ed. Montvale, NJ: Medical Economics Co.; 2001:288-95.
22. Amy Joy Lanou, Ph.D, et al, *Dairy Not Needed For Bone Health,* Physicians Committee for Responsible Medicine (PCRM), March 2005, US journal Pediatrics (2005;115(3):736-43).
23. Frank Oski, M.D., Chief of Pediatrics at john Hopkins Medical School, *Don't Drink Your Milk,* July 1994.
24. European Review Medical Pharmacological Science, 1998 May.
25. Michael Schmidt, Ph.D., *Brain-Building Nutrition,* 2001, Pub. Frog Ltd., ISBN 1583940480
26. Journal of Allergy & Clinical Immunology 1999 Jun, 103:6.
27. Lydia C. Medeiros, et al, *B-920R - Nutritional Content of Game Meat,* College of Agriculture, University of Wyoming, USA.
28. Karolinska Institute, Sweden, published in the Am. J. of Clinical Nutrition, Nov. 2004.
29. Journal of Dairy Science, 1999 Dec, 82:12.
30. Postgraduate Medical Journal, 1998 Sep, 104:3.
31. Journal of Clinical Gastroenterology, 1999 Apr, 28:3.
32. Digestive Science, 1998 Nov, 43:11.
33. Journal of the American College of Nutrition, Dec. 2005 (vol 23, no 6, 704S-711S).
34. Nutrition Action Healthletter, June, 1993.
35. Harvard study of 78,000 women, American Journal of Public Health, 1997:87.
36. Robert Cohen, Ph.D., author of "Not Milkman", website www.notmilk.com.
37. United Press International, March 11, 1983.
38. Sandra Steingraber, Ph.D., Living Downstream.
39. Amy Joy Lanou, Ph.D, *Physicians Committee for Responsible Medicine,* Dec. 2004.
40. Harvey and Marilyn Diamond, *Fit For Life.*
41. The Lancet, vol. 344, November 5, 1994.
42. Pediatric Allergy-Immunology, 1994, 5(5 supplement).
43. The National Mastitis Council, Inc., 1970, Washington, D.C.
44. Lincoln Lampert, Modern Dairy Products.

45. American Journal of Epidemiology, 1999; 150.
46. George Eisman, M.A., M.Sc., R.D., Vegetarian and Vegan Nutrition.
47. J. Moon, *The role of vitamin D in toxic metal absorption: a review.* J Am Coll Nutr. 1994 Dec;13(6):559-64.
48. Neal Barnard, M.D., Director of the *Physician's Committee for Responsible Medicine.* www.pcrm.org.
49. Endocrinology, 1999 Sep, 140:9
50. Frank Oski, M.D., *Don't Drink Your Milk*, Teach Services, Inc.
51. Miller V, et al, Mayo Clinic, Journal American College of Cardiology, March 2002.
52. Mayo Clin Proc. 2004;79:197-210, Mayo Foundation for Medical Education and Research.
53. Annemarie Colbin, MA, CCP, CHES, founder of Institute for Food and Health, N.Y., author of *Food and Our Bones*, Dutton Pub.
54. *A prospective study of dietary lactose and ovarian cancer*, Dept. of Medicine, Brigham and Women's Hospital, Harvard Medical School, Boston, MA, USA, June 2004.
55. *Nutrition Label Content*, page 163, The National Academies Press, Washington, USA.
56. The Journal of Proteome Research, vol. 4, no. 1, 2006.
57. Neva Ciftcioglu, *Screening of human gamma globulin products for nanobacteria markers*, 102nd meeting of the American Society for microbiology, Salt Lake City, May 2002.
58. John R. Lee, M.D. and Virginia Hopkins, *The Truth about Osteoporosis*, http://www.drgrisanti.com/osteopage.htm.
59. Lois Rogers, Medical Correspondent, *The Sunday Times*, www.sunday-times.co.uk/news/pages/sti/00/02/20/stinwenws03034.html?999, Feb. 21, 2000.
60. Robert Cohen, *Milk – The Deadly Poison*, Argus Publishing, January 1, 1998, ISBN: 0965919609.
61. Medical Hypothesis, 2000 May, 54:5.
62. Angela Dowden, *Are You Getting Enough?*, Orion, 1999, ISBN 0752817027.
63. *Pediatric Research*, December 7, 2004, and *Science Daily*, December 27, 2004.
64. *Physician's Committee for Responsible Medicine*, Washington DC, USA, www.pcrm.org.
65. *Nutrition*, 20(2004):200
66. *Cancer Research and the Journal of Endocrinology (*Cancer Research 1995, 1997).
67. *Life Sciences*, July 2000;66:1501-7.
68. *The Weekly Newsmagazine of Science*, Vol, 155, Number 26 (June 26, 1999).
69. *New England J. of Medicine*, Volume 327:302-30, July 30, 1992, Number 5.
70. *Marketplace*, Dec. 2001, www.cbc.ca/consumers/market/files/food/milk.
71. *American Journal of Clinical Nutrition*, Vol. 71, No. 6, 1525-1529, June 2000 (extract).
72. *Diabetologia*, 1994; 37(4).
73. *Diabetes Care* 1994, 17 (12).
74. Stephen Holt M.D., Igor Muntyan M.D., and Larisa Likyer, M.D. www.biopathics.com/diabetes_mellitus%5B1%5D.htm.
75. Bhathena SJ and Velasquez MT. *Beneficial role of dietary phytoestrogens in obesity and diabetes* Am J Clin Nutr 2002 76: 1191-1201.
76. Jayagopal V, Albertazzi P, Kilpatrick ES et al. *Beneficial effects of soy phytoestrogen intake in postmenopausal women with type 2 diabetes.* Diabetes Care. 2002 Oct;25(10):1709-14.
77. Eating your way to health, Soybean and Your health, www.picknpay.co.za.
78. Sandra R. Teixeira, University of Illinois at Urbana-Champaign, Aug. 2004.
79. *American Journal of Epidemiology*, January 2005.
80. *European J. of Clinical Nutrition*, volume 58,9:1211-6, September 2004.
81. *American Journal of Nutrition* (Nov. 2004).
82. Dr. Qing Jiang, Purdue University,l Indiana, USA, March, 2005.
83. Dr. Cedric Garland, The Calcium Diet, Penguin, 1988.
84. Robert O. Young Ph.D. and Shelley Redford Young, The pH Miracle, Time Warner 2002, ISBN 0751534064.
85. Report from the *Harvard School Of Public Health Nutrition Roundtable*, Section 3: Calcium: Too Much of a Good Thing? www.molliekatzen.com/harvard3.php.
86. US Department of Agriculture, Fluid Milk consumption selected Countries, www.fas.usda.gov/dlp2/circular/2001/01-12Dairy/mlkcons.pdf.
87. Kromhout D, et al, *Dietary saturated and trans fatty acids, cholesterol and 25-year mortality from coronary heart disease*, 1995, The Seven Countries study, 308-15.

88. Elaine Hardman, et al, Louisiana State University, *Mother's Prenatal and Lactational Diet May Protect Daughters from Breast Cancer*, presented to the American Association for Cancer Research, April 20, 2005.
89. Tim Griswold, former executive director of the Wisconsin Department of Commerce *'Dairy 2020 Initiative'* commenting in the Wisconsin State Journal, USA, April 25, 2005.
90. Willet, W.C. 1994. *Diet and Health: What should we eat?* Science 264:532-37.
91. Willcox, Bradley, M.D., et al. The Okinawa Way: How to improve your health and logevity dramatically, 2001, Michael Joseph, ISBN 0718144945.
92. *Including Walnuts in a Low Fat/Modified Fat Diet Improves HDL Cholesterol-to-Total Cholesterol Ratios in Patients With Type 2 Diabetes.* December 2004 issue of Diabetes Care, a journal of the American Diabetes Association (ADA).
93. Two articles published in the Journal of Proteome Research by Dr Andrei P. Sommer of the University of Ulm, Germany, and Professor Chandra Wickramasinghe of Cardiff University, UK show that nanobacteria are now accepted as being widely prevalent in the terrestrial environment and that their evidence is compelling for the existence of these nano-organisms, even in the stratosphere. In humans, nanobacteria have now been identified on four continents, according to the articles.
94. M. Park, MD, PhD, et al, *Consumption of milk and calcium in midlife and the future risk of Parkinson disease*, Neurology, 2005;64:1047-1051.
95. Email dated 5 May 2005 from The Dairy Council, www.milk.co.uk.
96. In the European Union about 20% – 25% of calcium in pasteurized milk gets absorbed into blood. In the USA about 32% – 35% gets absorbed. The difference is due to vitamin D3 which is added to milk in the USA. Most parts of the world do not add vitamin D3 so the rate is mostly 20% – 25%.
97. Deb Bromley, Science and Technology Researcher and President of *NatureGem Nontoxic Living*, an organization devoted to promoting awareness of toxins in food and the environment, www.naturegem.com.
98. Connie Weaver, Ph.D., *Meeting Calcium Needs for Optimal Bone Health* (Table 5, Food Sources of Bioavailable Calcium), Department of Foods and Nutrition, Purdue University.
99. Degorah E Sellmeyer, et al, *A high ratio of dietary animal to vegetable protein increases the rate of bone loss and the risk of fracture in postmenopausal women*, American Journal of Clinical Nutrition, Vol. 73, No. 1, 118-122, January 2001.
100. National Dairy Council, USA: email dated 9 May 2005 stating *'Phosphorus absorption efficiency in adults is approximately 60% - about twice as high as for calcium.'*
101. Daily Mail study into the effects of fish oil supplements in school children. study supervised by Dr. Madeleine Portwood, Senior Educational Psychologist at Durham LEA and principal investigator of the study. Published in The Daily Mail, p.34, May 10, 2005.
102. Margaret Neighbour, *Cubs breast-fed by woman die in zoo*, The Scotsman, 13 May 2005.
103. Guardiola, F. et al, Biological effects of oxysterols : Current status. Food Chem. toxicol. 1996 / 34 (2) / 193-211.
104. Guiwotta, C. et al, Prostaglandin F2-like compounds, F2 isoprostanes, are present in increased amounts in human atherosclerostic lesions. Atheroscler. Thromb. Vasc. Biol. 1997 / 17 (11) / 3236-3241.
105. Rise P, et al, Regulation of PUFA metabolism: pharmacological and toxicological aspects. Prostaglandins Leukot Essent Fatty Acids 2002 Aug;67(2-3):85.
106. O'Brien, K.O. et al, Increased efficiency of calcium absorption from the rectum and distal colon of humans. American Journal of Clinical Nutrition 1996 / 63 (4) / 579-583.
107. Peterson CA, et al, Alterations in calcium intake on peak bone mass in the female rat. J. Bone Miner. Res. 1995 / 10 (1) / 81-95.
108. Pazzaglia UE, Experimental osteoporosis in the rat induced by a hypocalcic diet. Ital. J. Orthop. Traumatol.1990 / 16 (2) / 257-265.
109. Davis JW, et al, Ethnic, anthropometric, and lifestyle associations with regional variations in peak bone mass. Calcif Tissue Int 1999 Aug;65(2):100-5. , Ulrich CM, et al, Lifetime physical activity is associated with bone mineral density in premenopausal women. J Womens Health 1999 Apr;8(3):365-75. , Boot AM, et al, Bone mineral density in children and adolescents: relation to puberty, calcium intake, and physical activity. J Clin Endocrinol Metab 1997 Jan;82(1):57-62. , Hu JF, et al, Dietary calcium and bone density among middle-aged and elderly women in China. Am J Clin Nutr 1993 Aug;58(2):219-27.

110. Bonofiglio D, et al, Critical years and stages of puberty for radial bone mass apposition during adolescence. Horm Metab Res 1999 Aug ;31 (8) : 478-82. , Maggiolini M, et al, The effect of dietary calcium intake on bone mineral density in healthy adolescent girls and young women in southern Italy. Int J Epidemiol 1999 Jun;28 (3): 479-84.
111. Bacon WE, et al, International comparison of hip fracture rates in 1988-89. Osteoporos Int. 199 / 6 (1) / 69-75.
112. Schwartz, A.V. et al, International variation in the incidence of hip fractures: cross-national project on osteoporosis for the World Health Organization Program for Research on Ageing. Osteoporosis Int. 1999 / 9 (3) / 242-253.Rowe, S.M. et al, An epidemiological study of hip fracture in Honan, Korea. Int. Orthop. 1993 / 17 (3) / 139-143.
113. Ghannam NN, et al, Bone mineral density of the spine and femur in healthy Saudi females: relation to vitamin D status, pregnancy, and lactation. Calcif Tissue Int 1999 Jul;65(1):23-8
114. Kung AW, Age-related osteoporosis in Chinese: evaluation of the response of intestinal calcium absorption and calcitropic hormones to dietary calcium deprivation. Am. J. Clin. Nutr. 1998 / 68 (6) / 1291-1297. Wang MC, et al, Associations of vitamin C, calcium & protein with bone mass in postmenopausal Mex. American women. Osteoporos Int 1997 / 7(6) / 533-8.
115. Taking extra vitamin D and calcium will not prevent fractures in seniors, Medical Research News, 28 April 2005, www.news-medical.net.
116. Michaelsson K, et al, Diet and hip fracture risk: a case-control study. Study Group of the Multiple Risk Survey on Swedish Women for Eating Assessment. Int. J. Epidemiol. 1995 / 24 (4) / 771-782.
117. Peter Axt, PhD and Michaela Axt-Gadermann, MD, *The Joy of Laziness: How to slow down and live longer*, Hunter House, Oct. 2003, ISBN: 0897934016.
118. Rutherford OM, et al, The relationship of muscle and bone loss and activity levels with age in women. Age Ageing 1992 / 21 (4) / 286-293.
119. Meyer T, et al, Identification of apoptotic cell death in distraction osteogenesis. Cell. Biol. Int.1999 / 23 (6) / 439-446. , Landry P, et al, Apoptosis is coordinately regulated with osteoblast formation during bone healing. Tissue Cell 1997 / 29 (4) / 413-419.
120. Rutherford OM., Is there a role for exercise in the prevention of osteoporotic fractures? Br J Sports Med 1999 / 33 (6) / 378-386.
121. Kerschan-Shindl K, et al, Long-term home exercise program: effect in women at high risk of fracture. Arch. Phys. Med. Rehabil. 2000 / 81 (3) / 319-323. , Greendale GA, et al, Lifetime leisure exercise and osteoporosis. The Rancho Bernardo study. Am. J. Epidemiol. 1995 / 141 (10) / 951-959. , Jaglal SB, et al, Past and recent physical activity and risk of hip fracture. Am. J. Epidemiol. 1993 / 138 (2) / 107-118.
122. *Handbook of Dairy Foods and Nutrition, Second Edition*, page 268 that the fractional absorption of calcium from milk is 32.1%. This data is from Weaver, CM Am J Clin Nutr 59 (Suppl) 1238s, 1994.
123. Ché Green, founder and director of *The Armedia Institute*, a nonprofit research and advocacy organization focusing on farm animal issues in the USA, 1 Aug. 2002.
124. Roswell Park Memorial Institute, USA, Cancer 64 (3): 605-612.
125. Karjalainen, *A bovine albumin peptide as a possible trigger of insulin-dependent diabetes mellitus*, N. Engl J Med, 1992, 327, pp. 302-307.
126. Fava, et al, *Relationship between dairy product consumption and the incidence of IDDM in childhood in Italy*, Diabetes Care, Dec. 1994, 17(12).
127. Catherine S. Berkey, ScD et al, *Milk, Dairy Fat, Dietary Calcium, and Weight Gain: A Longitudinal Study of Adolescents*, Arch Pediatr Adolesc Med. 2005;159:543-550.
128. Carolyn Becker, MD, New York Presbyterian Hospital-Columbia University, USA, *Prevention Of Osteoporosis: Maximizing Peak Bone Mass*, and other articles, webcasts, and published interviews.
129. Owusu W, et al, *Calcium intake and the incidence of forearm and hip fractures among men*, J Nutr. 1997 Sep;127(9):1782-7.
130. Feskanich D, et al, Milk, dietary calcium, and bone fractures in women: a 12-year prospective study, Am J Public Health. 1997 Jun;87(6):992-7.
131. Cramer, D.W., *Lactase persistence and milk consumption as determinants of ovarian cancer risk*, Am J Epidemiol. 1989 Nov;130(5):904-10.
132. Cramer, D.W. et al, *Galactose consumption and metabolism in relation to the risk of ovarian cancer*, Lancet. 1989 Jul 8;2(8654):66-71.

133. Jacobus CH, Holick MF, Shao Q, et al. Hypervitaminosis D associated with drinking milk. N Engl J Med 1992;326(18):1173-7.
134. Holick MF. Vitamin D and bone health. J Nutr 1996;126(4suppl):1159S-64S.
135. Email dated 9 June 2005 from Dr. Thomas Caceci, Ph.D, anatomist, electron microscopist, and biologist; Professor, Virginia-Maryland Regional College of Veterinary Med., USA.
136. Gillian Sanson, *The Myth of Osteoporosis*, 2003, MCD Century Publications, ISBN 0-9721233-4-2.
137. Email dated 24 June 2005 from www.calcify.com, a website dedicated to promoting the book 'The Calcium Bomb' and information about harmful calcification.
138. Mark J. Plotkin & Michael Shnayerson, *The Killers Within: The Deadly Rise of Drug Resistant Bacteria*, Back Bay Books (Sep. 2003), ISBN 0316735663.
139. Dr. George J. Georgiou, Ph.D., Clinical Nutritionist, *Milk - A Recipe for Disease*, Nov. 2002, worldwidehealthcenter.net.
140. Dr. Edward Giovannucci, Professor of Nutrition and Epidemiology, Harvard School of Public Health, *Qualified Health Claim (QHC): Calcium and various cancers*, May 2004 (published on FDA website, www.fda.gov/default.htm).
141. Rose DP, et al, International comparisons of mortality rates for cancer of the breast, ovary, prostate, and colon, and per capita food consumption, Cancer. 1986 Dec 1;58(11):2363-71.
142. Hartmann S, Natural occurrence of steroid hormones in food, *Food chem* 1998;**62**:7-20.
143. Ganmaa D, et al, Incidence and mortality of testicular and prostatic cancers in relation to world dietary practices. *Int.J.Cancer*, 2002;**98**:262-7.
144. Dr. Leo Galland's Drug-Nutrient Interactions Workshop Software from Allergy Research Group 800-545-9960 www.allergyresearchgroup.com
145. Seely S, Ischaemic heart failure: a new explanation of its cause and preventability, Int J Cardiol. 2002 Dec;86(2-3):259-63.
146. Couet C et al, J. of the American College of Nutrition 10(1):79-86, 1991.
147. Dr. David Gordon, *Milk and Mortality* (ISBN 0-9671605-0-2 $35), Gordon Books (925-443-6213), 567 Amber Court, Livermore California 94550, USA.
148. Huijuan Xu, et al, American Journal of Epidemiology, Vol. 139, No.3 1994.
149. **Karl S Roth, MD,** Professor, Department of Pediatrics, Creighton University School of Medicine, www.emedicine.com/ped/topic815.htm.
150. Eight sources as numbered. Note: the studies in item 5 refer to appetite suppression. **(1)** Chow, S.Y. et al, Brain oxytocin receptor antagonism disinhibits sodium appetite in preweanling rats. Regul. Pept. 1997 / 68 (2) / 119-124. , Arletti, R. et al, Influence of oxytocin on feeding behavior in the rat. Peptides 1989 / 10 (1) / 89-93. **(2)** Chua, S. et al, Influence of breastfeeding and nipple stimulation on postpartum uterine activity. Br. J. Obstet. Gynaecol. 1994 / 101 (9) / 804-805. **(3)** Moos, F.C. et al, Electrical recordings of magnocellular supraoptic and paraventricular neurons displaying both oxytocine- and vasopressin-related activity. Brain Res. 1995 / 669 (2) / 309-314. **(4)** Lindow, S.W. et al, Morphine suppresses the oxytocin response in breast-feeding women. Gynecol. Obstet. Invest. 1999 / 48 (1) / 33-37. **(5)** Bing, C. et al, The effect of moxonidine on feeding and body fat in obese Zucker rats: role of hypothalamic NPY neurones. Br. J. Pharmacol. 1999 / 127 (1) / 35-42. , Asakawa, A. et al, Urocortin reduces food intake and gastric emptying in lean and ob/ob obese mice. Gastroenterology 1999 / 116 (6) / 1287-1292. , Nishiyama, M. et al, Leptin effects on the expression of type-2 CRH receptor mRNA in the ventromedial hypothalamus in the rat. J. Endocrinol. 1999 / 11 (4) / 307-314. , Hakansson, M.L. et al, Leptin receptor immunoreactivity in chemically defined target neurons of the hypothalamus.J. Neurosci. 1998 / 18 (1) / 559-572. , Plamondon, H. et al, Anorectic action of bombesin requires receptor for corticotropin-releasing factor but not for oxytocin. Eur. J. Pharmacol. 1997 / 340 (2-3) / 99-109. **(6)** Brogan, R.S. et al, Suppression of leptin during lactation: contribution of the suckling stimulus versus milk production. Endocrinology 1999 / 140 (6) / 2621-2627. **(7)** Fortun-Lamothe, L. et al, Influence of prolactin on in vivo and in vitro lipolysis in rabbits. Comp. Biochem. Physiol. C. Pharmacol. Toxicol. Endocrinol. 1996 / 115 (2) / 141-147. **(8)** Dewey, K.G. et al, Maternal weight loss patterns during prolonged lactation. Am. J. Clin. Nutr. 1993 / 58 (2) / 162-166.
151. Souci, S.W. et al, Food Composition and Nutrition Tabels. Medpharm Scientific Publishers Stuttgart 1994 / 6-28.

152. Lang-Kummer J: Hypercalcemia. In: Groenwald SL, Goodman M, Frogge MH, et al., eds.: Cancer Nursing: Principles and Practice. 4th ed. Sudbury, Mass: Jones and Bartlett Publishers, 1997., pp 684-701.
153. Araki H, Watanabe H, Mishina T, Nakao M. High-risk group for benign prostatic hypertrophy. Prostate 1983;4:253-64.
154. Dr. Olavi Kajander, Nanobac Chief Science Officer, Nanobac Life Sciences, Inc: Announcement made on May 16-18, 2005, at the *PDA Viral and TSE Safety Conference* in Bethesda, MD, USA.
155. The Vitamin D Newsletter, Feb. 12, 2005, Racial Opportunities (John Jacob Cannell, MD, The Vitamin D Council Inc., 9100 San Gregorio Road, Atascadero, CA 93422, USA).
156. Jane A. Cauley, Dr.P.H., professor, epidemiology, University of Pittsburgh; Stephen Honig, M.D., director, Osteoporosis Center, Hospital for Joint Diseases, New York City; May 4, 2005, *Journal of the American Medical Association.*
157. The physician and sportsmedicine - vol 31 - no. 10 - october 2003.
158. Maciej S., *Dietary Calcium Intake in Lactose Maldigesting Intolerant and Tolerant African-American Women*, Journal of the American College of Nutrition, Vol. 21, No. 1, 47-54 (2002).
159. Bell, R.R. et al, *The influence of milk in the diet on the toxicity of orally ingested lead in rats.* Food and Cosmetics Toxicology 1981 / 19 / 429-436. , Lembeck, F. et al ,*Substance P as neurogenic mediator of antidromic vasodilation and neurogenic plasma extravasation.* Arch. Pharmacol. 1979 / 310 (2) / 175-183.
160. Shortt, C. et al, Effect of dietary lactose on salt-mediated changes in mineral metabolism and bone composition in the rat, British Journal of Nutrition, Volume 66, Number 1, July 1991, pp. 73-81(9).
161. Schuette, SA, et al, *Effect of lactose or its component sugars on jejunal calcium absorption in adult man.* Clinical Nutrition Research Unit, University of Chicago, IL 60637, USA.
162. Heller H.J. Effect of milk components on calcium bioavailability,J. Am. Coll. Nutr. 1999 ; 18 : 373S-378S.
163. Léon Guéguen, *The Bioavailability of Dietary Calcium*, J. of the Am. College of Nutrition, Vol. 19, No. 90002, 119S-136S (2000).
164. Dr. Anthony Cichoke, D.C., *Enzymes and enzyme therapy*, 1994, P.5, Pub. by Keats, Conneticut, USA.
165. Dr. Szekely EB, *The Chemistry of youth*, US International Biogenic Society, 1977.
166. American Journal of Epidemiology 1994;139.
167. Amanda Patenaude, et al, Inverse Relationship Between Simultaneously Measured Coronary Calcification and Bone Mineral Density in 12,000 Patients: Relationship to HDL Cholesterol. Paper presented at the American College of Cardiology Scientific Sessions, 2002.
168. Report submitted to the American Heart Association's Scientific Sessions 2004, stating that a test for nanobacteria is an accurate predictor of heart disease risk.

Appendix One:
Vitamins & Minerals

Vitamins

Vitamins are organic substances that are required in small amounts in the diet. They are necessary for numerous special functions in the body and are essential for good health. They can be affected by environmental conditions such as light, heat and air. Food storage, processing and cooking can all act to reduce the level of vitamins in food.

Vitamins may be either fat-soluble or water-soluble. The fat-soluble vitamins are vitamins A, D, E and K. Fat-soluble vitamins can be stored in the body and so dietary sources are not needed every day. The water-soluble vitamins are vitamin C and the B group of vitamins. The B group of vitamins includes B1, B2, B3, B6, B12, folic acid, biotin and pantothenic acid. The body is less able to store water-soluble vitamins (with the exception of vitamin B12 which is stored in the liver) and so they are needed daily. Water-soluble vitamins are more likely to be lost during cooking.

Vitamin A (retinol). For healthy skin, growth of bones, resistance to infection and night vision. Found in carrots, spinach, peppers, butter, margarine, watercress, dried apricots, full-fat dairy products. In plant foods it is present as its precursor, beta-carotene. Overdosing on vitamin A supplements has been associated with cancer and with the *aging* of the skin.

Vitamin B1 (thiamin). For breaking down carbohydrates for energy. Found in yeast extract, brazil nuts, peanuts, rice, bran, oatmeal, flour, wholemeal bread, sunflower seeds.

Vitamin B2 (riboflavin). Helps convert proteins, fats and carbohydrates into energy and for the growth and repair of tissues and healthy skin. Found in almonds, wholemeal bread, dried prunes, mushrooms, cashews, millet, avocados.

Vitamin B3 (niacin). For energy production, healthy skin, and the nervous system. Found in most foods including yeast extract, peanuts, wholemeal bread, mushrooms, sesame seeds.

Vitamin B6 (pyridoxine). For red blood cell formation and protein metabolism. Found in bran, wholemeal flour, yeast extract, hazelnuts, bananas, peanuts, currants.

Vitamin B12. For red blood cell formation, growth, and a healthy nervous system. Found in eggs and fortified plant foods including soy milks, breakfast cereals, veggie burger mixes, yeast extracts and some herbal soft drinks.

Folic acid or folate. For red blood cell formation, protein synthesis and DNA metabolism. Some functions are linked with vitamin B12. Found in yeast extract, spinach, broccoli, peanuts, almonds, hazelnuts.

Biotin. For energy production and healthy skin. Found in yeast extract, pulses, nuts, most vegetables.

Pantothenic acid. For energy production and antibody (immunity) formation. Widely found in most foods.

Vitamin C (Ascorbic acid). For healthy skin, bones, teeth and gums, resistance to infection and wound healing, energy production and growth. Found in citrus fruits, broccoli, spinach, berries, peppers. Overdosing on vitamin C supplements has been associated with decreased levels of vitamin B12 and with growth of tumors.

Vitamin D. For the absorption of calcium and phosphate and healthy bones and teeth. Found in margarine and some fortified foods. Also produced by the action of sunlight on the skin. Anyone confined indoors may need to consider a vitamin D supplement which is best taken formulated with calcium and magnesium rather than taken on its own, as this avoids possibility of vitamin D pulling calcium from the bones. Overdosing on vitamin D supplements has been associated with arteriosclerosis and bone deformities.

Vitamin E. Acts as an antioxidant protecting vitamins A and C and other important substances in the body. Helps prevent 'wear and tear' on the body. Found in vegetable oils, wheatgerm, hazelnuts, avocados. Overdosing on vitamin E supplements has been associated with bleeding in the brain, impaired immunity, cancer and arthritis.

Vitamin K. For effective blood clotting, and calcium assimilation. Found in spinach, cabbage, cauliflower. Vitamin K is also obtained from bacterial synthesis in the intestine. Deficiency is rare.

Minerals

Unlike many vitamins, the human body cannot make any minerals and they must all come from the diet. Overdosing on any mineral supplement is harmful to the body. Also, too much of one mineral can often decrease the levels of other minerals. The main minerals required in the diet are calcium, magnesium, sodium, potassium, chlorine, phosphorus and sulphur. Other minerals which are required in only tiny quantities (less than 100mg/day) are called trace elements. Inorganic minerals (obtained from soil or rocks instead of from plants) cannot be assimilated or used properly by the body.

Our bodies can only benefit from minerals that have been 'processed' by plants, referred to as 'elemental' minerals.

Sodium and Potassium. Both are important in maintaining the body's water balance controlling the composition of blood and other body fluids. Sodium chloride (salt) is present in dairy and processed foods and in small amounts in vegetables, fruits and grains. Most people consume too much sodium which can lead to high blood pressure. Potassium is widely found in plant foods, especially root vegetables and wholegrain cereals.

Calcium. For building and maintaining strong bones and teeth, muscle contraction and blood clotting. Found in leafy green vegetables, almonds, sesame seeds, dried fruit, pulses, fortified soya milks and other foods. Getting enough calcium in the diet is usually no problem as we only need a small amount for healthy bones. Calcium supplements are associated with osteoporosis because excess calcium acts to weaken bones in the long run. Also, excess calcium is associated with arthritis, muscle cramps, fibromyalgia, and harmful calcification of the arteries.

Magnesium. For strong bones and enzymes involved in energy production. Widely found in plant foods.

Phosphorus. Required with calcium for strong bones and teeth, muscle function, and as a vital component of all body cells. Found in nearly all foods and dietary deficiency is very rare.

Sulphur. Plays a role in some enzyme systems. Most dietary sulphur is in the sulphur-containing amino acids. There is no indication of sulphur deficiency except in association with protein deficiency.

Iron. An essential component of haemoglobin which transports oxygen in the blood through the body. Iron deficiency is one of the most common nutritional problems in a typical *First World* diet. Found in leafy green vegetables, pulses, wholemeal bread, dried fruit, pumpkin seeds, molasses. Vitamin C helps to absorb iron. Overdosing on iron is associated with heart attack, diabetes, colon cancer, Parkinson's disease, and infertility.

Zinc. Plays a role in a wide range of enzyme systems and is essential for DNA metabolism and growth. Found in sesame and pumpkin seeds, green vegetables, lentils, wholegrain cereals. Overdosing on zinc is associated with heart attack, diabetes, colon cancer, Parkinson's disease, and infertility.

Copper. For red blood cell formation and many enzyme functions. Found in green vegetables, yeast, nuts, wheatgerm. Overdosing on copper is associated with heart attack, diabetes, colon cancer, Parkinson's disease, and infertility.

Iodine. For the production of thyroid hormones important in body metabolism. Found in seafoods. Amount in plant foods depends upon the amount in soil in which plants were grown.

Selenium. For red blood cell function and acts as an antioxidant. Selenium in plant foods depends on selenium in the soil and can vary considerably. Overdosing associated with cancer.

Chromium. Necessary to maintain blood glucose level. Exact nutritional role is uncertain. Good sources include black pepper, yeast and wholemeal bread.

Manganese. For the function of many enzymes and also muscle function. Deficiency is very rare. Found in tea, green vegetables, wholegrain cereals, nuts, spices. Overdosing associated with heart attack, diabetes, colon cancer, Parkinson's disease, and infertility.

Molybdenum. Essential part of some enzyme systems though deficiency has never been observed. Amount in plant foods depends on the amount in the soil.

Boron. Essential for the efficient assimilation and retention of calcium in the bones. Found in most fruit, vegetables, nuts, and pulses. Also found in chocolate, coffee, beer and cereals.

Other minerals include vanadium, nickel, and silicon. *All minerals are toxic if taken in excess*. Some minerals such as aluminium, cadmium, mercury and arsenic have no known nutritional role and are toxic at very low levels. These toxic minerals are often environmental pollutants.

***

Appendix Two:
The Root Cause of Osteoporosis

Carolyn Becker, MD, USA, explains how bones are made:

Scattered throughout our bones are osteoclasts and osteoblasts. These cells perform the critical function of bone remodeling, in which old or damaged bone is taken away, or resorbed, and new, healthy bone is laid down in its place. The job of osteoclasts is to eat away the old bone, then osteoblasts come in to lay down the new bone. Throughout childhood and into our twenties, bone formation exceeds bone resorption, so that we are truly building stronger and healthier bones. After about age thirty, however, for reasons that are still unclear, this process starts to reverse, and bone resorption slightly outstrips bone formation. By age thirty, most of us have achieved our peak bone mass, and then we start to lose bone very slowly.

Every person has a biologically determined peak bone mass. By this I mean that gender, race, and other hereditary factors predetermine the maximum amount of bone that each of us can develop by the time we reach our thirties. Women tend to have lower peak bone masses than men. African Americans tend to have higher peak bone masses than Caucasians. About 80% of this peak bone mass is hereditary while the other 20% is affected by lifestyle and other factors.

A woman may be genetically "programmed" to have a normal peak bone mass at maturity. If she has an unhealthy lifestyle however, she may only achieve 80% of her potential peak bone mass, and end up with bones that are less dense than she might have had otherwise. In contrast, another woman may be destined to have a rather thin skeleton due to hereditary factors, so that even with an ideal lifestyle, her peak bone mass may measure significantly below [but be just as healthy] *as that of her peer group.* [128]

Osteoporosis is caused when bone cells cannot make enough new bone to keep up with the continual rate of bone decomposition, i.e. there is a gradual net loss of bone. In a healthy person, the net loss of bone is very gradual (not enough to cause weak bones in old age, but nevertheless, the bones do get weaker gradually however healthy you may be).

In a person with osteoporosis, the net loss of bone is sufficiently severe to cause weak bones that break easily. This can occur at any age in an adult person, but is more likely the older you get. Here we are not talking about osteoporosis caused by medical or hereditary factors, but **lifestyle** factors. This is often referred to as 'hormonal' or 'age related' osteoporosis even though it can strike at *any age*. The vast majority of cases of osteoporosis are caused by lifestyle factors, particularly the diet, and this is where milk comes in.

Dairy Milk

In the chapter *Dairy Milk Effect on Osteoporosis* dairy milk is shown to be the major *dietary* cause of osteoporosis so we will not repeat the information here. The point is this: the root cause of osteoporosis is a lack of bone-making cells. Some people may argue that the cause lies with osteoclasts, i.e. that bone decomposition is too high. However, all the research is showing that this is not the case because the rate of decomposition is a natural, steady and continual process. Certain hormones such as estrogen can affect the rate of decomposition, but it does not follow that osteoclasts are at the root of age-related osteoporosis.

Mounting evidence is showing that a lack of bone-*making* cells is at the root of osteoporosis and the question we need to answer is: *What causes bone-making cells to dwindle sufficiently to cause osteoporosis?*

Osteoblast lineage

Like the genealogy of a human being, a bone-making cell also has a genealogy called 'lineage'. The lineage of a bone-making cell goes roughly like this:

1. Stem cells ▶ 2. mesenchymal stem cells ▶ 3. Interphase progenitor cells ▶ 4. Active osteoprogenitor cells ▶ 5. osteoblast cells ▶ 6. osteocyte cells.

These six 'genealogy' points represent the main 'stages' in the lineage of bone-making cells (note: these are *dynamic* rather than static stages). There are other stages in bone-making cell lineage, but for simplicity we show just six. In general, some body cells divide (mitosis), others change (differentiation), while others do both or neither. So a bone-making cell originates from a stem cell, and in fact every cell in body originates from stem cells. In the case of bone-making cells, we are mainly interested in progenitor cells and osteoblast cells (stages 3, 4, and 5 in the above lineage), hence we talk about *osteoblast lineage*.

Osteoporosis is caused when bone-making cells dwindle, i.e. when *osteoblasts* dwindle. Osteoblasts make new bone around them until they become surrounded and encased in new bone. At this point the osteoblast is referred to as an osteocyte. It is estimated that 50% to 70% of osteoblasts die as osteocytes when bone material eventually decomposes (some osteocytes escape from their bone encasement and return to being osteoblasts).

Osteoprogenitor cells and osteoblast cells are spread throughout bone marrow, and as mentioned, whenever calcium goes into the bones about two thirds of the osteoblasts that attend to the newly arrived calcium are permanently lost to the bone-making process. Hence, the population of osteoblasts gets eroded every time new bone is made.

As far as is known, osteoblasts do not divide through mitosis. Rather, the osteoblast population is replenished from osteoprogenitor cells in bone marrow that divide and differentiate into osteoblasts. It is not thought that osteoprogenitor cells are in a *constant* state of mitosis. Rather, most progenitor cells probably spend their lives in 'interphase' during which they are more or less quiescent but not yet senescent (a kind of 'hibernation').

Chemical signals

As osteoblasts dwindle in number, some chemical trigger (hormones, cytokines, or substances released from an inflammation) causes *osteoprogenitor cells* to undergo 're-activation' and they divide to form a replacement population of progenitor cells and a second descendant lineage that differentiates into osteoblasts. So when the body 'detects' that the population of osteoblasts needs replenishing it calls on progenitor cells like a reserve army on stand-by. These progenitor cells are then mobilized by an appropriate signal when needed. [135]

So osteoblast production is likely to be controlled by localized chemical signals that alert progenitor cells to 'wake up' and differentiate into more osteoblasts (or go back into 'hibernation', i.e. stop dividing, stop producing osteoblasts, and re-enter the interphase quiescence).

If osteoblast production is controlled by localized chemical signals, *osteocytes* are the obvious candidate for the modulation signal. When osteocytes become 'trapped' in the new bone material they make around them, they stay in touch with neighbouring osteocytes and with osteoblasts on the surface of bone. They do this by sending chemical signals along thin tendrils that extend out from osteocytes to connect with other osteocytes and with osteoblasts. Osteocytes put these tendrils in place while making new bone.

The evidence

The precise mechanisms that control the population of osteoblasts are being intensely researched in efforts to prolong human life and find cures for osteoporosis. It could be that osteoprogenitor cells become less capable of replenishing osteoblasts because of changes in body chemistry or because the population of osteoprogenitor cells declines with age.

Whatever the underlying mechanism, it is known that with age osteoprogenitor cells become less capable of replenishing the body's population of bone-making osteoblasts. *The greater the erosion of osteoblasts, the greater the erosion of osteoprogenitor potential.*

In a major study on this subject scientists concluded that *'the data presented herein indicates that with age, the potential of marrow stromal cells [osteoprogenitor cells] to differentiate to osteoblasts may decrease. Thus bone loss could result from growing preponderance of osteoclasts relative to osteoblasts.'* Commenting on this study, one of the authors, Dr. Julie Glowacki, said: *'Skeletal aging is a consequence of aging of the marrow. With age, human marrow stromal cells [osteoprogenitor cells] appear to be less capable of becoming bone-forming cells, and more capable of supporting differentiation of bone-resorbing cells.'* [A]

Other studies show mounting evidence that a dwindling of bone-making cell potential in osteoblast lineage is at the root of osteoporosis:

Stem cells are progenitors for the tissue to be grown. For osteoblasts, mesenchymal stem cells (MSCs) are harvested from bone marrow. MSCs are present throughout life in bone marrow stroma, but numbers decline with age. [B]

Aging is associated with a marked decline in bone mineral density (BMD), an increased likelihood of falling and a much greater propensity for fracture. Several factors contribute to aging-related bone loss, including reduced bone formation. [C]

Age-related decrease in bone formation is well described [in medical literature]. *However, the cellular causes are not* [yet] *known. Aging* [of the bones] *is associated with decreased proliferative capacity of osteoprogenitor cells, suggesting that decreased osteoblastic cell* **number**, *and not function, leads to age-related decrease in bone formation.* [G]

It could be argued that osteoblasts decline in numbers as a natural and expected condition of aging. The challenge is to slow down the dwindling population of osteoblasts to an extent that will still keep bones healthy in old age. In some people this does not happen – in diet-related osteoporosis, osteoblasts (and their progenitors) are 'worn out' more quickly as a result of processing too much calcium in and out of bone too often. Hence, we can influence the health of bone-making cells by the way live, and in particular by the avoidance of dairy milk.

Calcium yo-yo effect

Two facts are known:

1. Osteoblasts (bone-making cells) get eroded whenever calcium from the bloodstream is processed into new bone.
2. The number of osteoblasts dwindles with human age.

In a healthy individual, these two facts do not present a problem because the bones outlive the person's life span before they become too porous and weak.

But in a person who regularly consumes acidic food high in calcium and lactose (i.e. dairy milk), this calcium is more likely to move in and out of bones causing greater erosion of osteoblassts than otherwise (the yo-yo effect, appendix four). When calcium is resorbed (pulled from the bones) in a *healthy* individual it is resorbed gently from 'exchangeable' bone, causing little or no erosion of osbteoblasts because osteocytes are mostly left intact.

So-called 'exchangeable' bone is used by the body to temporarily store calcium until it is needed by the bloodstream. This helps the bloodstream maintain a default level of calcium at all times.

When **dairy milk** is regulalrly consumed a combination of factors, as explained in ***Appendix Four***, conspire to overhwelm the bloodstream with too much calcium and then too little, causing wild swings that result in calcium being pulled from exchangeable *and* stable bone.

There is ample evidence to show that animal protein, such as in dairy milk, can readily pull calcium from stable bone. Here are some examples of the research:

- *Animal protein tends to leach calcium from the bones, leading to its excretion in the urine. Animal proteins are high in sulfur-containing amino acids, especially cystine and methionine. Sulfur is converted to sulfate, which tends to acidify the blood. During the process of neutralizing this acid, bone dissolves into the bloodstream and filters through the kidneys into the urine.* [D]

- *Increasing one's protein intake by 100% may cause calcium loss* [from the bones] *to double.* [J]

- *The body requires calcium for life and daily bodily repair. Since there is no usable calcium available* [in the bloodstream] *the brain instructs the bone matrix to release organic calcium into the blood stream. The net result is a loss of calcium from the bone matrix. This loss causes a weakening of the bone resulting in osteoporosis.* [E]

- *Dietary protein increases production of acid in the blood which can be neutralized by calcium mobilized from the skeleton.* [H]

- *We conclude that excessive dietary protein from foods with high potential renal acid load adversely affects bone, unless buffered by the consumption of alkali-rich foods or supplements.* [I]

- A 1994 study published in the American Journal of Clinical Nutrition (Remer T, Am J Clin Nutr 1994;59:1356-61) found that animal proteins cause calcium to be leached from the bones and excreted in the urine.

When calcium is pulled from the bones, this most likely erodes osteocytes,[F] and hence osteoblasts since osteocytes originate from osteoblasts. When this happens on a regular basis, the high erosion of osteoblasts eventually erodes osteoblast lineage cells. Here, we are using the word 'erosion' in its broadest sense to mean either a dwindling of osteoprogenitor cells or a curtailing of the capacity of osteoprogenitor cells to 'produce' osteoblasts.

This cascading effect of erosion from top down permanently reduces the available population of osteoblasts to a point where they can no longer keep up with the natural rate of bone decomposition. When this happens you are on the road to osteoporosis.

In this scenario, however much calcium you consume and absorb into the bloodstream, it will not help because there will be too few osteoblasts to keep up with osteoclasts and maintain a healthy level of bone density. (Osteoclasts, like pacman in the computer game, eat away at bone to make room for new bone material to be deposited). Throwing calcium and vitamin D supplements at the problem will only make matters worse because this will further erode osteoblasts as a consequence of the harmful calcium yo-yo effect.

In the future it may be possible to create/stimulate new osteoprogenitor cells by manipulating stem cells so as to give a boost to osteoblast lineage, and research in this area is well under way.

References:
A. Stefan Mueller and Julie Glowacki, Age-related decline in the osteogenic potential of human bone marrow cells cultured in three-dimensional collagen sponges, J. of Cellular Biochemistry, 82:583-590 (2000).
B. Karen Lyons, PhD, Dental Applications for Bone Morphogenetic Proteins (BMPs), MacDonald Research Laboratories, USA.
C. Drugs & Aging, June 1998, vol. 12, no. 6, pp. 477-484(8).
D. Breslau NA, et al, Relationship of animal protein-rich diet to kidney stone formation and calcium metabolism. J Clin Endocrinol 1988;66:140-6.
E. John McDougall, M.D (Physician and nutrition expert, USA).
F. Email dated 9 June 2005 from Dr. Thomas Caceci, Ph.D, anatomist, electron microscopist, and biologist; Professor, Virginia-Maryland Regional College of Veterinary Medicine, USA.
G. Stenderup K, et al, Aging is associated with decreased maximal life span and accelerated senescence of bone marrow stromal cells, J Bone Miner Res. 2003 Dec;33(6):919-26.
H. American Journal of Clinical Nutrition, 1995; 61 (4).
I. Uriel, S. et al, Excess Dietary Protein Can Adversely Affect Bone, The J. of Nutrition Vol. 128 No. 6 June 1998, pp. 1051-1053.
J. Journal of Nutrition, 1981; 111 (3).

Appendix Three:
Estrogen Myths

This appendix explains briefly the role of estrogen in the context of protecting the bones from osteoporosis, and the myths surrounding estrogen.

Estrogens are multi-functional hormones, and one of their functions involves the bones. A principal role of estrogen is to look after our bones throughout life. Sometimes confusion arises because reference is made to different types of osteoporosis such as hormonal, age-related, or postmenopausal osteoporosis. However, they are all the same because they are all caused by a lack of estrogen.

A variety of factors can make people run low on estrogen. Smoking, drinking alcohol, consuming dairy milk, having an early menopause, over-exercising, poor health, taking drugs, being over-weight, and certain medical conditions can all have an effect on whether the body can produce enough estrogen to keep bones healthy. For men the same applies: testosterone converts to a non-feminizing version of estrogen which in turn protects bones. When testosterone runs low bones are affected.

To get osteoporosis you need to run low on estrogen for many years, as the process is gradual. For example, when a postmenopausal woman aged over 50 gets osteoporosis (about 30% do!) the loss of bone actually started many years before the onset of her menopause.

Estrogen protects bones by slowing down the movement of calcium into and out of the bones. This in turn reduces the depletion of bone-making cells and keeps osteoporosis at bay. (This harmful calcium yo-yo effect is fully described in Appendix four).

How estrogen protects bones

The absorption of calcium requires the activity of bone-making cells called osteoblasts. These osteoblasts also compose pre-calcified bone-matrix, upon which the calcium can precipitate. Deportation of calcium from the bones requires the activity of osteoclasts. Osteoclast cells eat up old bone to make way for new bone to be put in the same space. If more calcium is absorbed into the bones, as happens when there is insufficient estrogen, [G] the production and activity of both osteoblasts and osteoclasts is increased. [H] When too much calcium is absorbed it gets deported (sent out of the bones). But 50 to 70% of the composing osteoblasts die in the composition of new matrix. [B] So the more their activity is stimulated, the more they die. [I] And since estrogen inhibits uptake of calcium, [D] estrogen prevents the death of osteoblasts. [J] Estrogen prevents apoptosis (death) of osteoblasts, in particular, because osteoblasts are more sensitive to aging phenomena than osteoclasts. [E] It is thought that estrogen supplements increase calcium influx into the bones, but this is only the case in the first few days of administration. [A] Hence the movement of calcium in and out bones is generally reduced.

To summarize: Hormones produced by the body induce circulation of calcium from the blood into the bones and vice versa, 'pumping' the calcium around. Estrogens act to slow down the movement of calcium into bones, thus preserving bone-making cells (osteoblasts) from erosion. [A, B, C]

The reason why osteoporosis risk is higher in women than in men is due to monthly estrogen and PTH fluctuations.[F] Estrogen levels in women strongly fluctuate monthly. When the estrogen level is at its lowest around menstruation, PTH levels shoot up, increasing deportation of calcium from the bones and uptake of calcium into the bones. PTH is a powerful hormone that increases the movement of calcium in and out of bones, thus eroding bone-making cells.

When a healthy person with a *normal level of estrogen* consumes dairy milk, this causes calcium to be pumped in and out of the bones (the harmful calcium yo-yo effect) in spite of the presence of estrogen. In a person with *depleted estrogen*, the calcium yo-yo effect is likely to be more pronounced and result in greater depletion of bone-making cells. For this reason, postmenopausal women in particular should avoid dairy milk.

Estrogen Misconceptions

Misconception no. 1: It is thought that that estrogen protects bones by correcting the imbalance between bone decomposition and bone creation, i.e. by slowing down bone decomposition and speeding up bone creation. This is not so for two reasons:

- Estrogen does not stimulate osteoblasts into making more bone. On the contrary, it inhibits this activity.

- New bone can only be made in the spaces made vacant by decomposition of old bone. Hence, when bone decomposition is slowed down by estrogen, the creation of new bone is also slowed down. (Otherwise there would be nowhere to put the newly create bone!). If bones are porous, they stay porous until they decompose and (hopefully) become replaced with more firm bone. Osteoblasts do not travel around the bones looking for porous holes to fill in.

Misconception no. 2: It is thought that estrogen protects bones by virtually stopping the decomposition of old bone. This is not so. If it were so, **little or no** new bone could be created to replace old bone. In this scenario, the bones would age through wear and tear, and become weaker and more brittle by not being gradually renewed.

Misconception no. 3: It is thought that estrogen makes bones stronger, i.e. denser. This is not so. Estrogen protects bones by ***not increasing bone density***. Whenever bone density is increased, valuable bone-making cells are depleted, bringing nearer the day that you may get osteoporosis. Remember: increased bone density does not necessarily equate with healthier bones.

Estrogen helps by keeping the rate at which bone is lost and replaced on a nice even keel (not too fast, not too slow, just enough to keep the bones sufficiently strong for normal everyday activities). This ensures you always have enough bone-making cells 'in the bank' to keep up with the rate of bone decomposition throughout life.

Estrogen (or testosterone) supplements do not increase bone density. This means that a woman with osteoporosis cannot hope to recover bone density by taking estrogen supplements. Estrogen helps by maintaining the status quo, i.e. by preventing further bone loss and by minimizing erosion of valuable bone-making cells. If it were possible to recover bone density by taking estrogen supplements osteoporosis would easily be eradicated.

Bone difference between men and women

Women experience an earlier, much more dramatic loss of bone density than men. The rapid loss of bone density, 1% to 3% loss per year, occurs at the time of menopause and continues for about the next 3 to 5 years. Several years after the menopause, the rate of bone loss slows down and then may increase again after age 70.

Note that 'bone loss' in the context of osteoporosis refers to a decrease in bone density due to insufficient bone-making cells. When this happens, you do not have enough bone-making cells to keep up with the rate of bone decomposition. This is a permanent and irreversible condition. In osteoporosis, the rate of bone loss can slow down if the rate of bone decomposition slows down.

Men do not have a rapid bone loss with age because they do not experience a dramatic decline in either estrogen or testosterone levels. This helps protect men from osteoporosis. Men experience greater bone loss later in life, around age 70 years or older, when estrogen and testosterone levels start to decline. When aged over 70, women are twice as likely as men to get osteoporosis.

The risk for fractures in the spine and hip increases after about age 50 in both men and women. The increase in the rate of hip fractures occurs later, after age 65. It is estimated that women are generally two to three times more likely to get osteoporosis compared to men. It seems to me that an estrogen test should always accompany a bone scan test to give a fuller picture.

Sources:

A. Qu Q, et al, Estrogen enhances differentiation of osteoblasts in mouse bone marrow culture. Bone '98 Mar;22(3):201-9.
B. Jilka RL, et al, Loss of estrogen upregulates osteoblastogenesis in the murine bone marrow. Evidence for autonomy from factors released during bone resorption. J. Clin. Invest. 1998 / 101 (9) / 1942-1950.
C. Westerlind KC, et al, Estrogen does not increase bone formation in growing rats. Endocrinology1993 / 133 (6) / 2924-2934.
D. Bryant HU, et al, An estrogen receptor basis for raloxifene action in bone. J Steroid Biochem Mol Biol 1999 / 69 (1-6) / 37-44. , Jilka RL, et al, Loss of estrogen upregulates osteoblastogenesis in the murine bone marrow. Evidence for autonomy from factors released during bone resorption. J. Clin. Invest. 1998 / 101 (9) / 1942-1950. , Sims NA, et al, Estradiol treatment transiently increases trabecular bone volume in ovariectomized rats. Bone1996 / 19 (5) / 455-461.Smith, G.R. et al, Inhibitory action of oestrogen on calcium-induced mitosis in rat bone marrow and thymus. J. Endocrinol. 1975 / 65 (1) / 45-53.
E. Eriksen EF, et al, The pathogenesis of osteoporosis. Horm. Res.1997 / 48 Suppl 5 / 78-82.
F. Zittermann A, et al, Physiologic fluctuations of serum estradiol levels influence biochemical markers of bone resorption in young women. J Clin Endocrinol Metab 2000 / 85 (1) / 95-101.
G. Erben RG, et al, Androgen deficiency induces high turnover osteopenia in aged male rats: a sequential histomorphometric study. J. Bone Miner. Res. 2000 / 15 (6) / 1085-1098. , Yeh JK, et al, Ovariectomy-induced high turnover in cortical bone is dependent on pituitary hormone in rats. Bone1996 / 18 (5) / 443-540. , Garnero P, et al, Increased bone turnover in late postmenopausal women is a major determinant of osteoporosis. J. Bone Miner. Res.1996 / 11 (3) / 337-349.
H. Taguchi Y, et al, Interleukin-6-type cytokines stimulate mesenchymal progenitor differentiation toward the osteoblastic lineage. Proc. Assoc. Am. Physicians 1998 / 110 (6) / 559-574. , Jilka RL, et al, Loss of estrogen upregulates osteoblastogenesis in the murine bone marrow. Evidence for autonomy from factors released during bone resorption. J. Clin. Invest. 1998 / 101 (9) / 1942-1950. , Tau KR, et al, Estrogen regulation of a transforming growth factor-beta inducible early gene that inhibits deoxyribonucleic acid synthesis in human osteoblasts. Endocrinology1998 / 139 (3) / 1346-1353. , Hietala EL, The effect of ovariectomy on periosteal bone formation and bone resorption in adult rats. Bone Miner. 1993 / 20 (1) / 57-65. , Egrise D, et al, Bone blood flow and in vitro proliferation of bone marrow and trabecular bone osteoblast-like cells in ovariectomized rats. Calcif. Tissue Int. 1992 / 50 (4) / 336-341.
I. Mogi M, et al, Involvement of nitric oxide and biopterin in proinflammatory cytokine-induced apoptotic cell death in mouse osteoblastic cell line MC3T3-E1. Biochem. Pharmacol. 1999 / 58 (4) / 649-654. , Kobayashi ET, et al, Force-induced rapid changes in cell fate at midpalatal suture cartilage of growing rats. J. Dent. Res.1999 / 78 (9) / 1495-1504.
J. Vegeto E, et al, Estrogen and progesterone induction of survival of monoblastoid cells undergoing TNF-alpha-induced apoptosis. FASEB J.1999 / 13 (8) / 793-803. , Tomkinson A, et al, The role of estrogen in the control of rat osteocyte apoptosis. J. Bone Miner. Res. 1998 / 13 (8) / 1243-1250.

Appendix Four:
The Calcium Yo-Yo Effect

This appendix describes how dairy milk causes calcium to go in and out of the bones (the yo-yo effect) thus eroding bone-making cells, causing bones to age and weaken prematurely. Whenever calcium goes into bone osteoblasts get used up. When this happens too often, the in-and-out movement of calcium can lead to osteoporosis.

The two chapters that relate to this appendix are: ***Dairy Milk Effect on Osteoporosis*** and ***Dairy Milk Effect on Calcification***. Also, see appendices two and three.

A *metaphorical* and a *technical* explanation is given for each movement of calcium going in or going out of the bones (the reader is invited to read both). This appendix is not intended to be a medical guide but an explanation for one of the major causes of osteoporosis.

As you read through each step keep in mind that in reality calcium is being pumped in and out of bones several times a day as part of the natural way the body works. The less vigorous this pumping (yo-yo) action the better for bones.

1. Metaphorical explanation – acidity pulls calcium from the bones.

Dairy milk is very acidic, caused by the high content of indigestible protein. So when consumed the high acidity quickly coats the digestive system. The body hates this as it much prefers alkalinity. Soon, the acidity creeps into the bloodstream and this cannot be tolerated as the blood always has to stay neutral, with acidity and alkalinity equally balanced. As a result, the bloodstream has to defend itself against the invading acidity, and it pulls calcium from the bones (calcium acts like a reserve army of alkaline soldiers). Soon, the alkaline soldiers take away the acidic invaders – they get stuck to each other and get expelled from the body, and the acidity goes down.

1. Technical explanation – acidity causes resorption of calcium.

The alkalinity of blood is pH 7.365. The body is required to keep alkaline/acidity levels of plasma tightly regulated. When dairy milk, which is acidic, is consumed PTH (parathyroid hormone) is released into the blood to raise levels of calcium and reduce levels of acidic protein molecules. In response to PTH, calcium is resorbed (from the bones) into blood. The alkaline calcium molecules then bind with the acidic protein molecules and get excreted in urine. This brings the level of acidity in the blood down to an acceptable level.

2. Metaphorical explanation – excess calcium pushes calcium into bones.

Now that the acidity caused by dairy milk is under control the bloodstream has to deal with the calcium from the milk which is beginning to come through from the digestive system, helped by the lactose in milk. As dairy milk is high in calcium it causes the level of calcium in the blood to get too high for comfort. This makes the blood think it is getting too much calcium from the digestive system so until things change it will get rid of as much calcium as possible. The bloodstream likes to have a good steady amount of calcium to carry around the body for feeding to body cells. It hates getting bombarded with large amounts of calcium because it makes the body grind to a halt. Muscles would not even move (the heart would stop beating!) if high levels of calcium were allowed to stay in the bloodstream.

To sort things out the bloodstream panics and gets rid of calcium however it can. It sends some of the calcium to the kidneys for excretion through urine, it dumps some of the calcium in nooks and crannies of the body causing harmful calcification, and the rest is parked in the bones to get it out of the way. Even though the calcium is now getting lower (phew!) the bloodstream continues to beaver away getting rid of as much calcium as possible in case more calcium is still being consumed. After all, who knows whether more calcium might be on its way!

2. Technical explanation – excess plasma calcium is deported to the bones:

As the plasma concentration of acidity comes down dietary calcium from dairy milk is absorbed, helped by milk lactose. Since calcium is essential, plasma levels must be tightly regulated. The normal range is 2.12-2.65 mmol/L. Dietary intake is variable, so the body must be able to adapt to raised or reduced plasma calcium. Calcium regulation involves the loss or gain of calcium from the kidneys, intestines, and bones. The increased plasma levels of calcium triggers the release of calcitonin, a hormone which acts to lower the level of calcium. Plasma calcium must be depleted for continued muscle function throughout the body. (Note that dairy milk itself contains calcitonin which serves to exacerbate the overall calcitonin effect on plasma calcium depletion).

In response to calcitonin, plasma calcium is deported to the kidneys for excretion, and to exchangeable bone. Also, some of the calcium is assimilated into arterial plaque where it gets used by nanobacteria leading to harmful calcification in parts of the body. Even though levels of plasma calcium are dropping, calcitonin continues to be released until it no longer feels the presence of calcium.

3. Metaphorical explanation - Too little calcium forces calcium to be pulled from the bones again.

Suddenly the bloodstream realizes there is no more calcium to get rid of and no more calcium is coming in from the outside world. The bloodstream had no way of knowing that this was going to happen so it got caught short. It now does not have enough calcium. This is bad news because it must always carry a certain level of calcium for feeding to body cells everywhere and keeping everything alive and well. The bloodstream now reverses engines and pulls calcium back from the bones (the yo-yo effect). In a frantic effort to recover more calcium than it intended to lose, the bloodstream also tells the kidneys to stop excreting calcium and return it. On top of that, it makes an extra big effort to squeeze as much calcium from the intestines as possible (let's hope there is still some left). Calcium now comes back into the bloodstream from these three sources.

Note: if the dairy milk has added vitamin D3, as in the USA, Canada, and some other countries, this gives a big boost to the bloodstream's efforts to recover calcium. Vitamin D3 helps the bloodstream get high amounts of calcium from just about everywhere (the bones, the kidneys, and the digestive system) thus adding to the harmful *calcium yo-yo effect*.

By now the bloodstream has succeeded in recovering *more than enough* calcium, just to make sure it got enough. As a result, the bloodstream now sends some of the surplus calcium back into the bones (the yo-yo effect) and to the kidneys. It also dumps some of the excess calcium in the arteries. This time round things are not so frantic as the bloodstream has the amount of calcium it likes to have. For the moment then everything is calm, until the next big wave of dairy milk causes havoc again when more is consumed.

3. Technical explanation – Low plasma calcium triggers resorption from bones.

When plasma calcium is low enough to not react with calcitonin, the release of calcitonin ceases. PTH (parathyroid hormone) is now released in response to low blood calcium. PTH acts to raise plasma calcium to its normal physiological concentration. Once blood calcium levels are restored, PTH production is inhibited. As a result of PTH secretion into plasma, calcium is resorbed from the bone, and kidney secretion is inhibited. Also, PTH precipitates calcium availability from the intestines.

When calcium levels go up sufficiently PTH secretion is inhibited and calcitonin is released to bring calcium down to a default level of concentration. So between PTH and calcitonin, calcium levels are brought 'under control'.

PTH stimulates uptake of calcium into the bones, osteoblast apoptosis (death), and deportation of calcium from the bones. This is exactly the opposite of the influence of estrogen, and since estrogen is protective, excessive PTH logically accelerates osteoporosis. In general PTH causes erosion of bone, releasing calcium and phosphate ions.

Note: some countries, such as the USA and Canada add vitamin D3 (cholicalciferol) to dairy milk. The amount added is 400 IU of D3 per quart - this is 100% of the US Recommended Daily Allowance (about 4 cupfuls provides the full RDA). This vitamin D3 acts to resorb calcium into plasma. This is so because vitamin D does not help the body absorb calcium until the vitamin D has first been absorbed into the bloodstream. *The vitamin D necessary to absorb calcium moving down the intestine must already have been in the bloodstream for a while – what is present with that calcium (in milk) is useless at that stage.*[46] As a consequence, vitamin D3 in dairy milk is available to resorb calcium from bone, and also absorb calcium from the intestines. This in turn adds to the harmful *calcium yo-yo effect*.

4. Metaphorical explanation – The yo-yo effect: Every time calcium goes in and out of the bones (the yo-yo effect) it uses up bone-making cells. This is so because bone-making cells sacrifice their lives in the process of making new bone. So as their numbers dwindle over time, their population becomes less and less capable of making enough new bone to keep up with the rate of decomposition of old bone. When this happens osteoporosis develops. Over-consumption of calcium combined with animal protein (as in the case of dairy milk) causes the *calcium yo-yo effect* which in turn leads to osteoporosis.

Note that in general the body hates any kind of yo-yo effect as it creates internal havoc and turmoil. For example, it is well known that yo-yo dieting (repeatedly losing and regaining weight) promotes cancer. People who keep their weight stable have at least a third more cancer-killing cells that help fight off disease.

4. Technical description – The yo-yo effect: Every time calcium is absorbed into bone osteoblast cells are eroded as they mature into osteocytes. 50% to 70% of osteoblasts differentiate into osteocytes and perish when bone decomposes.[135]

This erosion of osteoblasts eventually reduces the rate of bone replacement, increasing the risk of osteoporosis. Over-consumption of calcium combined with animal protein (as in the case of dairy milk) increases both uptake of calcium into bone and resorption from bone (the yo-yo effect), increasing the onset of osteoporosis. Note that if too little *calcitriol* (vitamin D3) is available, the secretion of PTH is not sufficiently inhibited.

The 'yo-yo' effect has other parallels in the body, albeit with different underlying mechanisms. For example, it is known that yo-yo dieting (repeatedly losing and regaining weight) promotes cancer. In the June 2005 issue of the *Journal of the American Dietetic Association* it was found that yo-yo dieting promotes long-term immune function decreases in proportion to how many times a woman reportedly intentionally loses weight. They also found that immune function as measured by natural-killer-cell activity was up to 40% higher among women who had been fairly weight stable over several years.

5. Metaphorical explanation – Avoiding the calcium yo-yo effect. The key is to give up dairy milk and eat little or no dairy products. It is best to follow a healthy *mixed* diet of fruit, vegetables, salads, nuts, seeds, and pulses. By doing this the body will get exactly the right amount of calcium it needs without the harmful calcium yo-yo effect.

Osteoporosis is caused when we keep consuming a cocktail of *excess calcium combined* with indigestible animal protein as contained in dairy milk. Very little vitamin D is needed for healthy bones. For example, studies show that women who always go outdoors wearing clothing that completely covers their body, do not suffer from a lack of vitamin D. [113]

If too little calcium is consumed a day (a very hard thing to do since virtually all fruit, vegetables, salads, seeds, and pulses contain calcium) *and* you get no vitamin D (by for example living in a cave), this can lead to osteoporosis as the bone-making cells will not have enough calcium to make new bone. To do this you would have to deliberately avoid foods containing calcium or vitamin D and always keep out of the sun!

5. Technical explanation – Avoiding the calcium yo-yo effect.

If dairy products are avoided or minimized and a balanced diet is consumed, the body will get the optimum amount of calcium it needs without the harmful calcium yo-yo effect.

Osteoporosis is caused as a consequence of frequent absorption of *excess calcium* into the bones. Each time calcium is absorbed (whether or not it is *excess calcium*) osteoblasts are eroded. Excess calcium always gets resorbed. Therefore the less frequent the absorption of calcium into bone, the less the osteoblasts get eroded. As with all minerals, the body normally absorbs just as much calcium from food as it needs. Only about 200 mg is absorbed into the blood, on the average, whether we consume 300 mg or 700 mg calcium daily, or sometimes even when we consume up to 1200 mg supplementary calcium daily. [114] In order to absorb the right amount of calcium, absorption rate decreases when we consume more calcium (unless *excess calcium* is consumed), and this avoids the calcium yo-yo effect. Also, note that very little vitamin D is needed for healthy bones. For example, studies show that women who always go outdoors wearing clothing that completely covers their skin exposure to sunlight, do not suffer from a lack of vitamin D. [113]

If too little calcium is consumed (less than 300 mg / day which is a very hard thing to achieve), and there is a lack of vitamin D / calcitriol, this can cause osteoporosis by making it impossible to increase calcium absorption.

Appendix Five:
Dairy Milk and Prostate Cancer

Prostate cancer is a major disease that is becoming more common in men, both young and old. Worldwide, it affects more *men* than any other type of cancer.

Although prostate cancer is more common in old age, the incidence is determined by lifestyle factors in *early* life. Scientists think that a poor diet is the biggest cause of prostate cancer, and many studies point in this direction.

In fact, virtually all the latest research is saying that dairy milk products are the principal *dietary* cause of prostate cancer. Strong evidence supports this: **Why do men in Japan have 90% less prostate cancer than men in the USA?** Because men in Japan consume much less dairy milk. **Why do Latvia, Denmark, and Romania have the highest per capita incidence of prostate cancer?** Because these three countries are among the highest milk-consuming countries in the world.

The evidence concerning prostate cancer and consumption of dairy milk is now so overwhelming that, for this reason alone, men of all ages should avoid dairy milk.

The following is a list of brief excerpts from the many studies into the causes of prostate cancer. Please do read the excerpts that follow as they paint a fascinating picture:

- *In conclusion, we found a positive association between **milk** consumption and prostate cancer.* Qin LQ, et al, Milk consumption is a risk factor for prostate cancer: meta-analysis of case-control studies, Nutr Cancer. 2004;48(1):22-7.

- *... higher calcium and **milk** intakes appear to increase risk of advanced prostate cancer.* Giovannucci E., The epidemiology of vitamin D and cancer incidence and mortality, Cancer Causes Control. 2005 Mar;16(2):83-95.

- *Dairy **milk** consumption may increase prostate cancer risk through a calcium-related pathway.* Tseng M, et al, Dairy, calcium, and vitamin D intakes and prostate cancer risk in the National Health and Nutrition Examination Epidemiologic Follow-up Study cohort, Am J Clin Nutr. 2005 May;81(5):1147-54.

- *These results support the hypothesis that dairy **milk** products and calcium are associated with a greater risk of prostate cancer.* Chan JM, et al, Dairy products, calcium, and prostate cancer risk in the Physicians' Health Study, Am J Clin Nutr. 2001 Oct;74(4):549-54.

- *A significantly increased risk of prostate cancer was associated with skim **milk** as compared to whole **milk**…suggesting that dietary animal fat is not associated with risk of prostate cancer.* Veierod MB, et al, Dietary fat intake and risk of prostate cancer: a prospective study of 25,708 Norwegian men, Int J Cancer. 1997 Nov 27;73(5):634-8.

- *Diet has long been recognized as a strong factor in prostate carcinogenesis. The most significant dietary factors in prostate carcinogenesis are energy, total fat, animal fat, **milk, calcium** and red meat.* Zhu G, et al, Role of dietary factors in prostate cancer development, Zhonghua Nan Ke Xue. 2005 May;11(5):375-8. (Chinese study in a country where dairy milk consumption is very low).

- *A significant trend of increasing risk with more frequent consumption was found for **milk** and dairy products. No strong association exists between any specific foods and prostate cancer, apart from an increased risk for **milk** and dairy products, and a possible protective effect of vegetables.* Bosetti C, et al, Food groups and risk of prostate cancer in Italy, Int J Cancer. 2004 Jun 20;110(3):424-8.

- *The strongest risk factor for prostate cancer mortality was animal products.* Grant WB, A multicountry ecologic study of risk and risk reduction factors for prostate cancer mortality, Eur Urol. 2004 Mar;45(3):271-9.

- *Among the food items examined, **milk** was most closely correlated with prostatic cancer incidence.* Li XM, et al, The effects of estrogen-like products in milk on prostate and testes, Zhonghua Nan Ke Xue. 2003 Jun;9(3):186-90.

- *For prostate cancer, epidemiologic studies consistently show a positive association with high consumption of **milk**…* Giovannucci E, Nutritional factors in human cancers, Adv Exp Med Biol. 1999;472:29-42.

- *These results support several cohort studies which found the non-fat portion of **milk** to have the highest association with prostate cancer, likely due to the **calcium**…* Grant WB, An ecologic study of dietary links to prostate cancer, Altern Med Rev. 1999 Jun;4(3):162-9.

- *Relative risks for prostate cancer were elevated for intake of beef and **milk**.* Le Marchand L, et al, Animal fat consumption and prostate cancer: a prospective study in Hawaii, Epidemiology. 1994 May;5(3):276-82.

- *Positive correlations between foods and cancer mortality rates were particularly strong in the case of meats and milk for breast cancer, **milk** for prostate and ovarian cancer.* Rose DP, et al, International comparisons of mortality rates for cancer of the breast, ovary, prostate, and colon, and per capita food consumption, Cancer. 1986 Dec 1;58(11):2363-71.

- *Suggestive positive associations were also seen between fatal prostate cancer and the consumption of **milk**, cheese, eggs, and meat.* Snowdon

DA, et al, Diet, obesity, and risk of fatal prostate cancer, Am J Epidemiol. 1984 Aug;120 (2):244-50.

- *A summary of studies of prostate cancer shows a repeated association between consumption of **dairy products** and an elevated risk of developing prostate cancer. For example, in one study consuming two glasses of **milk** per day was associated with a 50% greater risk.'* Report from the *Harvard School Of Public Health Nutrition Roundtable,* Section 3: Calcium: Too Much of a Good Thing? www.molliekatzen.com/harvard3.php.

- *Men who reported drinking three or more glasses of whole **milk** daily [average daily consumption in the USA is 2-3 glasses] had a relative risk [of prostate cancer] of 2.49 compared with men who reported never drinking whole **milk**...animal fat is related to increased risk of prostate cancer which is now the most common cancer diagnosed in U.S men.* Roswell Park Memorial Institute, USA, Cancer 64 (3): 605-612.

As you can see, virtually all the latest research into prostate cancer is pointing to *dairy milk* as being the principal dietary cause. But what is also becoming clear is that *calcium* in dairy milk is the culprit (rather than animal fat). When a cancerous prostate is examined, the cancerous growth inside the prostate is seen to be caused by calcification. Doctors are familiar with this and refer to it as 'calcified concretions in the prostate gland lumina.'

The question then is this: **What causes harmful calcification in the prostate?** The many studies into this subject usually have three factors in common:

1. Prostate cancer occurs as a result of calcification.
2. Prostate cancer incidence is highest in dairy milk consumers.
3. Calcium in dairy milk (rather than fat) is shown to be the instigator of prostate cancer.

With recent discoveries in nanobacteria a fourth factor can be added: scientists now widely accept that harmful calcification is caused by nanobacteria (see chapter ***Dairy Milk Effect on Calcification***).

For the first time, then, we can now begin to answer the question ***What causes harmful calcification in the prostate?*** The answer is that harmful calcification is likely to be caused by dairy milk which acts to feed calcium and phosphorus to nanobacteria lurking in the prostate. This explains why calcium rather milk-fat causes calcification. As is well known by medical scientists, when 'calcified concretions' develop in any part of the body this can interfere with the body's immunity and efficiency, and this in turn can lead to cancerous growth. The imperative for any man, young or old, is to avoid dairy milk as this reduces the risk of prostate cancer later in life.

Appendix Six: Milk Recipe List

A complete at-a-glance list of all the non-dairy milk recipes given in this book

For background information to each milk recipe: see *Part Two*.
For the milk recipes themselves: see *Part Three*.

Notes:

- The many sprouted seed milks that you can make are not listed in the table below as full details are given in the chapter *Sprouted seed milk* (**Part Two** of this book). Sprouted seed milk is delicious and super-nutritious, and well worth making.

- Asterisks (*) in the table indicate nut or seed based milks: these are usually regarded as the best tasting.

Basic ingredient (Alphabetical)	Corresponding non-dairy milk * Best tasting	Basic ingredient (Alphabetical)	Corresponding non-dairy milk * Best tasting
Almonds (dry almonds)	Dry Almond milk*	Macadamia nuts	Macadamia milk*
Almonds (soaked almonds)	Soaked Almond milk*	Oats, various	Oat milk
Blended milks	See 'Blended Milks' chapter in *Part Three*.	Peanuts	Peanut milk*
Brazil nuts	Brazil nut milk*	Peas – see Green Peas	See *Green pea milk*
Cashew nuts	Cashew nut milk*	Pecan nuts	Pecan milk*
Chestnuts	Chestnut milk*	Pine nuts	Pine nut milk*
Coconuts	Coconut milk*	Pumpkin seeds	Pumpkin seed milk*
Corn off the cob (sweet corn)	Corn milk	Sesame seeds	Sesame seed milk*

Grains: rice, millet, quinoa, amaranth, etc.	See 'Grain Milks' chapter in **Part Two**.	Soybeans	Soy milk
Green peas (frozen or fresh)	Green pea milk	Sprouted seeds	Sprouted seed milk (various)
Hazelnuts (dry hazelnuts)	Hazelnut milk*	Sunflower seeds	Sunflower seed milk*
Hazelnuts (soaked hazelnuts)	Hazelnut milk*	Tiger nuts	Tiger nut milk
Hemp seeds	Hempseed milk*	Walnuts	Walnut milk*

***

Appendix Seven: The Missing Link

This appendix addresses the missing link between osteoporosis on the one hand and diseases caused by calcification on the other hand. There is a strong correlation between the two, and to illustrate this we will look at heart disease. The question that arises is: *How can there be a common link between two diseases which, on the face of it, have nothing in common?* The evidence of a common link is clear from a number of studies:

1. *These results suggest that mitral* [heart] *annular calcification in elderly women can be attributed to ectopic calcium deposits* [harmful calcification] *related to the severe bone loss caused by postmenopausal osteoporosis.* Source: Sugihara N, et al, The influence of severe bone loss on mitral annular calcification in postmenopausal osteoporosis of elderly Japanese women, Jpn Circ J 1993;57:14–26.

2. *There is an association between age-related loss of bone mass and aortic/aortic valve calcification.* Source: Ouchi Y, et al, Age-related loss of bone mass and aortic/aortic valve calcification—reevaluation of recommended dietary allowance of calcium in the elderly. Ann N Y Acad Sci 1993;676:297–307.

3. *Women with aortic* [heart] *calcification had significantly lower... bone density compared to those without calcification. These women may be at increased risk for both osteoporosis and cardiovascular disease.* Source: Banks LM, et al, Effect of degenerative spinal and aortic calcification on bone density measurements in post-menopausal women: Links between osteoporosis and cardiovascular disease? Eur J Clin Invest 1994;12:813–17.

4. *Osteoporotic women had high serum cholesterol concentration which is unequivocally associated with peripheral vascular disease. Thus, our results are suggesting the relationship between atherosclerosis* [heart disease] *and osteoporosis.* Source: Broulik PD, et al, Interrelations between body weight, cigarette smoking and spine mineral density in osteoporotic Czech women. Endocr Regul 1993;27:57–60.

5. A study by Dr. R Boukhris showed a strong correlation between calcification of the aorta (heart artery) and osteoporosis. Source: Boukhris R, Becker KL. Calcification of the aorta and osteoporosis. JAMA 1972;219:1307–11.

6. *We conclude that aortic* [heart] *calcifications are a strong predictor for low bone density and fragility fractures.* Source: Eloy Schulz, et al, Aortic Calcification and the Risk of Osteoporosis and Fractures, The Journal of Clinical Endocrinology & Metabolism Vol. 89, No. 9 4246-4253.

7. *We have found a strong association between mitral annulus* [heart] *calcification and osteoporosis in women.* Source: Vedat Davutoglu MD, et al,

A Case of Massive Dystrophic Cardiac Calcinosis With Increased Bone Resorption Markers: A Novel Pathophysiologic Link? Cardiology in Review. 12(6):306-308, November/December 2004.

8. *In general, postmenopausal women are advised to take calcium supplements to prevent or treat osteoporosis, implying that bone loss is due to insufficient dietary calcium. Yet, in many patients with osteoporosis, loss of bone tissue from the skeleton occurs at the same time as formation of bone in the artery wall. This paradox suggests that dietary calcium is not the limiting factor. The association of osteoporosis with vascular calcification has been reported widely.* Source: Linda L Demer, Vascular calcification and osteoporosis: inflammatory responses to oxidized lipids, International Journal of Epidemiology 2002; 31:737-741.

9. *Coronary calcification in men appears to be directly related to bone mineral loss.* Source: Amanda Patenaude, et al, Inverse Relationship Between Simultaneously Measured Coronary Calcification and Bone Mineral Density in 12,000 Patients: Relationship to HDL Cholesterol. Paper presented at the American College of Cardiology Scientific Sessions, 2002.

The above studies and others show that the incidence of osteoporosis is much higher in people with heart disease and this has mystified doctors for many years – what is the common link between the two? When you look at breast cancer research a similar picture emerges. Here are just two quotes from the many studies that corroborate this:

Due to the high prevalence rates of both low bone mass and breast carcinoma in women, these two diseases commonly coexist in the same individuals. Source: Van Poznak, et al, Clinical management of osteoporosis in women with a history of breast carcinoma. Cancer. 2005 Aug 1;104(3):443-56.

Osteoporosis is one such problem that has been increasingly identified in cancer patients. Several studies have indicated that the prevalence of fractures is higher in breast and prostate cancer patients compared to the general population. Source: Hoff AO, et al, Osteoporosis in breast and prostate cancer survivors, Oncology (Williston Park). 2005 Apr;19(5):651-8. Review.

Doctors have known for many years that harmful calcification causes heart disease, breast cancer and a multitude of other diseases. Such calcification is sometimes referred to as being caused by *hypercalcemia* or calcinosis. But doctors have struggled to explain why diseases caused by calcification go hand in hand with a high incidence of osteoporosis. **It is now being recognized is that if you look at a cohort of patients with just about any calcification-based disease, you will find that the incidence of osteoporosis in the cohort is significantly higher than the average population.**

What is this missing link that causes both osteoporosis and calcification-based diseases? The answer is now becoming clear. Consider this:

A. Dairy milk ▶ calcium yo-yo effect ▶ loss of bone-making cells ▶ osteoporosis.

B. Dairy milk ▶ calcium yo-yo effect ▶ harmful calcification ▶ calcification-based disease.

The missing link that is common to both osteoporosis and calcification-based disease is the harmful calcium yo-yo effect caused by the regular consumption of dairy milk. As explained in appendix four, the calcium yo-yo effect wears out bone-making cells which ultimately increases the risk of osteoporosis. Equally, the calcium yo-yo effect galvanizes the bloodstream into inadvertently feeding calcium and phosphorus to nanobacteria – this in turn promotes harmful calcification and a multitude of diseases.

The missing link, then, is dairy milk. Some people have speculated that the missing link could be estrogen, but there is no evidence that estrogen or the lack of estrogen, promotes arterial plaque or harmful calcification. It could be argued that as estrogen acts to slow down the harmful calcium yo-yo effect (see appendix three), estrogen indirectly slows down the incidence of harmful calcification. This may be so, but estrogen is unlikely to be a common link since the dual presence of osteoporosis and calcification-based disease is apparent in both men and women.

Quite simply then, the missing link is the regular consumption of dairy milk. But this raises an interesting point: In July 2005 Katja Hansen, co-author of *The Calcium Bomb* stated on the book's website:

Calcification usually doesn't seem to have much to do with calcium intake, because most calcification happens when calcium levels in the blood are normal rather than too high. Some can happen when levels are too low, as with osteoporosis.

This is so because, as explained in this appendix, harmful calcification and osteoporosis go very much hand in hand. Clearly, harmful calcification is not related to calcium intake, but to the calcium yo-yo effect which triggers the availability of calcium and phosphorus for nanobacteria to feed on. It is also clear that calcification occurs whatever the level of calcium in the blood because, with the calcium yo-yo effect, the level of calcium can be just about anywhere, up or down. If a person *mostly* has a default level of calcium in the blood (i.e. a level that does not trigger unhealthy hormonal reactions and the calcium yo-yo effect), this person is likely to have optimum health. Such a person may harbour nanobacteria, but harmful calcification is unlikely to develop significantly in the absence of the calcium yo-yo effect. If this were **not so**, everybody, including super-healthy people, would suffer from calcification and clearly this is not the case.

About the Author

Russell Eaton lived in Ecuador as a child, and then moved back to England where he worked in the computer industry for many years. He has a *Higher National Diploma in Business Studies*, University of Wales, and is now an established author with books relating to travel, health, and property. With a life-long interest in health and nutrition he says: *'The Milk Imperative is a book I have always wanted to write because the truth about dairy milk is not so widely known. Also, I felt it was important to show a fuller picture about dairy milk given the new research that is coming to light '*

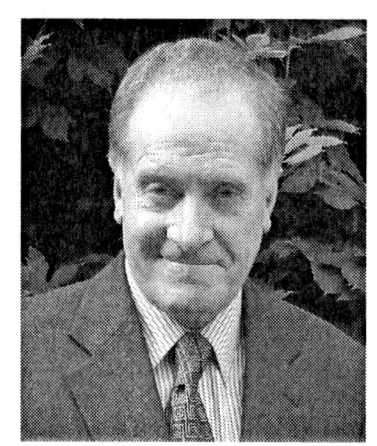

Other books by Russell Eaton include:

How To Avoid Stamp Duty

Shows how to avoid stamp duty and make substantial savings whether buying or selling property. Ideal for UK residential property. Buyers can avoid stamp duty and make big savings, prevent losing a property through lack of cash, and cover legal costs without using own money. Sellers can offer property at lower price or free of stamp duty without financial loss, and prevent losing a buyer over price. For more information go to www.stampduty.cc.

Air Travel Survival:
How to survive a plane crash and other flight dangers

Shows how to reduce the risk of injury and death in the event of a plane crash by using the unique **'S.I.N.G. Survival Method'**. It also shows how to stay well and avoid infection from re-circulated cabin air, how to avoid high altitude radiation, a foolproof way to avoid jetlag, best way to travel by air with children, and many other tips and tricks for air travellers. For more information go to www.airtravelsurvival.com.

Staying in touch with
The Milk Imperative

To stay in touch with all matters relating to this book, please visit the website www.milkimperative.com. Here you will find the latest news, comments and issues arising from the book, plus information to keep you up to date on dairy and non-dairy milk. Further copies of this book can be ordered from any good bookshop, from some health stores, and from online sources such as www.amazon.com. For more order information, please go to www.milkimperative.com. The author or publisher can be contacted through the website, or by email to: milkimperative@milkimperative.com.

Index

acidity, 50, 263
acne, 106
allergy, 12, 41
   nuts, 225
almond milk, 178
   recipe, 227
amino acids, 99, 162
animal milk, 136
antibiotics, 27
antigens, 117
arachidonic acid, 112
arteries clogged up, 87
atheromas, 87
baby formula, 117, 120
bleeding
   intestinal, 105
blended milks, 236
bloodstream, 71
BMD, 60, 69, 77
   fools paradise, 59
   low, 61
body growth, 103
   rate of, 104
bone density, 53
bone loss in women, 115
bone mass, 53
bone mineral density. *See* BMD
bones
   caring for, 53
boron, 78
brain building nutrition, 109
brain development, 111
brazil nut milk, 179
   recipe, 227
breast milk, 117
breastfeeding, 117, 120
butter, 135
calcification, 83, 274
   cause, 90
   definition, 83
calcification and milk, 90
calcium, 45, 46, 48, 57, 62, 69, 70, 148
   absorption, 75
   deposits, 88
   how used, 55

leaching, 156
leaching from bones, 257
loss in urine, 97
requirement, 63
terrible price, 58
yo-yo effect, 52, 90, 102, 256, 263
Calcium Bomb, 90
calcium warehouse, 55
calcium yo-yo effect, 276
calcium-rich foods, 61
calorie comparison, 129
calories, 123, 129
   in dairy & non-dairy, 129
calories in milk, 123
cancer, 11, 28, 29, 30, 32, 43, 50, 73, 83, 96, 98, 100, 125, 126, 133, 159, 160, 165
   breast, 28, 85
cardamom, 236
carob powder, 237
casein, 33
cashew nut milk, 182
   recipe, 227
chestnut milk, 184
   recipe, 228
chia seeds, 133
children, 69, 103
childrens bones, 67, 115
cholesterol, 86, 87, 174
   LDL, 108
   oxidized, 40
cinnamon, 236
circulatory disease, 89
coconut milk, 186
   recipe, 228
consumption by world region, 64
contamination, 19, 20
corn milk, 188
   recipe, 229
cows, dairy, 171
dairy milk. *See* relevant topic
DHA, 113

brain, 113
diet, 113
diabetes, 11, 22, 31, 39, 42, 97, 117, 133, 139, 163, 220
diet
   nutritious, 60
dieticians, 19
differentiation, 254
dioxins, 43
disease, 20
energy, 143
epithelial cells, 32
estrogen, 71, 79, 259
excess protein, 104
exchangeable bone, 257
exercise
   benefits of, 149
   harmful, 146
   how much, 149
   lack of, 147
   moderate, 149
   over-exercise, 147
   right way, 80
   what kind, 150
fat in milk, 123, 129
   types, 111
fats
   comparison, 170
   harmful, 33, 108
   low fat, 126
   milk content, 160
FDA, 30, 77, 177, 220
flavoured milks, 140
flax seeds, 132
food allergies, 120
formula, 110, 112, 116, 117, 163
free-radicals, 146
fruit, 237
galactose, 13, 24, 44, 125, 126, 136, 166
gamma linoleic acid, 111
goats milk, 135
green pea milk, 191, 229, 273
   recipe, 229
harmful fats, 108
hazelnut milk, 190, 192

recipe, 229
heart disease, 274
heart, bad for, 125
heat treatment of milk, 37
hemp seed milk, 194
hempseed milk
    recipe, 230
hip fracture rates, 68
hip fractures
    country comparisons, 67
homocysteine, 127
homogenization, 39
homogenized
    effect of, 92
homogenized fat, 104
homogenizing milk, 92
hormones, 28, 30
human breast milk, 118
human evolution, 103
hypercalcaemia, 93
hypocalcaemia, 93
IGF-1, 28
imperative
    avoid indigestible protein, 102
    avoid trap, 142
    breastfeeding, 121
    calcification, 95
    children, 115
    everybody benefits, 177
    not absorb calcium, 148
    prostate cancer, 271
    protect bones, 76
    switch to non-dairy, 44
indigestible protein, 37
industry(milk), 17
infant
    bleeding, 105
infant formulas, 110
infant milk, 116
infant milk feeding, 119
infant milk options, 119
infants
    low fat diet, 109
iron deficiency, 104
lactose intolerance, 13, 34, 143, 159

lecithin, 236
leukemia, 32
linoleic acid, 111
low fat milk, 124
Low G.I. Workout, 153
macadamia milk, 197
    recipe, 230
machines, making milk, 15
magnesium, 49
Mayo Clinic, 88
measurements, British & American, 222
medication of cows, 38
medicinal milks, 141
microfractures, 145
milk. *See* under relevant topic
minerals, 250
mother's milk, 114
mucus, 32, 144, 157
muscles, 145
myths, dairy milk, 155
nanobacteria, 11, 90, 92
NDM Plan, 122, 128, 130
non-dairy milk, 14
    choosing, 167
nut allergy, 119, 120, 177
nutmeg, 236
nutrients
    absorption, 36
nutritional content, 225
nutritional content, dairy milk, 36
nutritional loss, 37
oat milk, 199, 272
    recipe, 230
okara, 14, 171, 224
oleic acid, 111
omega 3, 112
omega 6, 112
omega-3 milk, 140
organic milk, 138
osteoblast lineage, 254
osteoblasts, 55, 64, 72, 146, 253, 255
osteoclasts, 253
osteocytes, 255

osteoporosis, 8, 10, 18, 45, 145, 149, 157, 253, 260, 263, 274
    aging, 47
    black people, 58
    dairy major cause, 48
    description, 45
    Harvard study, 71
    incidence, 68
    industry response, 72
    organizations, 77
    over-exercising, 146
    real cause, 253
    widespread, 76
    women, 77
osteoprogenitor, 254
over-exercising
    weaker bones, 147
pasteurization, 38, 125, 137, 143
pea milk. *See* green pea milk
peanut milk, 200
    recipe, 231
pecan nut milk, 202
    recipe, 231
physical activity
    effect of milk, 148
physical fitness, 143
phytates, 159
phytic acid, 214
pine nut milk, 204
    recipe, 231
plaque, 88
postmenopausal, 72, 78, 147
products, dairy, 135
prostate cancer, 29, 32, 85, 181, 269
protein, 12, 18, 23, 38, 50, 69, 74
    amino acids, 99
    bad for children, 101
    best sources, 99
    cancer, 96
    daily amount, 98
    effect of dairy, 96
    Eskimos, 97
    indigestible, 75, 100
    misconceptions, 107
    myth, 99
    negative food, 101

putrefaction, 101
RDA, 99
vegetarians, 107
weakens bones, 97
PTH, 265
puberty, 30
pumpkin seed milk, 206
   recipe, 231
pus, 26
rBGH, 31
recipes, 5, 14
   master recipe, 226, 234, 282
   table A, 227
   tips, 222
redundant calcium, 57
refrigeration, 224
salt, 237
saturated fat, 40, 110, 113, 175
serving volume, 222
sesame seed milk, 208
   recipe, 231

skim milk, 127
soy caution, 164
soy milk, 210
   recipe, 231
soybean milk, 120
   myth, 158
soybeans
   caution, 115
specialty milks, 140
Spock, 42, 114
sprouted seed milk, 212
   recipe, 232
sprouted seeds, 212
sterol, 176
straining the milk, 223
sunflower milk
   recipe, 232
sunflower seed milk, 215
sunlight, 65, 66, 67, 80
sweetener, 236
sweetening agent, 224
teeth, 74, 83

test yourself, 80
tiger nut milk, 216
   recipe, 233
toxins in milk, 39
trans fatty acids, 40, 175
tuberculosis, 24
ultrapasteurized, 37
unpasteurized
   organic, 137
   raw, 137
vegan, 62, 67, 107
vegetarian, 62, 107
vitamin D, 39, 52, 64
   harm caused, 67
vitamin D3, 65, 116, 266
vitamins, 249
walnut milk, 219
   recipe, 233
weaning, 116
weight loss, 122

[Photocopy this page for easy reference in kitchen]

The Master Recipe (Summary)

Makes approximate volume: 1 litre/2 pints/1 quart
1 CUP = 8 FL OZS = 1/2 PINT = 237ML

You will need:

Blender (Grinder/grain mill may also apply)	1 cup *basic ingredient*, i.e. raw ingredient, before being prepared/ground/soaked/cooked
Strainer	1/8 teaspoon salt
Drinking-quality water (at least 5 cups)	Sweetening agent, e.g. soaked prunes, maple syrup, stevia

Method:

1. **First blend:** Put all ingredients into the blender, i.e. salt and sweetener, plus ingredients in Table A – see *Part Three* of book. Also add just enough water for blending process to work. Use warm or hot water, but not too hot to touch. Blend until smooth.

2. **Add further water:** Gradually add further *cold* water until you reach the 6 cup mark (48 fl. oz or 1420 ml) on your blender. Blend for 1 to 3 minutes until smooth.

3. **Straining:** Strain the mixture to get as much milk as possible. Use special nylon stocking or large strainer over big bowl.

4. **Extra bonus:** To squeeze extra milk out of the recipe put the okara back into the blender and briefly blend with a little more water. This works particularly well with coconut and other nut-based milks.

5. **Tweaking the milk:** If after straining, the result is too thick, simply mix in a little extra water. If the taste is not sweet enough, add extra sweetener. Remember that when left standing, some of the milk recipes will separate from the water more readily. This is perfectly natural – simply shake or stir before serving!

6. **Refrigeration:** It is essential to keep the milk refrigerated at all times, and use up within five days maximum. Alternatively, freeze some of the milk for future use.

7. **Okara:** Depending on milk type, either discard left-over okara or keep/freeze for use in other recipes.

Printed in the United Kingdom
by Lightning Source UK Ltd.
105947UKS00001B/34-81